Radiation Medicine Rounds

Charles R. Thomas, Jr., MD

Editor-in-Chief

Professor and Chair
Department of Radiation Medicine
Professor, Division of Hematology/Oncology
Department of Medicine
Knight Cancer Institute
Oregon Health & Science University Cancer Institute
Portland, Oregon

Editorial Board

Forthcoming Issue

Hematologic Malignancies
Michael Tomblyn, Karen Winkfield, and Bouthaina Dabaja
Guest Editors

Radiation Medicine Rounds

VOLUME 3, ISSUE 2

Malignant Gliomas

Guest Editors

Arnab Chakravarti, MD
Chair and Professor, Department of Radiation Oncology
Max Morehouse Chair of Cancer Research
Co-Director, Brain Tumor Program
Arthur G. James Comprehensive Cancer Center
and Richard L. Solove Research Institute
The Ohio State University Medical School
Columbus, Ohio

Martin Fuss, MD
Professor and Vice Chair
Director, Program in Image-Guided Radiation Therapy
Department of Radiation Medicine
Oregon Health & Science University
Portland, Oregon

demosMEDICAL
New York

Acquisitions Editor: Richard Winters
Cover Design: Joe Tenerelli
Compositor: Newgen Imaging
Printer: Hamilton

Visit our website at www.demosmedpub.com

Radiation Medicine Rounds is published three times a year by Demos Medical Publishing.

Business Office. All business correspondence including subscriptions, renewals, and address changes should be sent to Demos Medical Publishing, 11 West 42nd Street, 15th Floor, New York, NY, 10036.

ISSN: 2151-4208
ISBN: 978-1-936287-76-5
E-ISBN: 978-1-617051-48-7

Library of Congress Cataloging-in-Publication Data

Malignant gliomas / guest editors, Arnab Chakravarti, Martin Fuss.
p. ; cm. — (Radiation medicine rounds, ISSN 2151-4208 v. 3, issue 2)
Includes bibliographical references and index.
ISBN 978-1-936287-76-5 — ISBN 978-1-61705-148-7 (e-ISBN)
I. Chakravarti, Arnab. II. Fuss, Martin, 1963 Oct. 3- III. Series: Radiation medicine rounds ; v. 3, issue 2. 2151-4208.
[DNLM: 1. Glioma — diagnosis. 2. Glioma — therapy. W1 RA162HD v.3 no. 2 2012 / QZ 380]

616.99'481 — dc23

2012032113

Printed in the United States of America
12 13 14 15 5 4 3 2 1

Contents

Foreword

FROM THE EDITOR-IN-CHIEF

Radiation Medicine Rounds is a hardcover periodical published three times a year that is designed to provide an up-to-date review of defined radiation medicine topics of interest to clinicians and scientists who are involved in the care of patients receiving radiotherapy. It is intended to serve as both a reference and instructional tool by students, housestaff, fellows, practicing clinicians, medical physicists, cancer biologists, radiobiologists, and interdisciplinary colleagues throughout the oncology spectrum.

For the current issue, *Malignant Gliomas,* our distinguished Guest Editors Drs. Arnab Chakravarti and Martin Fuss have shepherded the development of a series of very high-quality reviews on the role of radiotherapy in the management of one of the tumors most known to humans—primary brain gliomas. To their joint credit as well as to the credit of the panel of expert contributors, there is a balanced presentation of the current state of the art along with new directions that warrant further investigation. The contributions include much desired discussions on the multidisciplinary approach to malignant glioma. On behalf of the entire RMR editorial board, we sincerely believe that the pages to follow will provide a useful guide to the area of malignant glioma.

Dr. Charles R. Thomas, Jr.
Series Editor-in-Chief
Radiation Medicine Rounds
Portland, Oregon

Preface

Malignant gliomas are among the most devastating of all human malignancies, with median survival times remaining approximately 1 year despite aggressive surgery, radiation, and chemotherapy for grade IV tumors. The underlying molecular and genetic mechanisms predisposing the aggressive behaviors of these tumors are becoming better understood, although far from complete. It has been demonstrated that conventional treatments, including surgery, radiation, and chemotherapy, can be optimized to improve overall survival, with longer term survivors becoming more common in the modern era than in decades past. One of the important findings is that histopathologically identical malignant gliomas often demonstrate very distinct clinical behaviors. These observations serve to educate us that the future advances in the field will invariably be predicated upon a personalized care approach for this patient population. Therefore, this book *Malignant Gliomas* serves the dual mission of educating clinicians on the recent advances in the treatment of patients with malignant gliomas, at the same time educating them on future directions that will lead to more effective personalized care approaches for this patient population.

We dedicate this volume to our patients, who have taught us so much about courage and perseverance; our families, who have given us unconditional love and support to enable us to advance the frontiers of the field; our mentors and colleagues, who have given us due professional guidance; and our institutions, which have given us the foundation and framework to advance our academic careers.

We acknowledge the contributions of Ms. Allison Errett for her outstanding administrative support in the production and editing of this book. Without her efforts, this book would not have been possible.

Arnab Chakravarti, MD
Martin Fuss, MD

Contributors

Kenneth D. Aldape
Department of Pathology
University of Texas MD
Anderson Cancer Center
Houston, TX

Rolf F. Barth, MD
Department of Pathology
The Ohio State University
Columbus, OH

Aashish D. Bhatt, MD
Clinical Fellow in Proton Therapy
Department of Radiation Oncology
Massachusetts General Hospital
Harvard Medical School
Boston, MA

Peter Binns, PhD
Department of Radiation Oncology
Mt. Auburn Hospital
Cambridge, MA

Arnab Chakravarti, MD
Chair and Professor
Department of Radiation Oncology
Arthur G. James Comprehensive Cancer Center and Richard L. Solove Research Institute
The Wexner Medical Center at The Ohio State University
Columbus, OH

E. Antonio Chiocca, MD, PhD
Department of Neurological Surgery
Dardinger Laboratory for Neuro-Oncology and Neurosciences
Arthur G. James Comprehensive Cancer Center
The Wexner Medical Center at The Ohio State University
Columbus, OH

Adam P. Dicker, MD, PhD
Professor and Chair
Department of Radiation Oncology
Philadelphia, PA

Richard G. Everson, MD
Department of Neurosurgery
David Geffen School of Medicine at UCLA
Los Angeles, CA

Elena I. Fomchenko, PhD
Department of Neurosurgery
David Geffen School of Medicine at UCLA
Los Angeles, CA

David S. Foulad, MD
Department of Neurosurgery
David Geffen School of Medicine at UCLA
Los Angeles, CA

Anca-Ligia Grosu, MD
Chair
Department of Radiation Oncology
University Medical Center
Freiburg, Germany

Michael Guiou, MD
Chief Resident
Department of Radiation Oncology
Arthur G. James Comprehensive Cancer Center and Richard L. Solove Research Institute
The Wexner Medical Center at The Ohio State University
Columbus, OH

Deliang Guo, PhD
Assistant Professor
Department of Radiation Oncology
Comprehensive Cancer Center
The Ohio State University Medical Center
Columbus, OH

Otto K. Harling, PhD
Department of Nuclear Science & Engineering
Massachusetts Institute of Technology
Cambridge, MA

Erica Hlavin Bell, PhD
Research Assistant Professor
Department of Radiation Oncology
Comprehensive Cancer Center
The Wexner Medical Center at The Ohio State University
Columbus, OH

Shinji Kawabata, MD, PhD
Department of Neurosurgery
Osaka Medical College
Osaka, Japan

W. S. Kiger III, PhD
Department of Radiation Oncology
Beth Israel Deaconess Medical Center
Harvard Medical School
Boston, MA

Simon Kirste, MD
Department of Radiation Oncology
Comprehensive Cancer Center
The Ohio State University Medical Center
Columbus, OH

Linda M. Liau, MD, PhD
Professor and Vice Chair
Department of Neurosurgery
David Geffen School of Medicine at UCLA
Los Angeles, CA

Dominique N. Lisiero, PhD
UCLA Department of Neurosurgery
David Geffen School of Medicine at UCLA
Los Angeles, CA

Jay S. Loeffler, MD
Chief of Department
Department of Radiation Oncology
Massachusetts General Hospital
Herman and Joan Suit Professor of Radiation Oncology
Harvard Medical School
Boston, MA

Adam Maier, DO, MBA
Clinical Resident
Department of Radiation Oncology
Arthur G. James Comprehensive Cancer Center and Richard L. Solove Research Institute
The Wexner Medical Center at The Ohio State University
Columbus, OH

Ahmed Mohyeldin, MD, PhD
Department of Neurological Surgery
Dardinger Laboratory for Neuro-Oncology and Neurosciences
The James Comprehensive Cancer Center
The Wexner Medical Center
The Ohio State University
Columbus, OH

Christopher Pelloski, MD
Associate Professor
Department of Radiation Oncology
Department of Neurosurgery
Arthur G. James Comprehensive Cancer Center and Richard L. Solove Research Institute
The Wexner Medical Center at The Ohio State University
Columbus, OH

Aditya Raghunathan
Department of Pathology
University of Texas, MD
Anderson Cancer Center
Houston, TX

Kent J. Riley, PhD
Department of Radiation Oncology
Massachusetts General Hospital
Boston, MA

Wenyin Shi, MD, PhD
Assistant Professor
Department of Radiation Oncology
Jefferson Medical College of Thomas Jefferson University
Philadelphia, PA

Helen A. Shih, MD
Chief of Service
Central Nervous System and Eye Services
Department of Radiation Oncology
Massachusetts General Hospital
Assistant Professor of Radiation Oncology
Harvard Medical School
Boston, MA

M. Graca H. Vicente, PhD
Department of Chemistry
Louisiana State University
Baton Rouge, LA

Phyllis Wachsberger, PhD
Assistant Professor
Department of Radiation Oncology
Jefferson Medical College of Thomas Jefferson University
Philadelphia, PA

Wolfgang A. Weber, MD
Chair
Department of Nuclear Medicine
University Medical Center
Freiburg, Germany

Nicole Wiedenmann, MD
Department of Radiation Oncology
University Medical Center
Freiburg, Germany

demos MEDICAL

RADIATION MEDICINE ROUNDS

Recent Advances in the Treatment of Malignant Gliomas and Future Directions

Michael Guiou and Christopher Pelloski*

Department of Radiation Oncology, The Ohio State University, Columbus, OH

ABSTRACT

The vast majority of primary, intracerebral malignancies are derived from aberrant glial cells. The natural history, response to treatment, and overall prognosis of these lesions are highly variable and depend on tumor grade, cell type of origin, and molecular profile. In the following chapter, we discuss the clinical diagnosis, histological profile, current standard of care, and recent advances in the management of malignant gliomas including anaplastic oligodendroglioma, anaplastic astrocytoma, and glioblastoma.

Keywords: anaplastic oligodendroglioma, anaplastic astrocytoma, glioblastoma, radiation, chemotherapy

INTRODUCTION

Gliomas represent a broad range of central nervous system (CNS) neoplasms. A histological grading system created by the World Health Organization (WHO) classifies gliomas on a scale of I to IV (Table 1). Grade I and II lesions are low grade whereas grades III and IV are high grade. High-grade lesions are biologically more aggressive with a propensity to recur and lead to significant morbidity and/or mortality despite aggressive treatment. For the purposes of optimizing treatment strategies and designing

TABLE 1 WHO histological grading system for glioma

WHO Grade	Tumor Type
I	Pilocytic astrocytoma
II	Diffuse astrocytoma, oligodendroglioma
III	Anaplastic astrocytoma, anaplastic oligodendroglioma, anaplastic oligoastrocytoma
IV	Glioblastoma

Grades I and II are considered low grades, whereas grades III and IV are considered high grades.

*Corresponding author, Department of Radiation Oncology, The Ohio State University, 310 West 10th Ave, Columbus, OH 43210

E-mail address: Christopher.pelloski@osumc.edu

Radiation Medicine Rounds 3:2 (2012) 181–200.

DOI: 10.5003/2151–4208.3.2.181

demosmedpub.com/rmr

research trials, classification schemes based on pre- and post-treatment variables and their correlation to outcome have been developed for malignant glioma (Table 2). In the following chapter, we will discuss the diagnosis and management of high-grade glioma (WHO III and IV).

■ ANAPLASTIC OLIGODENDROGLIOMA

Introduction

Oligodendrogliomas (WHO grade II) are rare tumors accounting for 2% to 5% of intracranial neoplasms. Anaplastic oligodendroglioma (AO; WHO grade III) is a more aggressive variant that comprise 20% to 50% of oligodendroglial tumors (1). AO commonly occurs in adulthood with a peak in incidence between 40 and 60 years (2). The majority of AO arise in the white matter of the cerebrum, particularly in the frontal lobes. As with other malignant gliomas, metastasis is rare with spread outside the neuraxis typically reported at later stages of the disease. Likewise, leptomeningeal involvement is uncommon but has been reported in patients with recurrent disease. Median survival is approximately 4 to 5 years with a 5-year overall survival (OS-5yr) of approximately 40% (3). Patients with AO can present with global neurological symptoms such as seizure, headache, nausea, vertigo, and/or mental status changes as well as focal neurological deficits depending on the involved brain regions.

TABLE 2 Recursive Partitioning Analysis based on three clinical trials of patients with malignant glioma (WHO grade III/IV) treated with radiotherapy (RT) +/– chemotherapy from 1974 to 1989

Class	Definition
I	Age < 50, AA, normal MS
II	Age ≥ 50, AA, KPS 70–100, at least 3 months from symptom onset to start of treatment
III	Age < 50, AA, abnormal MS
	Age < 50, GBM, KPS 90–100
IV	Age < 50, GBM, KPS < 90
	Age ≥ 50, AA, KPS 70–100, 3 months or less from start of symptoms to treatment
	Age > 50, GBM, resection, good neurological function
V	Age ≥ 50, GBM, KPS 70–100, resection and unable to work, or biopsy only followed by at least 54.4 Gy of RT
	Age ≥ 50, KPS < 70, normal MS
VI	Age ≥ 50, GBM, KPS 70–100, biopsy only and RT < 54.4 Gy Age ≥ 50, KPS < 70, abnormal MS

Abbreviations: AA = anaplastic astrocytoma, MS = mental status, GBM = glioblastoma multiforme, KPS = Karnofsky Performance Scale, RT = radiotherapy, Gy = Gray.
Source: Modified from Curran et al. (1993).

Histology/Genetics

Histologically, AO is characterized by hypercellularity, marked atypia, frequent mitoses, endothelial proliferation, and necrosis (4–6). The most frequent chromosomal abnormality in oligodendroglioma is combined loss of chromosomal arms 1p and 19q. This is seen in approximately 60% to 90% of tumors. This combined loss is mediated by an unbalanced translocation of 19q to 1p (7). This loss is typically retained at the time of progression regardless of other changes in the cell suggesting that 1p/19q loss is an early genetic event in the evolution of malignant oligodendroglial cells. Patients harboring this mutation show a better response to therapy as well as significantly prolonged survival independent of treatment. This characteristic has led clinicians to consider AO as a low-grade lesion compared to other types of malignant glioma and as a separate biologic entity within the realm of clinical trials. Additional genetic abnormalities seen in AO include loss of heterozygosity at chromosome 9p, deletion of the CDKN2A gene (p16) (33%–50% tumors), deletion of chromosome 10 (20%–25% of cases), and O^6-methylguanine-DNA methyltransferase (MGMT) promoter hypermethylation in approximately 80% of patients (8). There is a strong correlation between MGMT promoter hypermethylation and chromosome 1p/19q codeletion. No specific immune histochemical markers exist for oligodendroglioma or AO though some tumors may exhibit staining for glial fibrillary acidic protein (GFAP), which is most often due to the presence of reactive astrocytes more than pure oligodendroglial cells. Often included in studies of patients with AO are patients with anaplastic oligoastrocytoma (AOA). Oligoastrocytic tumors are typically more aggressive, less responsive to therapy, and have poorer prognosis than their AO counterparts. In fact, the 2007 WHO classification of brain tumors now considers AOA with necrosis equivalent to GBM (9–11). The delineation between oligodendroglioma and mixed oligoastrocytoma is not entirely clear; however, as mixed-histology tumors generally have both oligodendroglioma foci and gemistocytic astrocytic components. Given the presence of astrocytes, AOA typically have areas that stain positive for GFAP within the substance of the tumor as opposed to pure oligodendrogliomas, which show higher GFAP activity in peritumoral tissue (2). AOA with necrosis typically have a lower percentage of 1p/19q codeletion and have genetic mutations more commonly seen in high-grade astrocytic tumors (like GBM) such as epidermal growth factor receptor (EGFR) overexpression and loss of chromosome 10 (12). For the purpose of clinical trials, large cooperative groups like the European Organizations for Research and Treatment of Cancer (EORTC) and Radiation Therapy Oncology Group (RTOG) have set arbitrary cutoff points as the presence of more than 25% astrocytic component to qualify a tumor as AOA though significant variability exists among pathologists in making this distinction (10).

Imaging

MRI is the gold standard for evaluation of intracranial neoplasms. AOs typically appear as heterogenous masses with both cyst-like and calcified components. On MRI, these lesions are hypointense on T1-weighted images, hyperintense on T2-weighted images, and may demonstrate ring-like enhancement seen in higher grade lesions like GBM. However, contrast enhancement should not be considered pathognomonic for high-grade glioma. In a study of 40 patients with nonenhancing supratentorial brain lesions on MRI, 40% were found to be high-grade lesions on histological analysis (13). Similar findings have been reported by other groups. Interestingly, patients with codeletion of 1p/19q may have lesions with ill-defined borders on T1-weighted sequences and intratumoral calcifications (14). Surrounding vasogenic edema is not common on fluid-attenuated inversion-recovery (FLAIR) sequences. Perfusion-based techniques typically show increased regional cerebral blood volume (rCBV) in high-grade versus low-grade neoplasms (15). Studies suggest that this parameter may be useful in monitoring treatment response (16). Metabolic-based modalities such as positron emission tomography (PET) can be useful in distinguishing between high-grade and low-grade lesions as well and, in the treatment setting, help guide surgical resection or radiotherapy planning (17). Likewise, magnetic resonance spectroscopy (MRS) has been proven to be useful in differentiating high- and low-grade lesions, with high-grade lesions showing significantly elevated choline/creatinine ratios reflective of increased cellular proliferation (15,18–20).

Treatment

Treatment of AO includes maximal safe resection followed by adjuvant radiotherapy to approximately 60 Gy in 30 fractions (21). AO has also been shown to be sensitive to chemotherapy both prior to and following brain radiotherapy. The most well-studied agent within this subset of glioma patients has been PCV (procarbazine/lomustine/vincristine). The response rate of patients with AO to PCV and other systemic cytotoxic agents is approximately 70%. Two landmark trials, one in the United States (RTOG 9402) and one in Europe (EORTC 26951), have demonstrated the improved response to treatment and outcome in this patient population. In RTOG 9402, 289 patients with AO and AOA were treated with either PCV (lomustine 130 mg/m^2 orally on day 1; procarbazine 75 mg/m^2 orally daily on days 8 to 21; and vincristine 1.4 mg/m^2 intravenously on days 8 and 29) for 4 cycles followed by radiation therapy to 59.4 Gy or radiation therapy alone. Although no differences in median OS (mOS) were seen (4.9 years for patients treated with combined modality therapy versus 4.7 years for patients treated with radiation therapy alone; $p = 0.26$), there was a significant difference in progression-free survival (PFS). Patients treated with PCV followed by radiation therapy had PFS of 2.6 versus 1.7 years; $p = 0.004$. Despite the lack of OS benefit for the group as a whole, subset analysis stratifying patients by 1p/19q deletion status showed that codeleted patients had an mOS of greater than 7 versus 2.8 years; $p \leq 0.001$ (Figure 1A). This difference was seen irrespective of treatment group indicating that 1p/19q status was a good prognostic factor but had relatively little value in predicting response to treatment (Figure 1B). However, it was noted that codeleted patients exhibited significantly decreased risk of tumor progression following treatment with PCV which led researchers to conclude that 1p/19q codeletion may have predictive value for chemotherapy responsiveness. A recent update of RTOG 9402 revealed 1p/19q codeletion is indeed predictive of response to treatment. In this updated analysis of 126 patients, the OS of codeleted patients in the radiotherapy plus PCV arm was 14.7 years versus 7.3 years in the radiotherapy-alone arm; $p = 0.03$. If patients were intact or only had deletion of one chromosome there was no difference between treatment arms with mOS of 2.6 versus 2.7 years; $p = 0.37$ (22). Although the progression-free and OS

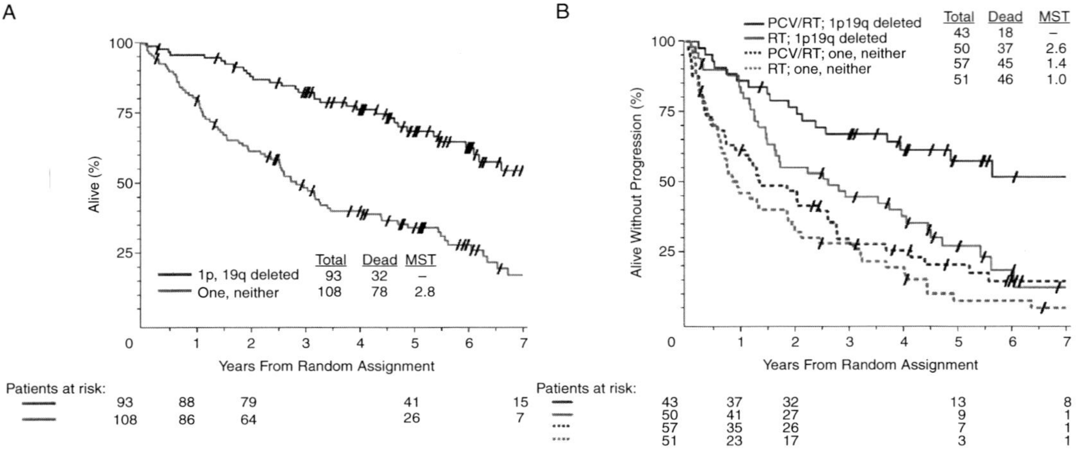

FIGURE 1 (A) OS stratified by 1p/19q deletion status. (B) PFS as stratified by 1p/19q deletion status and treatment group. Abbreviation: MST = median survival time.
Source: Cairncross et al., JCO 2006.

data in these patients is promising, PCV is not without its toxicities. In the initial report of RTOG 9402, 65% of patients experienced grade III or grade IV toxicity. One chemotherapy-related death was also recorded in the study (23). In a similar study performed in Europe, EORTC 26951, 368 patients with AO and AOA were treated with either radiation therapy (59.4 Gy) versus radiation therapy followed by 6 cycles of PCV (lomustine 110 mg/m^2 orally on day 1, procarbazine 60 mg/m^2 orally on days 8 to 21, and vincristine 1.4 mg/m^2 intravenous on days 8 and 29). With a median follow-up of 60 months, there was no significant difference in mOS between treatment groups (40.3 months combined modality versus 30.6 months radiation alone; p = 0.23). There was, however, a significant difference in PFS of 23 months for patients treated with radiation therapy followed by PCV versus 13.2 months for patients treated with radiation alone; p = 0.0018. (Figure 2A). Subgroup analysis of patients treated on EORTC 26951 showed that at 60 months, 74% of patients with 1p/19q codeletion were alive. Both 5-year overall survival (OS-5yr) and 5-year progression free survival (PFS-5yr) were significantly improved in codeleted patients. This was irrespective of treatment arm similar to that seen in the RTOG trial (Figure 2B) (24). As with the RTOG study, patients experienced moderate toxicity with the addition of PCV. MGMT hypermethylation has been shown to have significant prognostic value in patients with GBM. Given this, MGMT status was analyzed in 165 patients treated on EORTC 26951. MGMT promoter hypermethylation was observed in 80% of patients. This was strongly correlated with codeletion of chromosomes 1p and 19q; p = 0.00043. In subgroup analysis, patients that harbored MGMT hypermethylation had significantly improved OS and PFS, irrespective of treatment arm (RT + PCV versus RT alone). This led study leaders to conclude that, within this patient population, MGMT had significant prognostic value but was not predictive of response to treatment (25). A recent update of EORTC 26951 showed significant improvement in median progression free survival (mPFS) (24.3 versus 13.2 months; p = 0.003) and mOS (42.3 versus 30.6 months; p = 0.018) for patients receiving RT + PCV versus RT alone. The improvement in mOS was even more pronounced in patients with 1p/19q codeletion (not reached versus 113 months; p = 0.0487). No difference in mOS was observed for patients without 1p/19q codeletion. Subset analysis of the impact of MGMT methylation showed a slight trend toward improved mOS in the RT + PCV group; however, this difference was not significant (26).

Other agents have been tested in patients with AO including temozolomide (TMZ), an oral alkylating agent. Several phase II studies have demonstrated the response rate to TMZ (~33%) is similar to that of PCV but with significantly decreased toxicity. In a recent study stratifying patients by 1p/19q status, Mikkelsen et al. treated codeleted patients with TMZ alone (150 mg/m^2/d for cycles 1 and 2 with escalation to 200 mg/m^2/d if no myelosuppression occurred; repeat dosing was every 28 days following the first dose), whereas intact patients received TMZ (same initial dosing as codeleted patients) followed by concurrent RT (60 Gy) and TMZ (75 mg/m^2/d) followed by post-radiotherapy TMZ. Forty-eight patients

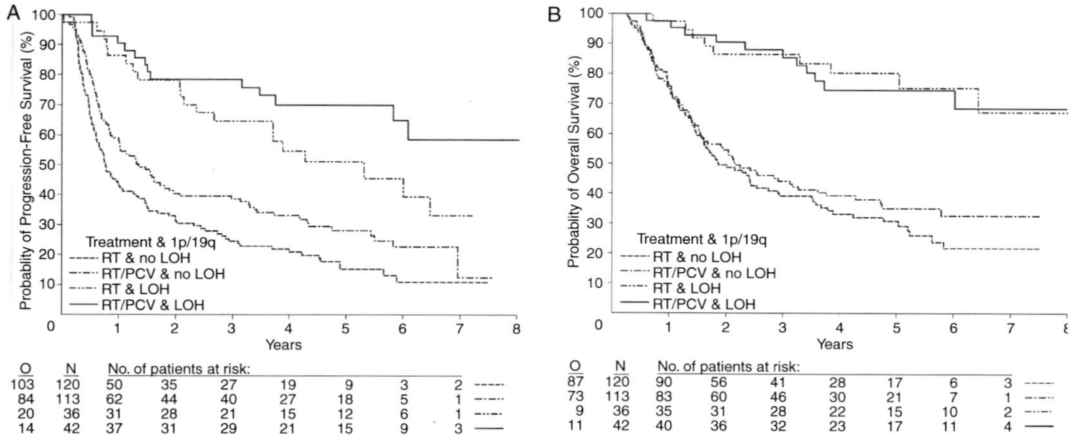

FIGURE 2 (A) PFS by 1p/19q status and treatment arm. (B) OS by 1p/19q status and treatment arm. Abbreviation: LOH = loss of heterozygosity.
Source: Van den Bent et al., JCO 2006.

with AO were treated, 75% of which were codeleted. Treatment response was documented in 94% of patients with mOS of 77.3 months. mPFS (28.7 versus 13.5 months), 1-year overall survival (OS-1yr) (97.2% versus 83.3%), and 2-year overall survival (OS-2yr) (90.1% versus 83.3%) were improved in the codeleted group; however, only OS-1yr and OS-2yr reached statistical significance; p = 0.016 (27). As with results from RTOG 9402 and EORTC 26951, these data highlight that the overriding variable in outcome in patients with AO is 1p/19q status. Other trials have reported a good response to TMZ with an acceptable toxicity profile. In the phase II trial RTOG BR0131, 42 patients with AO and AOA were treated with TMZ (150 $mg/m^2/d$, 7 days on/7 days off for up to 6 cycles) followed by concurrent RT (59.4 Gy) + TMZ (75 $mg/m^2/d$). The objective response rate was 32% with only 10% of exhibiting radiographic progression during pre-RT chemotherapy. A subgroup analysis showed that all patients with codeleted status (17 of 28 evaluable patients; 60.7%) and MGMT hypermethylation (16 of 20 evaluable patients; 80%) were progression free at 6 months (28).

TMZ alone in the treatment of AO has also been studied with promising results. In a study of 20 patients with AO treated with TMZ following surgical resection, Taliansky-Aronov et al. reported a radiographic response rate of approximately 75%. Time to progression of patients treated on this trial was 24 months. Patients with 1p/19q codeletion fared much better with a 6-month progression free survival (PFS-6m) of 100% versus 20% for intact patients; p = 0.057 (29).

Currently, two international, intergroup, randomized control trials are being conducted through the EORTC to help determine the optimal role of TMZ in patients with AO. EORTC 26081 is a phase III, three-arm trial in codeleted AO patients that randomizes to RT versus RT + TMZ followed by adjuvant TMZ versus TMZ alone. A second trial in noncodeleted patient is EORTC 26053, a phase III, 2 × 2 design that, following resection, randomizes initially to RT versus RT + TMZ followed by a second randomization to no further treatment versus continued TMZ. The results of these studies will be important in determining the optimal role of TMZ in both codeleted and intact patients with AO and AOA.

Targeted Therapy

Studies examining small, targeted agents have also shown some promise in recurrent AO following treatment with radiotherapy and chemotherapy. Based on reports of activity of imatinib mesylate (Gleevec), a selective receptor tyrosine kinase inhibitor, when combined with hydroxyurea, a ribonucleoside diphosphate reductase inhibitor, in recurrent GBM (30), Desjardins et al. examined the response in patients with recurrent grade III glioma at progression following standard radiotherapy and at least TMZ-based chemotherapy. Thirty-nine patients with anaplastic astrocytoma (AA), AO, and AOA initially treated with chemotherapy and radiotherapy were given Gleevec (500 mg twice daily for patients on enzyme inducing antiepileptic drugs [EIAEDs] and 400 mg daily if not on EIAEDs) and hydroxyurea (500 mg twice daily) at progression. The radiographic response rate was approximately 10%. Thirty-three percent of patients achieved stable disease. PFS-6m was approximately 24%. Subgroup analysis of responders versus nonresponders showed that if patients were scored as having stable disease at first evaluation, PFS-6m was 53% and at 12 months, it was 29% (31).

Trials of antiangiogenic drugs have also been completed. The most studied agent is bevacizumab (Avastin), a recombinant humanized monoclonal antibody that inhibits the activity of vascular endothelial growth factor (VEGF). In a study of 22 patients with recurrent, alkylator-resistant, codeleted AO, Chamberlain et al. demonstrated a 68% radiographic response, PFS-6m 68%, PFS-12m 23%, and mOS of 8.5 months in patients treated with bevacziumab alone. Minimal grade III or IV toxicity was recorded (32). The combination of bevacizumab and irinotecan has also shown efficacy. In a retrospective study of 25 patients with recurrent AO previously treated with RT and at least 1 cycle of TMZ, bevacizumab (10 mg/kg) and irinotecan (125 or 340 mg/m^2) every 14 days produced an objective response rate of 72% with PFS-6m of 42%. Despite these reasonably favorable outcome data, toxicity was moderate with an intratumoral hemorrhage rate of 24% and treatment discontinuation in 20% (33). Similar findings have been reported in studies of mixed grade III and grade IV gliomas. In a phase II study by Vredenburgh et al., 23 patients with malignant glioma (9 grade III glioma) were treated with bevacizumab (10 mg/kg every 2 weeks on a 6-week cycle) plus irinotecan (340 mg/m^2 or 125 mg/m^2 dependent on EIAED use) at the time of recurrence. A radiographic response was recorded in 63% of patients with grade III tumors indicating that this combination of agents has activity in recurrent high-grade glioma. PFS-6m for the entire cohort was 38% with OS-6m of 72%. There also appeared to be a trend towards improvement in OS in grade III tumors (30 weeks versus 23 weeks) though this difference was not significant (34).

■ ANAPLASTIC ASTROCYTOMA

Introduction

Anaplastic astrocytoma (AA), WHO grade III glioma, constitute approximately 4% of all malignant CNS tumors (35). Approximately 2,500 cases of AA are diagnosed annually in the Unites States (36). Peak incidence is seen between 45 and 60 years with approximately 1.5 times as many men affected as women. Overall, the prognosis for AA is quite poor with a median survival of 35 to 40 months (37). Many patients with AA will eventually progress to GBM (WHO grade IV) which portends an extremely poor prognosis with very few survivors past one year.

AA is a diffuse and infiltrative lesion which rarely metastasizes outside the CNS. Patients with AA often present with neurologic symptoms dependent on the functional brain region in which the tumor is located or from tumorogenic cerebral edema. Many patients present with headache and often, seizures. Patient characteristics associated with improved survival include age less than 50 years, good performance status, and intact neurological function (Table 2) (38).

Genetic risk factors for AA include neurofibromatosis type 1 (NF-1), neurofibromatosis type 2 (NF-2), tuberous sclerosis, and Li-Fraumeni syndrome (35). Environmental risk factors are not well understood though some studies suggest that exposure to electronic devices (cell phones in particular) (39,40), toxic chemical exposure (41), and work in factories (42) may bestow increased risk.

Imaging

On contrast-enhanced T1-weighted MRI, AA lesions demonstrate variable enhancement (43–45) with avidly enhancing tumors typically having a poorer prognosis (44,46). Significant tumor-related vasogenic edema is common on T2/FLAIR sequences. Other functional imaging modalities such as PET, MRS, and perfusion-weighted MRI (pMRI) can complement findings on conventional MRI. AA show high levels of metabolic activity secondary to elevated rates of cell proliferation. PET imaging utilizing the radiotracer fluorodeoxy glucose (FDG) has limited ability to characterize intracranial neoplasms given the many confounds of the technique (infection and nonmalignant processes can have increased FDG uptake) as well as the high basal metabolic activity of normal brain tissue. Other tracers, such as L-methyl-^{11}C-methionine (MET), have been shown to be more specific for malignant lesions (47). MET uptake reflects amino acid metabolism and serves as a surrogate marker for proliferative potential. As such, the signal from normal brain is low as the majority of cells in the CNS are terminally differentiated. In a study of 67 patients with intracranial gliomas (12 AA), Torii et al. found a strong correlation between areas of MET uptake and proliferative index by Ki-67 staining (48).

Magnetic resonance spectroscopy (MRS) exploits differences in cellular metabolism to distinguish tumor from normal brain. Multiple series in patients with AA have shown that the MRS profile can be used to distinguish tumor grade. In a study of 55 patients with glioma (including 8 AA, 11 GBM), Fayed et al. reported a strong correlation between choline/creatinine ratio and tumor grade (low- versus high-grade glioma) (49). Similar findings have been reported by other groups (50,51). MRS has also been shown to correlate with markers of tumor aggressiveness. In a study of 41 patients with astrocytoma (16 WHO grade I/II, 25 grade III/IV), significant elevations in choline/N-acetylaspartate and choline/creatinine were seen in high-grade versus low-grade lesions. In high-grade lesions, MRS signals correlated with elevated staining for matrix metalloproteinase-2 (MMP-2), a marker of tumor invasiveness. The same relationship was not seen for low-grade astrocytomas (52). Like MRS, perfusion MRI can distinguish between different grades of gliomatous lesions (53–55). Additionally, preoperative rCBV values appear to have prognostic value. In a study of 49 patients with high-grade glioma (18 AA, 23 GBM), OS-2yr was significantly longer in patients with lower (67%) versus higher (9%) rCBV values, irrespective of whether the tumor was AA or GBM; $p < 0.001$ (56).

Histology/Genetics

Progression from low- to high-grade glioma appears to be correlated with an increasing number of genetic mutations (Figure 3). Approximately 60% of low-grade gliomas carry mutations in platelet-derived growth factor receptor (PDGF-R) leading to overexpression (57). TP53 (commonly seen in low-grade glioma) mutations are seen in approximately 65% of patients (58,59). Mutations in TP53 can lead to defective apoptosis and uncontrolled proliferation. Although TP53 mutations are also seen in patients with GBM, it is more frequent in patients with AA (59). Other genetic abnormalities that appear to be more frequent in high-grade astrocytic tumors involve multiple cell cycle regulatory pathways such as deletion or mutation in cyclin-dependent kinase (CDK) inhibitor $p16^{INK4}$, pRB1 (retinoblastoma susceptibility locus), phosphate and tensin homology (PTEN), and amplification or overexpression of CDK4 as well as HDM2 (human double minute 2) (60). Studies have demonstrated that patients with these mutations have an overall poorer prognosis as compared to AA patients without them (61,62).

Treatment

The standard treatment of AA includes maximal safe resection followed by partial brain radiotherapy (60 Gy in 30 fractions) (21). Extent of surgery is an important prognostic factor for OS. In a retrospective review of 102 patients with AA, Keles et al. found that the volume of residual disease on postoperative MRI was a significant predictor of time to progression ($p < 0.001$) as well as OS ($p = 0.003$) despite adjuvant treatment with radiation (100% of patients) and chemotherapy (94% of patients) (43). Similar benefits of gross total resection have been reported in other series as well (63,64). However, recurrence is quite common (43). Following maximal safe resection, radiation therapy has been shown to have a significant impact on both OS and PFS. In the Brain Treatment Study Group (BTSG) studies 78 and 80, patients with high-grade glioma showed improved OS when postoperative, whole brain RT was delivered alone or with combination chemotherapy as compared to chemotherapy alone or best supportive care (65,66). Given the toxicities of WBRT (especially to higher doses), the use of partial brain radiation was evaluated. BTSG study 83 evaluated WBRT to 60.2 Gy versus WBRT to 43 Gy followed by a cone-down to the postsurgical cavity of 17.2 Gy. Results of this study showed no difference in OS (67). Given these findings, partial brain irradiation became standard of care. Unfortunately, attempts at optimizing RT including altered fractionation as well as dose escalation have shown no benefit. In a study conducted in Europe by the Medical Research Council (MRC), 474 patients with grade III or IV astrocytoma were treated with partial brain RT to either 60 Gy in 30 fractions versus 45 Gy in 20 fractions following maximal safe resection. The group receiving 60 Gy had a superior outcome (mOS 12 versus 9 months; $p = 0.007$) indicating little role for altered fractionation (68). Studies of dose escalation have similarly shown no benefit. In a joint randomized trial between the RTOG and the Eastern Cooperative Oncology Group (ECOG), 626 patients with high-grade glioma were treated with traditional fractionation (60 Gy in 30 fractions) versus 60 Gy plus a 10 Gy boost to the postsurgical cavity versus chemoradiotherapy (60 Gy plus BCNU or CCNU). Patients in the boost arm showed no improvement with regard to PFS or OS (69). Given these findings, the current recommended adjuvant RT schedule is 60 Gy in 30 fractions provided the patient has a good performance status.

To date, the role of adjuvant chemotherapy in the treatment of AA is unclear with many studies reporting conflicting results. Another factor making interpretation of this data difficult is the fact that many older studies included both grade III and grade IV patients leaving them underpowered to make

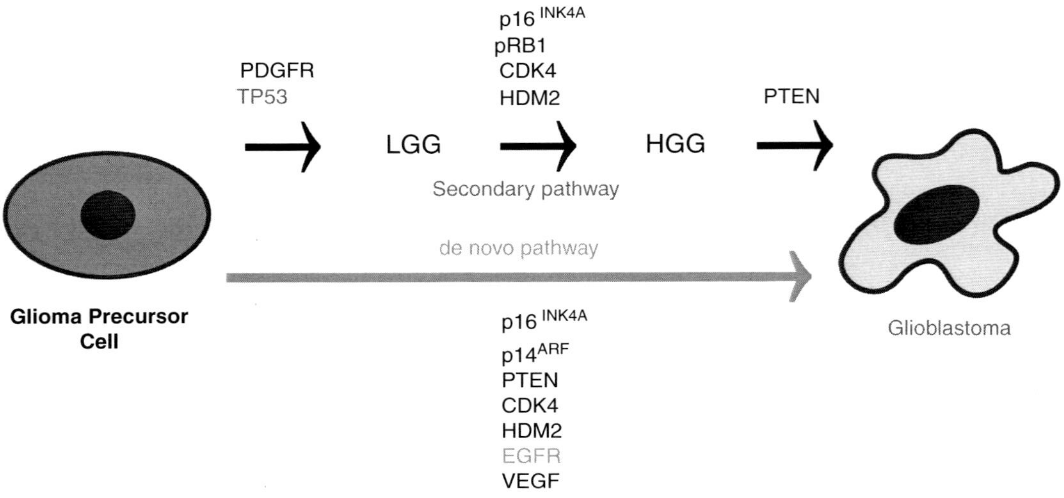

FIGURE 3 Primary (de novo) and secondary pathway and associated genetic mutations for development of GBM. Mutations that predominate to a specific pathway are indicated in grey (de novo) or black (secondary). Adapted from Sathornsumetee et al., 2007 (70).

definitive conclusions regarding AA patients specifically. In 1994, an EORTC Brain Tumor Group trial reported favorable outcomes in patients with AA treated with adjuvant concurrent chemoradiotherapy with dibromodulcitriol (DBD) followed by BCNU + DBD. In this study, 269 patients (grade III and IV gliomas) were randomized to either RT (60 Gy in 30 fractions) versus the same radiotherapy regimen plus concurrent DBD (700 mg/m^2) for 6 weekly cycles followed by every 6 weeks BCNU (150 mg/m^2) + DBD (1,000 mg/m^2) for 1 year. Improvements were noted in mOS (10.4 versus 13 months; p = 0.04), OS-2yr (12% versus 21%), and PFS-2yr (5% versus 16%). Subgroup analysis showed that patients with AA had greater response to chemotherapy than patients with GBM; however, due to the small sample size, the difference was not significant (71). Given these findings, a follow-up trial was initiated looking only at AA patients. Published in 2008, EORTC 26882 examined 193 AA patients treated on the previous regimen. mOS for the entire study was 23.9 months with no statistically significant difference in OS (23.9 months RT alone versus 27.3 months RT + DBD/BCNU) (72). In addition to BCNU, trials have investigated the effect of PCV chemotherapy in the upfront treatment of AA. Levin et al. reported a trend toward improved survival when combining adjuvant PCV with DFMO (α-difluoromethyl ornithine; eflornithine), an irreversible inhibitor of ornithine decarboxylase (involved in accumulation of polyamines leading to stabilization of DNA), versus PCV alone in a study of 249 patients with anaplastic glioma (~70% AA). Neither mOS (71 months [PCV + DFMO] versus 52 months [PCV]; p = 0.10) nor PFS (56 months [DFMO + PCV] versus 34 months [PCV]; p = 0.13) were statistically significant for all patients in this study by intention to treat analysis. Subgroup analysis of patients with AA showed a similar, albeit nonsignificant trend for both PFS and mOS in favor of DFMO + PCV (PFS 43 versus 17 months; p = 0.15, mOS 64 versus 41 months; p = 0.11). Toxicity in the combination chemotherapy arm was greater with more cases of grade III diarrhea and anemia (73). Given the variability across different chemotherapy trials, several meta-analyses have been conducted. In 1990, data from the Northern California Oncology Group protocol 6G61 for patients treated with 60 Gy adjuvant RT and either BCNU or PCV between 1977 and 1983 were reported. Both patients with GBM and AA had improvement in PFS and OS with PCV versus BCNU; however, this was only statistically significant in the AA group (n = 73) (74). A subsequent retrospective pooled analysis of patients treated with BCNU (RTOG 70–18, 83–02, and 90–06; n = 257) versus PCV (RTOG 94–04; n = 175) failed to confirm these findings. No difference in OS was noted between the two different treatment regimens (37). A prospective randomized trial performed by the MRC Brain Tumour Working Party investigating adjuvant PCV (every 6 weeks for maximum of 12 cycles) + RT versus RT alone in patients with high-grade glioma (n = 674) treated between 1988 and 1997 showed no benefit to adjuvant PCV. Patients in the combined modality arm had mOS of 10 versus 9.5 months; p= 0.50 (75). A large meta-analysis published in 2002 of 12 adjuvant chemotherapy trials (multiple regimens of both single- and multiagent chemotherapy) incorporating 3,004 patients with malignant glioma (24% AA) performed between 1965 and 1997 reported a small but significant benefit in OS at 1 and 2 years (5% and 6%, respectively) with the addition of chemotherapy to standard adjuvant radiotherapy (76). Although no toxicity data was provided in the report, many of the agents included in the study have well-documented high rates of treatment-related morbidity and mortality (23,24). Given the equivocal findings in the chemotherapy literature, the current standard of care outside of a clinical trial is surgical resection followed by involved field radiation therapy to 60 Gy in 30 fractions.

Incorporation of TMZ into the upfront treatment of GBM has resulted in significant improvement in OS when combined with radiation (77,78). As such, much interest has been generated in its incorporation into the treatment of AA. Multiple phase II studies have demonstrated the safety and efficacy of TMZ in the treatment of AA. In a multicenter trial of neoadjuvant TMZ in patients with newly diagnosed supratentorial malignant glioma (37% AA), a 39% objective response rate (11% complete (CR), 28% partial (PR)) was reported. An additional 32% of patients had stable disease. In a subset analysis of patients with AA, the response rate was 34% (10% complete (CR), 24% partial (PR)) with 30% patients demonstrating stable disease. mPFS and mOS in AA patients was 7.6 and 23.5 months, respectively. Grade III and IV adverse events were 28% and 12% for all patients, respectively, indicating that TMZ is relatively well tolerated (79). In a neoadjuvant, phase II study of newly diagnosed patients with malignant glioma (27% AA) published in 2005, Brada et al. reported an objective response rate of 20% and PFS prior to standard radiotherapy of 64% for patients receiving 2 cycles of TMZ (200 mg/m^2 for 5 days every 28 days). mOS was 10 months and OS-1yr was 41%. Response to TMZ was an important factor as mOS of responders was significantly greater than that of nonresponders (16 versus 9 months; $p < 0.001$). Subgroup analysis showed that patients with AA had longer mOS than patients with GBM (14 versus 8 months; $p = 0.005$) (80). Of note, patients in this study had only biopsy (91%) or partial excision (9%) of their tumor which may explain the general overall poorer results when compared to historical controls. These data support the activity of TMZ in the upfront setting. Recent studies have addressed the optimal sequencing of initial treatment. The NOA-04 randomized phase III trial of sequential radiochemotherapy in patients with grade III anaplastic glioma showed no difference in PFS or OS whether patients were treated with radiation or chemotherapy up front. In this study, following surgical resection or biopsy, 318 patients were randomized to receive RT (60 Gy in 1.8–2 Gy fractions) versus one of two chemotherapy regimens: PCV versus TMZ. At the time of radiographic progression, patients who initially received RT then received either PCV or TMZ, whereas patients initially randomized to chemotherapy went on to receive RT. mOS for all patients in this study was 72 versus 83 months in favor of patients who received chemotherapy upfront though this difference was not significant. No difference in survival was noted between PCV and TMZ. Likewise, no difference was noted with regard to PFS (30.6 months for RT, 31.9 months for chemotherapy; $p = 0.87$). Subgroup analysis of patients with AA showed improved PFS in the upfront chemotherapy arm (18.2 versus 10.8 months) though no difference was noted between chemotherapy regimens. Interestingly, patients who received RT upfront were less likely to undergo treatment at recurrence leading authors to posit if patients with grade III glioma should be treated with chemotherapy upfront holding radiotherapy in reserve for recurrence.

Recurrent Disease

Despite maximal treatment, failure is frequent in AA. Therefore, much effort has been placed in maximizing treatment approaches in the recurrent setting. Unfortunately, definitive data is lacking to guide treatment choices. Studies examining agents such as paclitaxel and gemcitabine have shown no significant activity in the recurrent setting (81). Irinotecan has been shown to be active in up to 15% of recurrent patients (82). Phase I trials investigating irinotecan plus temozolomide have shown response rates from 25% to 36% (83–85) TMZ alone has shown promising results. In a phase II study of 162 patients with recurrent high-grade glioma (97 AA, 14 AO), treatment with TMZ (200 mg/m^2/d if TMZ naïve versus 150 mg/m^2/d if previously treated with TMZ) resulted in an objective response rate of 35%. PFS at 6 and 12 months was 46% and 24%, respectively. mOS was 13.6 months. Progression-free status and objective radiographic response were both associated with improvements in quality of life. Treatment was well tolerated. Adverse side effects were mild to moderate with hematologic side effects being reported in less than 10% of patients.

Targeted Agents in Recurrent Setting

Studies of targeted therapies have shown mixed results in patients with recurrent AA. Many AA show overexpression of PDGF-R. The small molecule inhibitor, imatinib (Gleevec) inhibits PDGF-R and c-kit. Gleevec has been studied in recurrent high-grade glioma with mixed results. In a phase I/II trial of recurrent high-grade glioma (34 GBM, 21 anaplastic glioma), 5 stable disease and 0 partial responses were recorded in the anaplastic glioma group. PFS-6m in this group was only 10% and dose reductions were required in 15 of 21 patients due to hemorrhage (86). Results from a phase II study combining imatinib with hydroxyurea in recurrent grade III glioma demonstrated a PFS-6m of 24% with improved 6- and 12-month PFS (53% and 29%, respectively) in responders versus nonresponders (31). AA also exhibit high levels of neoangiogenesis. In patients with recurrent AA, bevacizumab-based regimens (either alone or in combination with systemic agents) have shown stabilization of performance status, decreased steroid use, and mOS ranging from 4 to 9 months (87–89).

■ GLIOBLASTOMA

Introduction

Glioblastoma multiforme (GBM) accounts for roughly 75% of all high-grade gliomas with approximately 9,500 new cases per year diagnosed in the United States alone (90). GBM is the most aggressive glial neoplasm with very poor prognosis. Median survival for patients with GBM is 15 months even with intensive intervention. Average age at diagnosis is typically in the sixth or seventh decade of life with a male to female ratio of 1.6:1. Common presenting symptoms include headache, nausea, vomiting, seizure, and localized neurological symptoms dependent on the location of the tumor. The majority of GBM are supratentorial though they can occur throughout the neuraxis. Several stratification schemes have been applied to the original RPA for malignant glioma to identify variables that predict outcome. A modified RPA was proposed by Shaw et al. in 2003 in the pre-TMZ era that correlated patient groups (based on age, performance status, extent of resection, and neurologic function) with OS (91). This stratification can be seen in Table 3. The RPA has been shown to maintain its prognostic significance in patients receiving RT +/– TMZ (Table 4) (92).

Histology/Genetics

Histologically, GBM is characterized by marked cellular atypia, necrosis, pseudopallisading, and neoangiogenesis. GBM can develop from lower grade lesions (secondary GBM) or arise de novo (primary GBM). Primary tumors constitute 90% of GBM and are typically seen in older patients, have a shorter clinical history (typically less than 3 months), and poorer overall prognosis compared to secondary lesions. At the genetic level, primary and secondary lesions demonstrate similar mutations but recent studies show each has a unique profile that may underlie their different natural course (93) (Figure 3). A characteristic mutation in primary lesions is amplification (40% of lesions) and overexpression (>60% of lesions)

TABLE 3 Modified RPA classification for GBM as proposed by Shaw et al.

Class	Definition	Med OS (mos)	OS-1yr (%)	OS-2yr (%)	OS-5yr (%)
III	Age < 50, KPS ≥ 90	17.1	70	20	14
IV	Age < 50, KPS < 90	11.2	46	7	4
	Age ≥ 50, KPS ≥ 70, G/STR, W+				
V+VI	Age ≥ 50, KPS ≥ 70, G/STR, W–	7.5	28	1	0
	Age ≥ 50, KPS ≥ 70, Biopsy				
	Age ≥ 50, KPS < 70				

Abbreviations: G/STR = gross or subtotal resection, W+ = neurological function (working), W– = neurological function (not working).
Source: Modified from Shaw et al. (2003).

TABLE 4 Modified RPA for patients with GBM treated with RT +/– TMZ

Class	Definition	Med OS (mos)	OS-2yr (%)	*p*
III	Age < 50, WHO PS 0	21 vs. 15	43 vs. 20	0.006
IV	Age < 50, WHO PS 1–2 Age ≥ 50, G/STR, MMSE ≥ 27	16 vs. 13	28 vs. 11	0.0001
V	Age ≥ 50 MMSE < 27, biopsy only	10 vs. 9	17 vs. 6	0.054

Values for Med OS and OS-2yr in each cell represent TMZ as part of treatment versus no TMZ, respectively. Abbreviations: G/STR = gross or subtotal resection, MMSE = Mini-Mental State Examination, WHO PS = World Health Organization Performance Status.
Source: Modified from Mirimanoff et al. (2006).

of epidermal growth factor receptor (EGFR) that results in enhanced proliferation and cell survival by blocking apoptosis (93,94). A second mutation seen almost exclusively in primary GBM is mutation in the PTEN gene that leads to increased cell migration and invasion (93). Secondary GBM exhibits many of the genetic mutations seen in lower grade lesions (AA, AO). One such mutation, TP53, is seen in nearly two-thirds of precursor, low-grade lesions and is present in ~75% of secondary GBM but less than 30% of primary GBM (59,95). Mutations in TP53 can result in abnormal cell cycle regulation and differentiation, enhanced survival, and neovascularization associated with malignancy. Mutations in TP53 are thought to be an important step in the initiation of glial malignancies.

The genetic profile of GBM has also been shown to be an important factor in response to treatment and overall prognosis (96,97). MGMT is a DNA repair protein that removes alkyl adducts from DNA. Alkylating agents such as TMZ are first-line treatment for newly diagnosed GBM. High levels of MGMT expression lead to enhanced repair of such lesions and decreased responsiveness to chemoradiotherapy utilizing alkylating chemotherapies. Hypermethylation of the MGMT promoter (and thus decreased levels of MGMT and increased responsiveness to treatment) is seen in approximately 75% of secondary and 35% of primary GBM (98).

Advances in molecular biology have allowed high throughput expression analysis of large numbers of genes. Using these techniques, researchers have identified four unique subtypes of GBM: proneural, neural, classical, and mesenchymal (99). Patients with the proneural subtype are typically younger in age, show homology with predominantly oligodendritic tumors and, like those tumors, have longer OS. Conversely, patients with the mesenchymal subtype are older with poorer survival. Efforts are currently underway to identify gene profiles within GBM that predict survival and response to treatment in hopes of optimizing current therapies and identifying new targets for intervention (96).

Imaging

On T1-weighted, contrast-enhanced, MRI images, GBM commonly present as ring-enhancing lesions with variable areas of central necrosis. Surrounding this region of central enhancement is a variable amount of hyperintense T2/FLAIR signal. The extent of T2/FLAIR activity is largely dependent on lesion size but clinically is felt to represent areas of active, infiltrative tumor. These MRI volumes form the basis for radiotherapy target delineation. As discussed earlier, though MRI is the current clinical gold standard for the assessment of intracranial pathology, it is limited by the fact the origins of its signal are merely surrogate markers of tumor presence (tumor-associated breakdown of the blood–brain barrier and cerebral edema) versus a direct measure of neoplastic involvement. Functional imaging techniques have helped clinicians better delineate tumor from normal brain but these techniques are also not without their limitations. The most commonly used PET radiotracer, [^{18}F]-fluorodeoxyglucose, is relatively insensitive at differentiating malignancy from normal brain due to the inherent high basal metabolic demands of normal brain function (100). Clinically available radiotracers such as L-methyl-^{11}C-methionine (MET) and O-(2-[^{18}F]fluoroethyl)-L-tyrosine (FET) have shown promise in more precisely localizing high-grade gliomas. Recent studies have shown that MET-PET can more accurately identify areas of active tumor versus traditional MRI (101,102). MET is actively taken up by glioma but shows only low uptake in normal brain. In a study of 14 patients with high-grade glioma, MET-PET was highly correlated with areas of endothelial proliferation and mitotic activity (103) a more direct marker of tumor activity. In a study of 26 patients with GBM, Lee et al. (101) demonstrated that 5 of 26 patients had areas of MET-PET positivity outside radiotherapy volumes defined by MRI. All of these patients had noncentral failures. In 14 patients where MET-PET positive areas were covered in the high-dose radiotherapy volume none had noncentral failures. One limitation of MET-PET is that it is actively taken up in areas of inflammation, somewhat limiting its use in the postoperative setting. FET-PET also correlates with areas of active tumor but shows relatively low signal in inflammatory tissues. In a study of 31 patients with GBM, FET-PET was highly correlated with areas of active tumor on biopsy (104). Like with MET-PET, FET-PET studies have been shown to identify tissue outside of areas active on MRI. In a study comparing FET-PET and MRI, Piroth et al (105) showed that areas active on FET-PET not covered by MRI-based radiotherapy target volumes predicted a shorter disease-free survival (5.1 versus 9.6 months) and OS 6.9 versus 20 months) suggesting that radiation treatment planning may be further optimized by the integration of metabolically based imaging techniques. Functional imaging is also proving valuable in the recurrent setting. The specificity of FET-PET and MET-PET to detect recurrent disease is approximately 90% and 70%, respectively (105). Areas active on FET-PET show a high correlation with biopsy proven areas of active disease (104) and regions of enhancing tissue on MRI are often negative on FET-PET.

MRS, which measures the differential concentrations of metabolites in the brain, can aid in the diagnosis and planning for radiotherapy (106–110). Spectroscopically, GBM shows a high choline to creatinine ratio (reflecting cellular proliferation and cell membrane turnover), high lactate signal, high lipid signal, and low or absent N-acetyl aspartate (measure of neuronal integrity) (111). MRS profiles have been shown to correlate with tumor grade (49,51) and invasiveness (52). MRS has also proven to be valuable in distinguishing recurrent disease and, in some studies, has demonstrated improved accuracy versus MRI (71% versus 55%) (112).

GBM demonstrate high levels of neoangiogenesis leading to significant alterations in regional cerebral blood flow (rCBV). As such, perfusion-sensitive techniques like perfusion-weighted MRI (pMRI) show elevated signal in areas involved with tumor (113,114). In a study of 51 patients with intracranial glioma, Arvinda et al. demonstrated that preoperative pMRI values in tumor regions showed a significant correlation with final tumor grade (113). Other groups have reported a similar relationship between rCBV and glioma grade (55,114,115) and some suggest that rCBV maps are more accurate than contrast-enhanced scans for identification of tumor, which could help improve surgical targeting as well as radiotherapy target delineation (114).

Treatment

Initial therapy in the treatment of GBM is safe maximal resection (21). The extent of resection is significantly correlated with OS (116–118). In a retrospective study of 416 patients with GBM, Lacroix et al. found a significant survival advantage for patients with 98% resection of gross tumor volume (mOS 13 months) versus those with lesser resection (mOS 8.8 months; $p < 0.001$) (116). Despite the benefits of maximal resection, surgery alone is inadequate given the diffusely infiltrative nature of GBM. With surgery as the only treatment modality, OS-1yr is less than 30% with very few survivors at 2 years (119). The benefit of adjuvant radiotherapy to doses of 50 to 60 Gy was demonstrated in several studies conducted by the BTSG in the 1970s (120,121). Initially, patients were treated using whole brain fields but analysis of patterns of recurrence showed most patients recurred within 2 cm of the original tumor. This combined with the toxicity of whole brain radiotherapy to high doses led to trials comparing whole brain and involved-field radiation. No significant difference in survival was noted between the two techniques (122); therefore, the standard for radiation therapy became involved-field only to 60 Gy. Given that most patients recur very close to the original tumor, attempts have been made to escalate radiation doses in attempt to improve tumor control. Unfortunately, studies of hyperfractionation (123), brachytherapy (122,124), stereotactic radiosurgery (SRS) (125), or fractionated stereotactic radiotherapy (FSRT) (126) have shown no significant benefit in OS.

Historically, the addition of chemotherapy to adjuvant radiation led to only modest improvements in OS. A meta-analysis of studies published between 1993 and 2007 showed a 6% increase in 1-year survival and 2-month increase in median survival for patients receiving chemotherapy (76). The bulk of chemotherapy studies during this era employed alkylating agents like Carmustine (BCNU). Studies of BCNU wafers (Gliadel) placed in the surgical cavity at the time of resection show improved mOS (13.1 versus 11.4 months; $p = 0.017$) versus placebo (127). The major breakthrough in the management of GBM has been the introduction of TMZ in the adjuvant setting. In 2005, the EORTC 26981–22981/National Cancer Institute of Canada Clinical Trials Group CE3 (NCIC) published the results of a phase III randomized control trial of 573 patients with GBM treated postoperatively with either RT alone (60 Gy in 30 fractions) versus RT + TMZ (75 mg/m^2, 7 days per week) followed by 6 cycles of TMZ (150 to 200 mg/m^2 for 5 days of each 28-day cycle). The addition of TMZ to adjuvant radiotherapy improved mOS (14.6 versus 12.1 months) and OS-2yr (26.6% versus 10.4%) (78). The survival curves are depicted in Figure 4. When the data from this landmark trial were assessed using the EORTC RPA criteria, a significant survival benefit was seen in RPA classes III and IV. A smaller and borderline significant difference was seen in RPA class V (92). The modified RPA classification is shown in Table 4. A secondary analysis of the relationship between MGMT silencing and OS was also performed for patients treated on this trial. MGMT was found to be an independent favorable prognostic factor. A significant survival benefit was seen in those patients with hypermethylated MGMT promoter (21.7 versus 15.3 months; $p = 0.007$) (97). Survival curves for MGMT hypermethylated patients are shown in Figure 5. There was a similar improved survival in those patients treated with RT alone though the values were not statistically significant. A 5-year update of patients treated on this study was published in 2009. The survival benefit in patients treated with RT + TMZ was maintained (9.8 versus 1.9%; $p < 0.0001$) (77). This benefit was seen across all prognostic diagnostic groups. The survival curves are shown in Figure 6. As in the original 2005 study, MGMT methylation status was the strongest predictor of outcome and response to TMZ-based chemoradiotherapy (77). Given these results, the current standard of care for newly diagnosed GBM is maximal safe resection followed by concurrent chemoradiation with TMZ.

Recent advances in molecular techniques have led to the advent of therapies that allow clinicians to target specific aspects of tumor biology involved in abnormal cell growth, survival, invasion, and neoangiogenesis. GBMs are rapidly proliferating tumors with high levels of neovascularization. However, the vessels are highly disorganized and inefficient leading

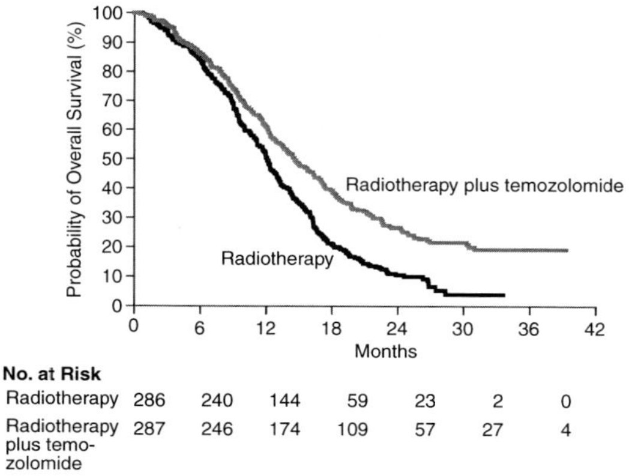

FIGURE 4 OS curves for patients treated with adjuvant RT +/– TMZ.
Source: Stupp et al., NEJM 2005.

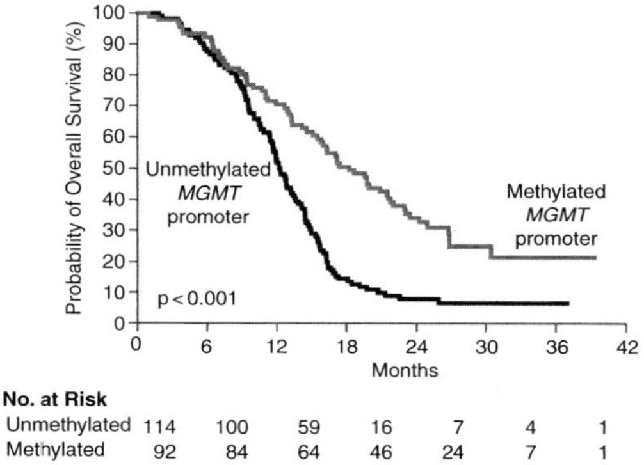

FIGURE 5 OS stratified by MGMT methylation status.
Source: Hegi et al., NEJM 2005.

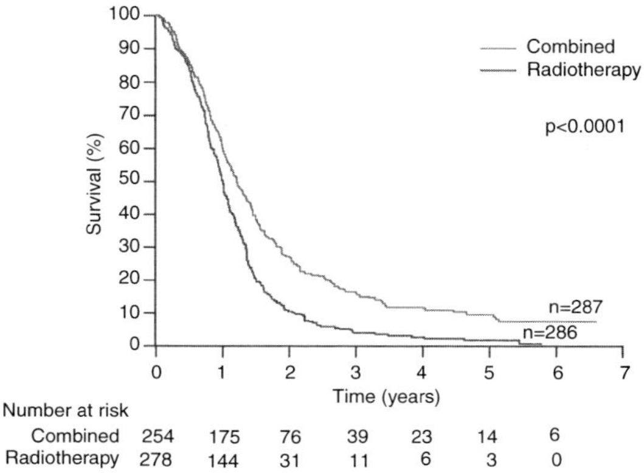

FIGURE 6 Five-year update of group treated on original Stupp trial from 2005. OS gains between groups were maintained at 5 years.
Source: Stupp et al., Lancet 2009.

to tumor hypoxia and increased levels of hypoxia-inducible factor 1 alpha (HIF-1α). This activates proangiogenic pathways such as vascular endothelial growth factor (VEGF) that initiate a cascade of events leading to cell proliferation, survival, and formation of new blood vessels. VEGF-A is the predominant factor secreted by GBM and its effect is mediated through the VEGFR-2 receptor. Bevacizumab is a monoclonal antibody against VEGF-A. It has been approved for treatment of a variety of cancers including recurrent GBM (as discussed in the next section) (128). Its use in the upfront setting is also currently being tested in multi-institution, phase III, randomized control trial being conducted through the RTOG. RTOG 0825 randomized newly diagnosed GBM patients to adjuvant chemoradiotherapy with TMZ +/– bevacizumab. Patients received an initial 3 weeks of chemoradiation (30 Gy in 2 Gy fractions) with daily TMZ. They were then stratified by MGMT methylation status and molecular profile (favorable versus unfavorable) to either an additional 3 weeks of radiotherapy (30 Gy in 2 Gy fractions) + daily TMZ + placebo every 2 weeks versus radiotherapy + daily TMZ + bevacizumab every 2 weeks. Four weeks following completion of chemoradiotherapy, maintenance TMZ (days 1–5 for a 28-day cycle) + bevacizumab every 2 weeks versus placebo every 2 weeks was given for a maximum of 12 cycles. This trial closed in 2011. The outcome of the trial is being eagerly awaited. If bevacizumab shows benefit in the newly diagnosed setting it may shift the standard of care for GBM.

Recurrent Disease

The majority of patients with GBM recur within 8 to 12 months following completion of adjuvant therapy thus optimizing treatment options in the recurrent setting is of great importance. Depending on the magnitude of the recurrence, options include re-resection, radiotherapy (SRS versus FSRT), chemotherapy, targeted agents, or combinations thereof. Re-irradiation with or without chemotherapy has shown the most promise. The majority of patients fail within 2 cm of the primary site, thus highly focused and conformal radiotherapy techniques, such as SRS, have been widely studied (129–131). SRS provides the benefit of minimizing further radiation exposure to areas of normal brain treated to high dose within a short-time interval. Studies of SRS in the recurrent setting suggest a modest improvement in outcome; however, the risk of radionecrosis within the retreatment field is significant and often requires surgical resection. The results of patients treated with FSRT have been more promising with mOS ranging from approximately 7 to 14 months but with reduced rates of morbidity (129,132–134) as compared to SRS. Dosing regimens with a cumulative dose exceeding 40 Gy appear to be associated with a greater degree of radiation necrosis (135,136). Response on post-procedure MRI appears to be an important prognostic factor for either SRS or FSRT. In a study of 36 patients (26 SRS, 10 FRST) patients showing response on post-treatment MRI had median survival of 15.8 versus 7.3 months for nonresponders (129).

Combination chemoradiotherapy has shown some efficacy in the recurrent setting. In a study of 25 patients with recurrent high-grade glioma (20 GBM, 4 AA) treatment with FSRT (30 Gy in 5 fractions) plus concurrent bevacizumab resulted in a median survival of 12.5 months following treatment (137) with toxicity rates comparable to studies of GBM patients treated with bevacizumab alone. A recent phase I, dose escalation trial of gefitinib, an EGFR tyrosine kinase inhibitor, plus FSRT (18 to 36 Gy in 1 to 3 fractions) in 15 patients (11 GBM, 4 AA) showed this combination was well tolerated at all dose levels. mPFS was 7 months with a PFS-6m of 63% and OS-1yr of 40% (138). Studies combining cytotoxic chemotherapy with FSRT agents have shown similar response rates with acceptable toxicity profiles (139,140).

Recurrent disease can also be managed with chemotherapy alone. Modifications in the dosing regimen of TMZ show modest improvements in PFS. Standard dosing regimens of TMZ (200 mg/m^2) produce a PFS-6m of 21% (141). TMZ delivered in a low dose, protracted schedule (75 mg/m^2 for 21 days of a 28-day cycle) in an attempt to deplete MGMT has resulted in PFS-6m of 30% (142). Other single-agent studies have failed to show significant durable response. Patients treated on combination regimens fare better than those treated on single-agent regimens. For example, in a recent phase II study, treatment with irinotecan (a topoisomerase inhibitor) plus bevacizumab produced a PFS-6m of 46% (34) as compared to studies of single-agent irinotecan alone which show response rates of 0% to 17% (82,143,144) A recent phase II trial of 167 patients with recurrent GBM comparing bevacizumab plus irinotecan versus bevacizumab alone demonstrated promising results in both groups. PFS-6m was 50.3% in the combination treatment arm versus 42.6% in those treated with bevacizumab alone (145). These data plus other similar studies have led to FDA approval of bevacizumab for use in recurrent GBM. Treatment with antiangiogenic agents alone is not without its pitfalls. In a study comparing recurrent patients with no prior antiangiogenic exposure to those with prior antiangiogenic treatment retreated with bevacizumab, the PFS-6m and OS was 36% versus 14% and 18 months versus 4 months, respectively (146). Other studies looking at treatment following exposure to bevacizumab with other agents show similar poor results. Some postulate that exposure to bevacizumab selects for a treatment-resistant, highly infiltrative phenotype not readily visible on contrast-enhanced MRI (147). However, definitive data on this issue and the underlying mechanism are lacking.

REFERENCES

1. Engelhard HH, Stelea A, Mundt A. Oligodendroglioma and anaplastic oligodendroglioma: clinical features, treatment, and prognosis. *Surg Neurol.* 2003;60(5):443–456.
2. van den Bent MJ. Anaplastic oligodendroglioma and oligoastrocytoma. *Neurol Clin.* 2007;25(4):1089–109, ix.
3. Shaw EG, Scheithauer BW, O'Fallon JR. Supratentorial gliomas: a comparative study by grade and histologic type. *J Neurooncol.* 1997;31(3):273–278.
4. Cairncross JG, Ueki K, Zlatescu MC, et al. Specific genetic predictors of chemotherapeutic response and survival in patients with anaplastic oligodendrogliomas. *J Natl Cancer Inst.* 1998;90(19):1473–1479.
5. Macdonald DR. Low-grade gliomas, mixed gliomas, and oligodendrogliomas. *Semin Oncol.* 1994;21(2):236–248.
6. Kros JM, Gorlia T, Kouwenhoven MC, et al. Panel review of anaplastic oligodendroglioma from European Organization for Research and Treatment of Cancer Trial 26951: assessment of consensus in diagnosis, influence of 1p/19q loss, and correlations with outcome. *J Neuropathol Exp Neurol.* 2007;66(6):545–551.
7. Jenkins RB, Blair H, Ballman KV, et al. A t(1;19)(q10;p10) mediates the combined deletions of 1p and 19q and predicts a better prognosis of patients with oligodendroglioma. *Cancer Res.* 2006;66(20):9852–9861.
8. Möllemann M, Wolter M, Felsberg J, Collins VP, Reifenberger G. Frequent promoter hypermethylation and low expression of the MGMT gene in oligodendroglial tumors. *Int J Cancer.* 2005;113(3):379–385.
9. Louis DN, Ohgaki H, Wiestler OD, et al. The 2007 WHO classification of tumours of the central nervous system. *Acta Neuropathol.* 2007;114(2):97–109.
10. Bromberg JE, van den Bent MJ. Oligodendrogliomas: molecular biology and treatment. *Oncologist.* 2009;14(2):155–163.
11. Miller CR, Dunham CP, Scheithauer BW, Perry A. Significance of necrosis in grading of oligodendroglial neoplasms: a clinicopathologic and genetic study of newly diagnosed high-grade gliomas. *J Clin Oncol.* 2006;24(34):5419–5426.
12. Dehais C, Laigle-Donadey F, Marie Y, et al. Prognostic stratification of patients with anaplastic gliomas according to genetic profile. *Cancer.* 2006;107(8):1891–1897.
13. Ginsberg LE, Fuller GN, Hashmi M, Leeds NE, Schomer DF. The significance of lack of MR contrast enhancement of supratentorial brain tumors in adults: histopathological evaluation of a series. *Surg Neurol.* 1998;49(4):436–440.
14. Megyesi JF, Kachur E, Lee DH, et al. Imaging correlates of molecular signatures in oligodendrogliomas. *Clin Cancer Res.* 2004;10(13):4303–4306.
15. Spampinato MV, Smith JK, Kwock L, et al. Cerebral blood volume measurements and proton MR spectroscopy in grading of oligodendroglial tumors. *AJR Am J Roentgenol.* 2007;188(1):204–212.
16. Cha S, Knopp EA, Johnson G, et al. Dynamic contrast-enhanced T2-weighted MR imaging of recurrent malignant gliomas treated with thalidomide and carboplatin. *AJNR Am J Neuroradiol.* 2000;21(5):881–890.
17. Derlon JM, Chapon F, Noël MH, et al. Non-invasive grading of oligodendrogliomas: correlation between *in vivo* metabolic pattern and histopathology. *Eur J Nucl Med.* 2000;27(7):778–787.
18. Hlaihel C, Guilloton L, Guyotat J, Streichenberger N, Honnorat J, Cotton F. Predictive value of multimodality MRI using conventional, perfusion, and spectroscopy MR in anaplastic transformation of low-grade oligodendrogliomas. *J Neurooncol.* 2010;97(1):73–80.
19. Chang SM, Nelson S, Vandenberg S, et al. Integration of preoperative anatomic and metabolic physiologic imaging of newly diagnosed glioma. *J Neurooncol.* 2009;92(3):401–415.
20. Oshiro S, Tsugu H, Komatsu F, et al. Quantitative assessment of gliomas by proton magnetic resonance spectroscopy. *Anticancer Res.* 2007;27(6A):3757–3763.
21. Network, NCCN Guidelines Version 1.2012, Central nervous system cancers. NCCN, 2012.
22. Cairncross G, Wang M, Shaw E, et al. Chemotherapy plus radiotherapy (CT-RT) versus RT alone for patients with anaplastic oligodendroglioma: long-term results of the RTOG 9402 phase III study. *J Clin Oncol.* 2012;30(suppl; abstr 2008b).
23. Cairncross G, Berkey B, Shaw E, et al.; Intergroup Radiation Therapy Oncology Group Trial 9402. Phase III trial of chemotherapy plus radiotherapy compared with radiotherapy alone for pure and mixed anaplastic oligodendroglioma: Intergroup Radiation Therapy Oncology Group Trial 9402. *J Clin Oncol.* 2006;24(18):2707–2714.
24. van den Bent MJ, Carpentier AF, Brandes AA, et al. Adjuvant procarbazine, lomustine, and vincristine improves progression-free survival but not overall survival in newly diagnosed anaplastic oligodendrogliomas and oligoastrocytomas: a randomized European Organisation for Research and Treatment of Cancer phase III trial. *J Clin Oncol.* 2006;24(18):2715–2722.

25. van den Bent MJ, Dubbink HJ, Sanson M, et al. MGMT promoter methylation is prognostic but not predictive for outcome to adjuvant PCV chemotherapy in anaplastic oligodendroglial tumors: a report from EORTC Brain Tumor Group Study 26951. *J Clin Oncol.* 2009;27(35):5881–5886.
26. Van den Bent M, Hoang-Xuan K, Brandes A, et al. Long-term follow-up results of EORTC 26951: a randomized phase III study on adjuvant PCV chemotherapy in anaplastic oligodendroglial tumors (AOD). *J Clin Oncol.* 2012;30 (suppl; abstr 2).
27. Mikkelsen T, Doyle T, Anderson J, et al. Temozolomide single-agent chemotherapy for newly diagnosed anaplastic oligodendroglioma. *J Neurooncol.* 2009;92(1):57–63.
28. Vogelbaum MA, Berkey B, Peereboom D, et al. Phase II trial of preirradiation and concurrent temozolomide in patients with newly diagnosed anaplastic oligodendrogliomas and mixed anaplastic oligoastrocytomas: RTOG BR0131. *Neuro-oncology.* 2009;11(2):167–175.
29. Taliansky-Aronov A, Bokstein F, Lavon I, Siegal T. Temozolomide treatment for newly diagnosed anaplastic oligodendrogliomas: a clinical efficacy trial. *J Neurooncol.* 2006;79(2):153–157.
30. Reardon DA, Egorin MJ, Quinn JA, et al. Phase II study of imatinib mesylate plus hydroxyurea in adults with recurrent glioblastoma multiforme. *J Clin Oncol.* 2005;23(36):9359–9368.
31. Desjardins A, Quinn JA, Vredenburgh JJ, et al. Phase II study of imatinib mesylate and hydroxyurea for recurrent grade III malignant gliomas. *J Neurooncol.* 2007;83(1):53–60.
32. Chamberlain MC, Johnston S. Bevacizumab for recurrent alkylator-refractory anaplastic oligodendroglioma. *Cancer.* 2009;115(8):1734–1743.
33. Taillibert S, Vincent LA, Granger B, et al. Bevacizumab and irinotecan for recurrent oligodendroglial tumors. *Neurology.* 2009;72(18):1601–1606.
34. Vredenburgh JJ, Desjardins A, Herndon JE 2nd, et al. Phase II trial of bevacizumab and irinotecan in recurrent malignant glioma. *Clin Cancer Res.* 2007;13(4):1253–1259.
35. Stupp R, Reni M, Gatta G, Mazza E, Vecht C. Anaplastic astrocytoma in adults. *Crit Rev Oncol Hematol.* 2007;63(1):72–80.
36. Chang S, Theodosopoulos P, Sneed P. Multidisciplinary management of adult anaplastic astrocytomas. *Semin Radiat Oncol.* 2001;11(2):163–169.
37. Prados MD, Scott C, Curran WJ Jr, Nelson DF, Leibel S, Kramer S. Procarbazine, lomustine, and vincristine (PCV) chemotherapy for anaplastic astrocytoma: A retrospective review of radiation therapy oncology group protocols comparing survival with carmustine or PCV adjuvant chemotherapy. *J Clin Oncol.* 1999;17(11):3389–3395.
38. Curran WJ Jr, Scott CB, Horton J, et al. Recursive partitioning analysis of prognostic factors in three Radiation Therapy Oncology Group malignant glioma trials. *J Natl Cancer Inst.* 1993;85(9):704–710.
39. Hardell L, Carlberg M, Mild KH. Case-control study of the association between the use of cellular and cordless telephones and malignant brain tumors diagnosed during 2000–2003. *Environ Res.* 2006;100(2):232–241.
40. Thomas TL, Stolley PD, Stemhagen A, et al. Brain tumor mortality risk among men with electrical and electronics jobs: a case-control study. *J Natl Cancer Inst.* 1987;79(2):233–238.
41. Heineman EF, Cocco P, Gómez MR, et al. Occupational exposure to chlorinated aliphatic hydrocarbons and risk of astrocytic brain cancer. *Am J Ind Med.* 1994;26(2):155–169.
42. Andersson E, Nilsson R, Torén K. Gliomas among men employed in the Swedish pulp and paper industry. *Scand J Work Environ Health.* 2002;28(5):333–340.
43. Keles GE, Chang EF, Lamborn KR, et al. Volumetric extent of resection and residual contrast enhancement on initial surgery as predictors of outcome in adult patients with hemispheric anaplastic astrocytoma. *J Neurosurg.* 2006;105(1):34–40.
44. Matar E, Cook RJ, Fowler AR, et al. Post-contrast enhancement as a clinical indicator of prognosis in patients with anaplastic astrocytoma. *J Clin Neurosci.* 2010;17(8):993–996.
45. Scott JN, Brasher PM, Sevick RJ, Rewcastle NB, Forsyth PA. How often are nonenhancing supratentorial gliomas malignant? A population study. *Neurology.* 2002;59(6):947–949.
46. Tortosa A, Viñolas N, Villà S, et al. Prognostic implication of clinical, radiologic, and pathologic features in patients with anaplastic gliomas. *Cancer.* 2003;97(4):1063–1071.
47. De Witte O, Goldberg I, Wikler D, et al. Positron emission tomography with injection of methionine as a prognostic factor in glioma. *J Neurosurg.* 2001;95(5):746–750.
48. Torii K, Tsuyuguchi N, Kawabe J, Sunada I, Hara M, Shiomi S. Correlation of amino-acid uptake using methionine PET and histological classifications in various gliomas. *Ann Nucl Med.* 2005;19(8):677–683.
49. Fayed N, Modrego PJ. The contribution of magnetic resonance spectroscopy and echoplanar perfusion-weighted MRI in the initial assessment of brain tumours. *J Neurooncol.* 2005;72(3):261–265.
50. Majós C, Alonso J, Aguilera C, et al. Proton magnetic resonance spectroscopy ((1)H MRS) of human brain tumours: assessment of differences between tumour types and its applicability in brain tumour categorization. *Eur Radiol.* 2003;13(3):582–591.
51. Meyerand ME, Pipas JM, Mamourian A, Tosteson TD, Dunn JF. Classification of biopsy-confirmed brain tumors using single-voxel MR spectroscopy. *AJNR Am J Neuroradiol.* 1999;20(1):117–123.
52. Zhang K, Li C, Liu Y, et al. Evaluation of invasiveness of astrocytoma using 1H-magnetic resonance spectroscopy: correlation with expression of matrix metalloproteinase-2. *Neuroradiology.* 2007;49(11):913–919.
53. Calli C, Kitis O, Yunten N, Yurtseven T, Islekel S, Akalin T. Perfusion and diffusion MR imaging in enhancing malignant cerebral tumors. *Eur J Radiol.* 2006;58(3):394–403.

54. Maia AC Jr, Malheiros SM, da Rocha AJ, et al. MR cerebral blood volume maps correlated with vascular endothelial growth factor expression and tumor grade in nonenhancing gliomas. *AJNR Am J Neuroradiol.* 2005;26(4):777–783.

55. Lee SJ, Kim JH, Kim YM, et al. Perfusion MR imaging in gliomas: comparison with histologic tumor grade. *Korean J Radiol.* 2001;2(1):1–7.

56. Hirai T, Murakami R, Nakamura H, et al. Prognostic value of perfusion MR imaging of high-grade astrocytomas: long-term follow-up study. *AJNR Am J Neuroradiol.* 2008;29(8):1505–1510.

57. Nozaki M, Tada M, Kobayashi H, et al. Roles of the functional loss of p53 and other genes in astrocytoma tumorigenesis and progression. *Neuro-oncology.* 1999;1(2):124–137.

58. Chawengchao B, Petmitr S, Ponglikitmongkol M, et al. Detection of a novel point mutation in the p53 gene in grade II astrocytomas by PCR-SSCP analysis with additional Klenow treatment. *Anticancer Res.* 2001;21(4A):2739–2743.

59. Ohgaki H, Dessen P, Jourde B, et al. Genetic pathways to glioblastoma: a population-based study. *Cancer Res.* 2004;64(19):6892–6899.

60. Rivera AL, Pelloski CE, Sulman E, Aldape K. Prognostic and predictive markers in glioma and other neuroepithelial tumors. *Curr Probl Cancer.* 2008;32(3):97–123.

61. Smith JS, Tachibana I, Passe SM, et al. PTEN mutation, EGFR amplification, and outcome in patients with anaplastic astrocytoma and glioblastoma multiforme. *J Natl Cancer Inst.* 2001;93(16):1246–1256.

62. Bäcklund LM, Nilsson BR, Liu L, Ichimura K, Collins VP. Mutations in Rb1 pathway-related genes are associated with poor prognosis in anaplastic astrocytomas. *Br J Cancer.* 2005;93(1):124–130.

63. Donahue B, Scott CB, Nelson JS, et al. Influence of an oligodendroglial component on the survival of patients with anaplastic astrocytomas: a report of Radiation Therapy Oncology Group 83–02. *Int J Radiat Oncol Biol Phys.* 1997;38(5):911–914.

64. Nitta T, Sato K. Prognostic implications of the extent of surgical resection in patients with intracranial malignant gliomas. *Cancer.* 1995;75(11):2727–2731.

65. Walker MD, Alexander E Jr, Hunt WE, et al. Evaluation of BCNU and/or radiotherapy in the treatment of anaplastic gliomas. A cooperative clinical trial. *J Neurosurg.* 1978;49(3):333–343.

66. Walker MD, Green SB, Byar DP, et al. Randomized comparisons of radiotherapy and nitrosoureas for the treatment of malignant glioma after surgery. *N Engl J Med.* 1980;303(23):1323–1329.

67. Deutsch M, Green SB, Strike TA, et al. Results of a randomized trial comparing BCNU plus radiotherapy, streptozotocin plus radiotherapy, BCNU plus hyperfractionated radiotherapy, and BCNU following misonidazole plus radiotherapy in the postoperative treatment of malignant glioma. *Int J Radiat Oncol Biol Phys.* 1989;16(6):1389–1396.

68. Bleehen NM, Stenning SP. A Medical Research Council trial of two radiotherapy doses in the treatment of grades 3 and 4 astrocytoma. The Medical Research Council Brain Tumour Working Party. *Br J Cancer.* 1991;64(4):769–774.

69. Chang CH, Horton J, Schoenfeld D, et al. Comparison of postoperative radiotherapy and combined postoperative radiotherapy and chemotherapy in the multidisciplinary management of malignant gliomas. A joint Radiation Therapy Oncology Group and Eastern Cooperative Oncology Group study. *Cancer.* 1983;52(6):997–1007.

70. Sathornsumetee S, Rich JN, Reardon DA. Diagnosis and treatment of high-grade astrocytoma. *Neurol Clin.* 2007 Nov;25(4):1111–1139.

71. Hildebrand J, Sahmoud T, Mignolet F, Brucher JM, Afra D. Adjuvant therapy with dibromodulcitol and BCNU increases survival of adults with malignant gliomas. EORTC Brain Tumor Group. *Neurology.* 1994;44(8):1479–1483.

72. Hildebrand J, Gorlia T, Kros JM, et al.; EORTC Brain Tumour Group investigators. Adjuvant dibromodulcitol and BCNU chemotherapy in anaplastic astrocytoma: results of a randomised European Organisation for Research and Treatment of Cancer phase III study (EORTC study 26882). *Eur J Cancer.* 2008;44(9):1210–1216.

73. Levin VA, Hess KR, Choucair A, et al. Phase III randomized study of postradiotherapy chemotherapy with combination alpha-difluoromethylornithine-PCV versus PCV for anaplastic gliomas. *Clin Cancer Res.* 2003;9(3):981–990.

74. Levin VA, Silver P, Hannigan J, et al. Superiority of post-radiotherapy adjuvant chemotherapy with CCNU, procarbazine, and vincristine (PCV) over BCNU for anaplastic gliomas: NCOG 6G61 final report. *Int J Radiat Oncol Biol Phys.* 1990;18(2):321–324.

75. Medical Research Council Brain Tumor Working Party. Randomized trial of procarbazine, lomustine, and vincristine in the adjuvant treatment of high-grade astrocytoma: a Medical Research Council trial. *J Clin Oncol.* 2001;19(2):509–518.

76. Stewart LA. Chemotherapy in adult high-grade glioma: a systematic review and meta-analysis of individual patient data from 12 randomised trials. *Lancet.* 2002;359(9311):1011–1018.

77. Stupp R, Hegi ME, Mason WP, et al.; European Organisation for Research and Treatment of Cancer Brain Tumour and Radiation Oncology Groups; National Cancer Institute of Canada Clinical Trials Group. Effects of radiotherapy with concomitant and adjuvant temozolomide versus radiotherapy alone on survival in glioblastoma in a randomised phase III study: 5-year analysis of the EORTC-NCIC trial. *Lancet Oncol.* 2009;10(5):459–466.

78. Stupp R, Mason WP, van den Bent MJ, et al.; European Organisation for Research and Treatment of Cancer Brain Tumor and Radiotherapy Groups; National Cancer

Institute of Canada Clinical Trials Group. Radiotherapy plus concomitant and adjuvant temozolomide for glioblastoma. *N Engl J Med*. 2005;352(10):987–996.

79. Gilbert MR, Friedman HS, Kuttesch JF, et al. A phase II study of temozolomide in patients with newly diagnosed supratentorial malignant glioma before radiation therapy. *Neuro-oncology*. 2002;4(4):261–267.
80. Brada M, Ashley S, Dowe A, et al. Neoadjuvant phase II multicentre study of new agents in patients with malignant glioma after minimal surgery. Report of a cohort of 187 patients treated with temozolomide. *Ann Oncol*. 2005;16(6):942–949.
81. Kortmann RD, Jeremic B, Weller M, Plasswilm L, Bamberg M. Radiochemotherapy of malignant glioma in adults. Clinical experiences. *Strahlenther Onkol*. 2003;179(4):219–232.
82. Friedman HS, Petros WP, Friedman AH, et al. Irinotecan therapy in adults with recurrent or progressive malignant glioma. *J Clin Oncol*. 1999;17(5):1516–1525.
83. Gruber ML, Buster WP. Temozolomide in combination with irinotecan for treatment of recurrent malignant glioma. *Am J Clin Oncol*. 2004;27(1):33–38.
84. Loghin ME, Prados MD, Wen P, et al. Phase I study of temozolomide and irinotecan for recurrent malignant gliomas in patients receiving enzyme-inducing antiepileptic drugs: a North American brain tumor consortium study. *Clin Cancer Res*. 2007;13(23):7133–7138.
85. Reardon DA, Quinn JA, Rich JN, et al. Phase I trial of irinotecan plus temozolomide in adults with recurrent malignant glioma. *Cancer*. 2005;104(7):1478–1486.
86. Wen PY, Yung WK, Lamborn KR, et al. Phase I/II study of imatinib mesylate for recurrent malignant gliomas: North American Brain Tumor Consortium Study 99–08. *Clin Cancer Res*. 2006;12(16):4899–4907.
87. Hofer S, Elandt K, Greil R, et al. Clinical outcome with bevacizumab in patients with recurrent high-grade glioma treated outside clinical trials. *Acta Oncol*. 2011;50(5):630–635.
88. Verhoeff JJ, Lavini C, van Linde ME, et al. Bevacizumab and dose-intense temozolomide in recurrent high-grade glioma. *Ann Oncol*. 2010;21(8):1723–1727.
89. Narayana A, Kelly P, Golfinos J, et al. Antiangiogenic therapy using bevacizumab in recurrent high-grade glioma: impact on local control and patient survival. *J Neurosurg*. 2009;110(1):173–180.
90. CBTRUS Statistical Report. Primary brain and central nervous system tumors diagnosed in the United States in 2004–2008. Accessed February 3, 2012
91. Shaw E, et al. Reexamining the Radiation Therapy Oncology Group (RTOG) Recursive Partitioning Analysis (RPA) for glioblastoma multiforme (GBM) patients. *Int J Radiat Oncol Biol Phys*. 2003;57(2, suppl):S135–S136.
92. Mirimanoff RO, Gorlia T, Mason W, et al. Radiotherapy and temozolomide for newly diagnosed glioblastoma: recursive partitioning analysis of the EORTC 26981/22981-NCIC CE3 phase III randomized trial. *J Clin Oncol*. 2006;24(16):2563–2569.
93. Ohgaki H, Kleihues P. Genetic pathways to primary and secondary glioblastoma. *Am J Pathol*. 2007;170(5):1445–1453.
94. Mischel PS, Shai R, Shi T, et al. Identification of molecular subtypes of glioblastoma by gene expression profiling. *Oncogene*. 2003;22(15):2361–2373.
95. Watanabe K, Tachibana O, Sata K, Yonekawa Y, Kleihues P, Ohgaki H. Overexpression of the EGF receptor and p53 mutations are mutually exclusive in the evolution of primary and secondary glioblastomas. *Brain Pathol*. 1996;6(3):217–23; discussion 23.
96. Colman H, Zhang L, Sulman EP, et al. A multigene predictor of outcome in glioblastoma. *Neuro-oncology*. 2010;12(1):49–57.
97. Hegi ME, Diserens AC, Gorlia T, et al. MGMT gene silencing and benefit from temozolomide in glioblastoma. *N Engl J Med*. 2005;352(10):997–1003.
98. Nakamura M, Watanabe T, Yonekawa Y, Kleihues P, Ohgaki H. Promoter methylation of the DNA repair gene MGMT in astrocytomas is frequently associated with G:C –> A:T mutations of the TP53 tumor suppressor gene. *Carcinogenesis*. 2001;22(10):1715–1719.
99. Verhaak RG, Hoadley KA, Purdom E, et al.; Cancer Genome Atlas Research Network. Integrated genomic analysis identifies clinically relevant subtypes of glioblastoma characterized by abnormalities in PDGFRA, IDH1, EGFR, and NF1. *Cancer Cell*. 2010;17(1):98–110.
100. Pauleit D, Stoffels G, Bachofner A, et al. Comparison of (18)F-FET and (18)F-FDG PET in brain tumors. *Nucl Med Biol*. 2009;36(7):779–787.
101. Lee IH, Piert M, Gomez-Hassan D, et al. Association of 11C-methionine PET uptake with site of failure after concurrent temozolomide and radiation for primary glioblastoma multiforme. *Int J Radiat Oncol Biol Phys*. 2009;73(2):479–485.
102. Kawai N, Maeda Y, Kudomi N, et al. Correlation of biological aggressiveness assessed by 11C-methionine PET and hypoxic burden assessed by 18F-fluoromisonidazole PET in newly diagnosed glioblastoma. *Eur J Nucl Med Mol Imaging*. 2011;38(3):441–450.
103. Sadeghi N, Salmon I, Decaestecker C, et al. Stereotactic comparison among cerebral blood volume, methionine uptake, and histopathology in brain glioma. *AJNR Am J Neuroradiol*. 2007;28(3):455–461.
104. Pauleit D, Floeth F, Hamacher K, et al. O-(2-[18F]fluoroethyl)-L-tyrosine PET combined with MRI improves the diagnostic assessment of cerebral gliomas. *Brain*. 2005;128(Pt 3):678–687.
105. Piroth MD, Pinkawa M, Holy R, et al. Prognostic value of early [18F]fluoroethyltyrosine positron emission tomography after radiochemotherapy in glioblastoma multiforme. *Int J Radiat Oncol Biol Phys* 2011;80(1):176–184.
106. Ballangrud AM, Lymberis S, Thakur SB, et al. Magnetic resonance spectroscopy imaging in radiotherapy planning for recurrent glioma. *Med Phys*. 2011;38(5):2724–2730.

107. Chang J, Thakur SB, Huang W, Narayana A. Magnetic resonance spectroscopy imaging (MRSI) and brain functional magnetic resonance imaging (fMRI) for radiotherapy treatment planning of glioma. *Technol Cancer Res Treat.* 2008;7(5):349–362.

108. Laprie A. [Proton magnetic resonance spectroscopic imaging and other types of metabolic imaging for radiotherapy planning in adult and pediatric high-grade gliomas]. *Cancer Radiother.* 2009;13(6–7):556–561.

109. Nelson SJ, Graves E, Pirzkall A, et al. *In vivo* molecular imaging for planning radiation therapy of gliomas: an application of 1H MRSI. *J Magn Reson Imaging.* 2002;16(4):464–476.

110. Pirzkall A, McKnight TR, Graves EE, et al. MR-spectroscopy guided target delineation for high-grade gliomas. *Int J Radiat Oncol Biol Phys.* 2001;50(4):915–928.

111. Fellows GA, Wright AJ, Sibtain NA, et al. Combined use of neuroradiology and 1H-MR spectroscopy may provide an intervention limiting diagnosis of glioblastoma multiforme. *J Magn Reson Imaging.* 2010;32(5):1038–1044.

112. Hollingworth W, Medina LS, Lenkinski RE, et al. A systematic literature review of magnetic resonance spectroscopy for the characterization of brain tumors. *AJNR Am J Neuroradiol.* 2006;27(7):1404–1411.

113. Arvinda HR, Kesavadas C, Sarma PS, et al. Glioma grading: sensitivity, specificity, positive and negative predictive values of diffusion and perfusion imaging. *J Neurooncol.* 2009;94(1):87–96.

114. Chaskis C, Stadnik T, Michotte A, Van Rompaey K, D'Haens J. Prognostic value of perfusion-weighted imaging in brain glioma: a prospective study. *Acta Neurochir (Wien).* 2006;148(3):277–85; discussion 285.

115. Emblem KE, Scheie D, Due-Tonnessen P, et al. Histogram analysis of MR imaging-derived cerebral blood volume maps: combined glioma grading and identification of low-grade oligodendroglial subtypes. *AJNR Am J Neuroradiol.* 2008;29(9):1664–1670.

116. Lacroix M, Abi-Said D, Fourney DR, et al. A multivariate analysis of 416 patients with glioblastoma multiforme: prognosis, extent of resection, and survival. *J Neurosurg.* 2001;95(2):190–198.

117. Vecht CJ, Avezaat CJ, van Putten WL, Eijkenboom WM, Stefanko SZ. The influence of the extent of surgery on the neurological function and survival in malignant glioma. A retrospective analysis in 243 patients. *J Neurol Neurosurg Psychiatr.* 1990;53(6):466–471.

118. Simpson JR, Horton J, Scott C, et al. Influence of location and extent of surgical resection on survival of patients with glioblastoma multiforme: results of three consecutive Radiation Therapy Oncology Group (RTOG) clinical trials. *Int J Radiat Oncol Biol Phys.* 1993;26(2):239–244.

119. Quick A, Patel D, Hadziahmetovic M, Chakravarti A, Mehta M. Current therapeutic paradigms in glioblastoma. *Rev Recent Clin Trials.* 2010;5(1):14–27.

120. Stage WS, Stein JJ. Treatment of malignant astrocytomas. *Am J Roentgenol Radium Ther Nucl Med.* 1974;120(1):7–18.

121. Uihlein A, Colby MY Jr, Layton DD, Parsons WR, Carter TL. Comparison of surgery and surgery plus irradiation in the treatment of supratentorial gliomas. *Acta Radiol Ther Phys Biol.* 1966;5:67–78.

122. Shapiro WR, Green SB, Burger PC, et al. Randomized trial of three chemotherapy regimens and two radiotherapy regimens and two radiotherapy regimens in postoperative treatment of malignant glioma. Brain Tumor Cooperative Group Trial 8001. *J Neurosurg.* 1989;71(1):1–9.

123. Lutterbach J, Weigel P, Guttenberger R, Hinkelbein W. Accelerated hyperfractionated radiotherapy in 149 patients with glioblastoma multiforme. *Radiother Oncol.* 1999;53(1):49–52.

124. Selker RG, Shapiro WR, Burger P, et al.; Brain Tumor Cooperative Group. The Brain Tumor Cooperative Group NIH Trial 87–01: a randomized comparison of surgery, external radiotherapy, and carmustine versus surgery, interstitial radiotherapy boost, external radiation therapy, and carmustine. *Neurosurgery.* 2002;51(2):343–55; discussion 355.

125. Souhami L, Seiferheld W, Brachman D, et al. Randomized comparison of stereotactic radiosurgery followed by conventional radiotherapy with carmustine to conventional radiotherapy with carmustine for patients with glioblastoma multiforme: report of Radiation Therapy Oncology Group 93–05 protocol. *Int J Radiat Oncol Biol Phys.* 2004;60(3):853–860.

126. Cardinale R, Won M, Choucair A, et al. A phase II trial of accelerated radiotherapy using weekly stereotactic conformal boost for supratentorial glioblastoma multiforme: RTOG 0023. *Int J Radiat Oncol Biol Phys.* 2006;65(5):1422–1428.

127. Westphal M, Ram Z, Riddle V, Hilt D, Bortey E; Executive Committee of the Gliadel Study Group. Gliadel wafer in initial surgery for malignant glioma: long-term follow-up of a multicenter controlled trial. *Acta Neurochir (Wien).* 2006;148(3):269–75; discussion 275.

128. Chi AS, Sorensen AG, Jain RK, Batchelor TT. Angiogenesis as a therapeutic target in malignant gliomas. *Oncologist.* 2009;14(6):621–636.

129. Patel M, Siddiqui F, Jin JY, et al. Salvage reirradiation for recurrent glioblastoma with radiosurgery: radiographic response and improved survival. *J Neurooncol.* 2009;92(2):185–191.

130. Hsieh PC, Chandler JP, Bhangoo S, et al. Adjuvant gamma knife stereotactic radiosurgery at the time of tumor progression potentially improves survival for patients with glioblastoma multiforme. *Neurosurgery.* 2005;57(4):684–92; discussion 684.

131. Biswas T, Okunieff P, Schell MC, et al. Stereotactic radiosurgery for glioblastoma: retrospective analysis. *Radiat Oncol.* 2009;4:11.

132. Fogh SE, Andrews DW, Glass J, et al. Hypofractionated stereotactic radiation therapy: an effective therapy

for recurrent high-grade gliomas. *J Clin Oncol.* 2010;28(18):3048–3053.

133. Fokas E, Wacker U, Gross MW, Henzel M, Encheva E, Engenhart-Cabillic R. Hypofractionated stereotactic reirradiation of recurrent glioblastomas: a beneficial treatment option after high-dose radiotherapy? *Strahlenther Onkol.* 2009;185(4):235–240.

134. Combs SE, Thilmann C, Edler L, Debus J, Schulz-Ertner D. Efficacy of fractionated stereotactic reirradiation in recurrent gliomas: long-term results in 172 patients treated in a single institution. *J Clin Oncol.* 2005;23(34):8863–8869.

135. Shepherd SF, Laing RW, Cosgrove VP, et al. Hypofractionated stereotactic radiotherapy in the management of recurrent glioma. *Int J Radiat Oncol Biol Phys.* 1997;37(2):393–398.

136. Vordermark D, Kölbl O, Ruprecht K, Vince GH, Bratengeier K, Flentje M. Hypofractionated stereotactic re-irradiation: treatment option in recurrent malignant glioma. *BMC Cancer.* 2005;5:55.

137. Gutin PH, Iwamoto FM, Beal K, et al. Safety and efficacy of bevacizumab with hypofractionated stereotactic irradiation for recurrent malignant gliomas. *Int J Radiat Oncol Biol Phys.* 2009;75(1):156–163.

138. Schwer AL, Damek DM, Kavanagh BD, et al. A phase I dose-escalation study of fractionated stereotactic radiosurgery in combination with gefitinib in patients with recurrent malignant gliomas. *Int J Radiat Oncol Biol Phys.* 2008;70(4):993–1001.

139. Glass J, Silverman CL, Axelrod R, Corn BW, Andrews DW. Fractionated stereotactic radiotherapy with cis-platinum radiosensitization in the treatment of recurrent, progressive, or persistent malignant astrocytoma. *Am J Clin Oncol.* 1997;20(3):226–229.

140. Lederman G, Wronski M, Arbit E, et al. Treatment of recurrent glioblastoma multiforme using fractionated stereotactic radiosurgery and concurrent paclitaxel. *Am J Clin Oncol.* 2000;23(2):155–159.

141. Yung WK, Albright RE, Olson J, et al. A phase II study of temozolomide vs. procarbazine in patients with glioblastoma multiforme at first relapse. *Br J Cancer.* 2000;83(5):588–593.

142. Brandes AA, Tosoni A, Cavallo G, et al.; GICNO. Temozolomide 3 weeks on and 1 week off as first-line therapy for recurrent glioblastoma: phase II study from gruppo italiano cooperativo di neuro-oncologia (GICNO). *Br J Cancer.* 2006;95(9):1155–1160.

143. Cloughesy TF, Filka E, Kuhn J, et al. Two studies evaluating irinotecan treatment for recurrent malignant glioma using an every-3-week regimen. *Cancer.* 2003;97(9 Suppl):2381–2386.

144. Prados MD, Lamborn K, Yung WK, et al.; North American Brain Tumor Consortium. A phase 2 trial of irinotecan (CPT-11) in patients with recurrent malignant glioma: a North American Brain Tumor Consortium study. *Neuro-oncology.* 2006;8(2):189–193.

145. Friedman HS, Prados MD, Wen PY, et al. Bevacizumab alone and in combination with irinotecan in recurrent glioblastoma. *J Clin Oncol.* 2009;27(28):4733–4740.

146. Beal K, Abrey LE, Gutin PH. Antiangiogenic agents in the treatment of recurrent or newly diagnosed glioblastoma: analysis of single-agent and combined modality approaches. *Radiat Oncol.* 2011;6:2.

147. Iwamoto FM, Abrey LE, Beal K, et al. Patterns of relapse and prognosis after bevacizumab failure in recurrent glioblastoma. *Neurology.* 2009;73(15):1200–1206.

demos MEDICAL

RADIATION MEDICINE ROUNDS

Metabolic Imaging: Amino Acid (AA) Positron Emission Tomography (PET) Imaging in Malignant Glioma

Nicole Wiedenmann,[1] Simon Kirste,[2] Wolfgang A. Weber,[3] and Anca L. Grosu[1*]

[1]*Department of Radiation Oncology, University Medical Center, Freiburg, Germany*

[2]*Department of Radiation Oncology, Comprehensive Cancer Center, The Ohio State University Medical Center, Columbus, OH*

[3]*Department of Nuclear Medicine, University Medical Center, Freiburg, Germany*

ABSTRACT

Amino acid positron emission tomography (PET) imaging of the brain is a valuable addition to morphological imaging (CT, MRI) within the field of neurooncology. Due to independence from unspecific changes of the blood–brain barrier, amino acid tracers offer increased specificity in identifying tumor cells. PET imaging of brain tumors has evolved from imaging glucose metabolism (FDG-PET) to amino acid PET, as amino acids are avidly and selectively taken up by glioma cells in contrast to normal cerebral tissues. Commonly applied radiolabeled amino acids used in the diagnosis of gliomas are carbon-11-labeled methionine (MET), iodine-123-labeled α-methyl-tyrosine (IMT), and fluorine-18-labeled O-(2)-fluoroethyl-L-tyrosine (FET). Amino acid tracers are sensitive markers for viable tumor tissue extension in both high- and low-grade gliomas. In the clinical setting, PET tracers 11C-MET or 18F-FET PET are applied at initial diagnosis, follow-up, evaluation of treatment-related changes, detection of residual tumor or tumor recurrence, and for differentiation between vital tumor cells and radiation necrosis. In radiation oncology, 11C-MET PET or 18F-FET PET is used for tumor delineation, for example, radiation treatment planning of recurrent glioma.

Keywords: glioma, IMT SPECT, amino acid PET, FET, MET

THE NEED FOR CEREBRAL POSITRON EMISSION TOMOGRAPHY (PET) IMAGING: LIMITATIONS OF MORPHOLOGICAL IMAGING METHODS

The diagnosis of brain tumors is generally based on morphological imaging methods such as MRI and CT. These methods have a high accuracy in the visualization of the brain morphology and offer significant information about tumor architecture and the anatomy of the surrounding normal tissues. The integration of both, CT and MRI in the radiation treatment planning process was a revolution 30 years ago and had a huge impact in the development of modern radiation therapy. Newer radiation techniques, such as 3-D rad three-dimensional therapy, stereotactic radiotherapy and radiosurgery, intensity modulated radiotherapy, and image guided radiotherapy are all based on CT and MRI data. However, over the years, it became also clear that these techniques have their limits. The

*Corresponding author, Department of Radiation Oncology, University Medical Center, Freiburg, Germany

E-mail address: anca.grosu@uniklinik-freiburg.de

Radiation Medicine Rounds 3:2 (2012) 201–208.

DOI: 10.5003/2151–4208.3.2.201

contrast enhancement on CT or T1-weighted MRI sequences does not correlate exactly with the extension of the tumor tissue. This drawback is especially pronounced after therapy: surgery, radiation therapy or chemotherapy, where treatment-related changes can not be differentiated from residual or recurrent tumor. To describe this phenomenon correctly, concepts like pseudoprogression after radiochemotherapy in glioblastoma multiforme (GBM) or pseudoremission after treatment of GBM with targeted therapies were introduced (1).

Pseudoprogression describes the finding of contrast enhancement and edema on MRI after radiochemotherapy, without true tumor progression. This is most likely due to a breakdown of the blood–brain barrier (BBB) following an inflammatory reaction. This outcome can be found in 20% to 30% of patients after radiochemotherapy (2). It occurs more frequently in combination with temozolamide chemotherapy than without (3). In the clinical setting, it is important to separate pseudoprogression from radio necrosis or tumor recurrence since these conditions make further treatment necessary. Figure 1 shows an example of pseudoprogression. MRI shows very low-contrast enhancement whereas FET-PET shows a

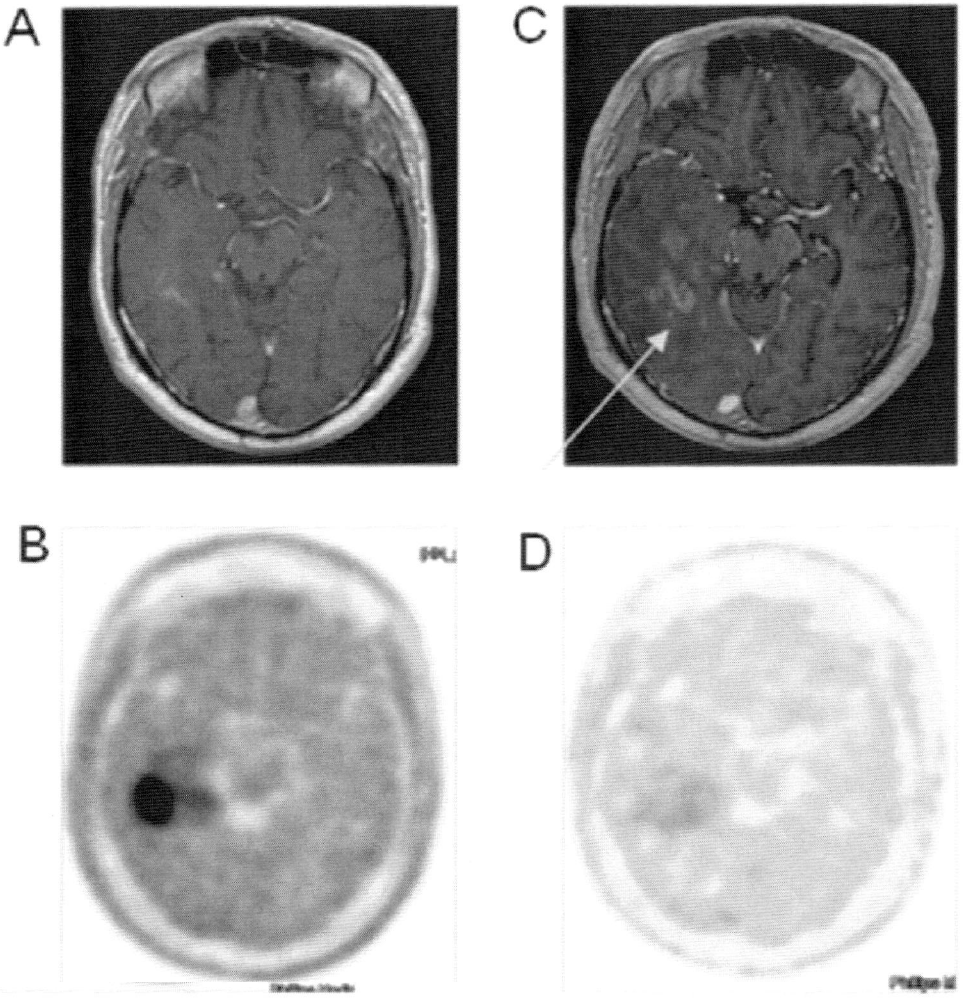

FIGURE 1 MRI T1 images with contrast (gadolinium) and FET-PET images before and after stereotactic fractionated radiation therapy (reirradiation, 39 Gy, 3 Gy/d) in a patient with recurrent glioblastoma (after 60 Gy + TMZ). (A) T1—MRI before therapy with low-contrast enhancement at the site of recurrence. (B) FET-PET before therapy showing strong amino acid uptake in the corresponding area. (C) T1—MRI 6 weeks after therapy. Contrast enhancement and edema could still be seen indicating tumor. (D) FET-PET 6 weeks after therapy shows no uptake, making pseudoprogression likely.

strong amino acid (AA) uptake in the corresponding area before treatment. In the follow-up MRI images 6 weeks after stereotactic reirradiation, a contrast enhancement in the T1-weighted MRI images can be seen indicating a tumor whereas the FET-PET shows no uptake making pseudoprogression very likely.

The term pseudoremission refers to the finding of decreased contrast enhancement and edema on MRI without a true tumor regression. This can be caused by anti-inflammatory treatment with corticosteroids or as a consequence of treatment with targeted therapies like bevacizumab (1,4).

In a series of studies in the 1980s CT, MRI, and MET-PET were compared with stereotactic biopsies. Bergström et al. (5), Mosskin et al. (6), Ogawa et al. (7), and Braun et al. (8) compared CT, MRI, and MET-PET with stereotactic biopsies suggesting that MET-PET has a higher accuracy in defining the extent of gliomas than either CT or MRI.

With modern radiation treatment techniques like stereotactic radiotherapy or radiosurgery, which deliver a very high dose of radiation to a small well-defined area to spare the normal tissues, it becomes even more important to exactly delineate the tumor-integrating morphological as well as metabolic information.

■ EVOLUTION FROM FDG-PET TO AA-PET

The radiolabeled AAs most frequently used in the diagnosis of gliomas are carbon-11-labeled methionine (MET), iodine-123-labeled α-methyl-tyrosine (IMT), and fluorine-18-labeled O-(2)-fluoroethyl-L-tyrosine (FET). The accumulation of FDG in the brain is closely related to glucose metabolism. Unlike other tissues, the brain utilizes glucose almost exclusively to meet its energy demands. Consequently, the accumulation of FDG in normal brain tissue, especially in the gray matter, is very high. Therefore, brain tumors with increased FDG uptake may be indistinguishable from normal brain tissue, limiting the usefulness of FDG for brain tumor imaging. The value of FDG-PET in three-dimensional treatment planning was systematically analyzed by Gross et al. (9). In 18 patients with malignant brain gliomas, the tumor volume defined by FDG-PET was compared with the tumor volume defined by PET/MRI fusion images. Additional information was derived from FDG-PET for only a few patients for radiation treatment planning due to the low contrast between viable tumor and normal brain tissue. However, FDG uptake is regionally related to anaplasia areas (10). DiChiro et al. (11) and Alavi et al. (12) showed that the amount of FDG uptake in the tumor tissue correlates to the histological grading and has prognostic implications. Analyzing 160 biopsies in 20 patients with low- and high-grade gliomas and comparing the results with FDG-PET findings, Goldman et al. demonstrated that FDG uptake is anatomically heterogeneous and regionally related to the presence of anaplasia (10).

■ EVOLUTION FROM SINGLE-PHOTON EMISSION COMPUTED TOMOGRAPHY (SPECT) TO POSITRON EMISSION TOMOGRAPHY (PET)

SPECT, as a scintigraphic method to visualize AAs pathways in brain tumors, was introduced at the end of the 1980s (13,14). IMT is used as tracer for SPECT. The uptake of IMT is supposed to reflect AA transport into the cell rather than the increased AA demand needed for protein synthesis. IMT is not incorporated into proteins but is an indicator of increased metabolic demand by the cell (15).

Several authors showed that MET-PET and IMT-SPECT are comparable in the ability to identify tumor tissue (16–20). IMT-SPECT as an integrated part of the radiation treatment planning process was assessed in a study of our own group (21). It was shown that target volumes for radiation therapy based on SPECT differed in a significant number of patients from the target volumes derived from MRI information alone in the postoperative setting. In another study, it was shown that radiation treatment planning with either MET-PET or IMT-SPECT can improve survival time in patients with recurrent high-grade gliomas (22). These results need to be confirmed in a study with a higher patient number.

Although IMT-SPECT has some advantages over MET-PET, such as easier radiosynthesis, there are several disadvantages. The most prominent of them is the decreased spatial resolution (7–8 mm) compared to PET (3–4 mm) making it difficult to discriminate certain anatomic structures as well as a worse tumor-to-brain contrast (23). A high resolution is especially important for the radiation treatment planning process. As a consequence, PET and PET/CT imaging is considered superior to SPECT regarding the imaging characteristics.

■ EVOLUTION FROM MET-PET TO FET-PET

The short physical half-life (about 20 min) of C11-MET limits its clinical usefulness to centers with on-site cyclotrons. The advantage of the AA analog FET is that it can be radiolabeled with fluorine-18, an isotope with a longer physical half-life (about 110 min) than that of C11, so that it can be distributed to PET centers without an on-site cyclotron. Weber et al. showed that MET-PET and FET-PET were equal in their ability to diagnose vital glioma tumor tissue (24). The similarity between MET- and FET-PET for tumor visualization was demonstrated in many studies (17,24). In a study conducted by Grosu et al., 42 patients with gliomas and metastases were imaged by MET- and FET-PET, consecutively. Sensitivity and specificity of both tracers were found to be nearly identical (25). For glioma patients the intensity of tracer uptake and the tumor extension in FET-PET and MET-PET were closely correlated. Based on these and similar studies, MET-PET and FET-PET are considered to be equivalent for detection of glioma extension.

■ MECHANISM OF INCREASED AA UPTAKE IN GLIOMA

By radio labeling AAs it has been shown that AAs are avidly taken up by glioma cells, while only a low uptake in normal cerebral tissues occurs. It is hypothesized that AAs are required by tumor cells to meet their increased demand due to a higher proliferation rate. The uptake in tumor cells is mediated by specific L and A AA transporters at the level of the BBB, independent of the BBB disturbance (26,27). It has been shown that the increase in AA uptake is caused by increased AA transport rather than increased protein synthesis.

Several transport systems for AA transport have been identified, among these are the transport systems A and L. The transport systems LAT1 and LAT2 have been further characterized regarding the transport of radiolabeled AAs used in glioma imaging (28,29).

■ CORRELATION OF AA UPTAKE WITH HISTOLOGICAL TUMOR TYPE AND TUMOR GRADING

Herholz et al. showed a sensitivity and specificity of MET-PET in differentiating between nontumoral tissue and low-grade gliomas of 76% and 87%, respectively (30). Several studies reported that tumor MET uptake is significantly different between low- and high-grade gliomas (31). A significant correlation between tumor uptake of MET and survival has also been found in low-grade gliomas (32). A higher IMT uptake in high-grade gliomas than in low-grade gliomas was described (33,34). However, IMT-SPECT does not significantly add to the accuracy of MRI in determining the tumor grade (35). A number of studies provided controversial findings regarding the impact of AA tracers on determination of the tumor grade in various brain tumors (27,36). In summary, AA tracers are sensitive markers for viable tumor tissue extension in both high- and low-grade gliomas. However, several conceptual inconsistencies in determining tumor grading currently limit any definite conclusions about the ability of AA-PET to predict the tumor grade and its clinical value in this setting.

■ CLINICAL APPLICATION—AA-PET AS A DIAGNOSTIC TOOL: INITIAL DIAGNOSIS, FOLLOW-UP, EVALUATION OF TREATMENT-RELATED CHANGES, DETECTION OF RESIDUAL TUMOR AND TUMOR RECURRENCE, DIFFERENTIATION BETWEEN TUMOR RECURRENCE AND RADIATION NECROSIS

MET-PET is an established tool for diagnosis of brain neoplasia. In malignant glioma, AA-PET is used for initial diagnosis and for follow-up examinations. In the diagnostic setting, AA-PET can be used to identify the optimal site for stereotactic biopsies. Voges et al. reported MET-PET as a diagnostic tool for gliomas and as a monitoring tool for brachytherapy with 125I seeds (37). Forty-six patients with suspected brain tumors were investigated with MET-PET. In 67% of the cases, the spatial extent of increased tracer uptake in gliomas was larger than that of the contrast enhancement on CT/MRI images, while in the remaining 33% of the cases, the extent of tumor tissue was diagnosed with comparable accuracy. A significant decline of MET uptake was noticed 12 months after seed implantation. The authors concluded that MET-PET may improve the definition of brain tumor extension and provide valuable information regarding therapeutic effects. Several trials followed, and by 2007, 45 trials with a total of 1,721 patients analyzing the role of MET-PET in the diagnosis of glioma were published. Eleven studies including 706 patients were based on stereotactical biopsies after PET, MRI, and CT imaging. The sensitivity of MET-PET for malignant gliomas was found to be comparable to MRI (85%–95%). The specificity was reported between 80% and 100%, which is considerably superior to the specificity found for MRI for detection of malignancy (about 50%). In summary,

MET-PET was found to allow a more accurate delineation of tumor extension compared to CT and MRI, to allow differentiation of residual tumor or tumor recurrence against treatment-related or unspecific changes and to allow differentiation between radiation necrosis and viable tumor tissue (Table 1).

■ CLINICAL APPLICATION—AA-PET FOR RADIATION TREATMENT PLANNING

The superior diagnostic accuracy of AA-PET and improved detection of residual tumor is the rationale for using this technique in target volume delineation of gliomas. Beneficial effects have been shown especially in the postsurgical situation and after first-line treatment when reirradiation is considered.

Tumor Delineation Based on AA-PET

AA imaging may have a significant impact on radiation treatment planning by revealing additional information on tumor extension. AA uptake is independent from BBB disruption, allowing the visualization of vital tumor tissue with and without BBB disruption (Table 2).

In 2000, Grosu et al. investigated the value of IMT-SPECT for radiation treatment planning of brain gliomas compared to MRI in respect to gross target volume (GTV), planning target volume (PTV), and biological volume (BV), that is, the volume based on SPECT definition (42). On MRI/SPECT fusion images, the GTV defined on SPECT was compared with the volume of hyperintensity regions on T2-weighted MRI and with the volume of gadolinium (Gd) enhancement on T1-weighted MRI. PTV and BV were delineated accordingly based on either MRI alone or on MRI/SPECT-fused images (21,42). When nonoperated low- and high-grade glioma patients were analyzed, the hyperintensity area on T2-MRI included the area with increased IMT uptake in SPECT for most patients, confirming that T2 changes incorporate both tumor tissue and perifocal edema (42). However, in high-grade glioma patients, tumor uptake of IMT extended beyond T2 changes in MRI. In 7/30 patients, IMT uptake was found up to 20 mm beyond T2 changes. By adding IMT-SPECT information to the T2-MRI a mean relative increase of GTV of 33% was obtained. On T1-MRI/SPECT-fusion images, the IMT tumor uptake incorporated the contrast enhancement regions in all cases and extended beyond the Gd-enhancing regions.

Another question that remains to be answered is if treatment planning integrating PET imaging has an impact on overall survival. In one study including 44 patients with recurrent high-grade gliomas, the addition of MET-PET resulted in an increased survival compared to the group with treatment planning based on MRI/CT only (22). Further investigations to clarify this question are ongoing.

Detection of Residual Tumor in the Postsurgical Situation

The interpretation of postsurgical MRI scans is often equivocal. Postsurgical alterations can cause unspecific contrast enhancement on T1 scans as well as edema on T2 scans. An unequivocal differentiation between residual tumor and unspecific postsurgical alterations is generally regarded as impossible by most radiologists with the exception of scans obtained within 48 hours after surgery. In contrast to Gd enhancement, tumor-related AA uptake is not affected by a postsurgical BBB disruption. Therefore, AA-PET imaging can be used to identify residual tumor and to image the tumor extension. The impact of IMT-SPECT on GTV, PTV, and BV delineation was analyzed in 66 patients with low- and high-grade gliomas after surgical resection (21). Size and location

TABLE 1 Sensitivity and specificity of amino acid (AA) PET, SPECT, and MRI for discrimination of radiation necrosis and tumor recurrence

	FET-PET	MET-PET	IMT-SPECT	MRI
Number of patients	45	21	78	45
Sensitivity (%)	94	78	94	97
Specificity (%)	93	100	100	50
References	39	40	41	39

Source: Ref. (38).

of IMT uptake differed considerably from abnormalities in postoperative T1-Gd and T2-MRI. In 29% of patients, IMT uptake was located outside of the changes in MRI whereas areas of the pathologic IMT uptake were located up to 2 cm outside of the regions altered on T2 scans. Contrast enhancement and edema were significantly extended compared to IMT uptake as a consequence of postoperative BBB disturbances and edema. These data imply that IMT-SPECT can visualize tumor tissue with a higher specificity and sensitivity than anatomic imaging modalities due to its independence from the integrity of the BBB.

MET-PET has a superior resolution in comparison to IMT-SPECT. Therefore, other trials analyzed the impact of MET-PET in GTV delineation of operated gliomas (46,47). Only in a minority of patients (18%) did the uptake of MET correspond exactly to Gd enhancement, whereas in 79% of patients the region of MET uptake was larger than that of Gd enhancement and MET uptake was detected up to 45 mm beyond Gd enhancement. The area of Gd enhancement extended beyond the area of MET enhancement in 74% of patients. AA uptake also did not correspond exactly to hyperintensity areas on T2, as MET uptake was extended beyond the hyperintensity on T2 in 50% of patients (up to 40 mm). For all patients investigated at least some hyperintensity on T2 was located outside of the MET enhancement area.

An analysis of an AA-SPECT– or PET-planned group of patients with recurrent gliomas reirradiated using stereotactic fractionated radiotherapy suggests that the integration of AA-PET or -SPECT in target volume definition might contribute to an improved outcome (48). Nuutinen et al. reported about the feasibility of MET-PET for radiation treatment planning and for monitoring patients with low-grade gliomas. In comparison with MRI, MET-PET was helpful in outlining the GTV in 3/11 cases (27%), whereas it was complementary to MRI in 46% of the cases and less distinctive in 27% (48).

■ OUTLOOK: OTHER TRACERS

While FDG and AA tracers depict glucose and AA metabolism, there are a variety of tracers under investigation to image additional metabolic pathways or biological characteristics. Among these are tracers for proliferation, the tumor microenvironment (e.g., hypoxia, fatty acid metabolism), or cell-to-cell interaction proteins. To image proliferation, which is a basic mechanism for malignant cell growth, the tracer [^{18}F]-fluorine labeled thymidine analogue 3′-deoxy-3′-[^{18}F]-fluorothymidine (FLT) was developed. FLT is retained in the cell after phosphorylation by thymidin kinase 1, whose levels were shown to correlate with cell proliferation. The kinetic of FLT uptake in malignant gliomas correlates with the cell proliferation measured by Ki-67 a nuclear protein associated with cell proliferation (49).

Tumor hypoxia has been identified as a factor negatively correlated with prognosis and local control after radiation therapy for several tumor types, including squamous cell cancer of the head and neck, the cervix and with growing evidence also in glioma. First reports showing that malignant gliomas have a diminished level of oxygenation were already published in the early 1990s (50) using FMISO-PET. To date, the real impact of hypoxia imaging in the diagnosis and treatment of high-grade gliomas is under investigation.

A target for visualization of cell-to-cell interaction and cell adhesion is the $\alpha v\beta 3$ integrin receptor. F18-labeled RDG-containing glycopeptide, which binds on the $\alpha v\beta 3$ receptor, is currently used to image the expression of $\alpha v\beta 3$ integrin (51). Besides cell adhesion, $\alpha v\beta 3$ is also involved in tumor-induced angiogenesis and metastasis. On the therapeutic stage, the $\alpha v\beta 3$ integrin receptor can be blocked by cilengitide, a new drug that is currently under investigation for treatment of high-grade gliomas.

TABLE 2 Sensitivity and specificity of AA-PET and MRI for brain tumor delineation—comparison with gold standard (histologic evaluation)

References	Patients	Imaging Method	Sensitivity (%)	Specificity (%)
8	32	MET-PET	87	75
43	32	MET-PET	100	100
44	30	MET-PET	87	89
45	31	FET-PET	93	94
		MRI	96	53

Source: Ref. (38).

■ REFERENCES

1. Brandsma D, van den Bent MJ. Pseudoprogression and pseudoresponse in the treatment of gliomas. *Curr Opin Neurol.* 2009;22(6):633–638.
2. Taal W, Brandsma D, de Bruin HG, et al. Incidence of early pseudo-progression in a cohort of malignant glioma patients treated with chemoirradiation with temozolomide. *Cancer.* 2008;113(2):405–410.
3. Brandsma D, Stalpers L, Taal W, Sminia P, van den Bent MJ. Clinical features, mechanisms, and management of pseudoprogression in malignant gliomas. *Lancet Oncol.* 2008;9(5):453–461.
4. Clarke JL, Chang S. Pseudoprogression and pseudoresponse: challenges in brain tumor imaging. *Curr Neurol Neurosci Rep.* 2009;9(3):241–246.
5. Bergström M, Collins VP, Ehrin E, et al. Discrepancies in brain tumor extent as shown by computed tomography and positron emission tomography using [68Ga]EDTA, [11C]glucose, and [11C]methionine. *J Comput Assist Tomogr.* 1983;7(6):1062–1066.
6. Mosskin M, Ericson K, Hindmarsh T, et al. Positron emission tomography compared with magnetic resonance imaging and computed tomography in supratentorial gliomas using multiple stereotactic biopsies as reference. *Acta Radiol.* 1989;30(3):225–232.
7. Ogawa T, Shishido F, Kanno I, et al. Cerebral glioma: evaluation with methionine PET. *Radiology.* 1993;186(1):45–53.
8. Braun V, Dempf S, Weller R, Reske SN, Schachenmayr W, Richter HP. Cranial neuronavigation with direct integration of (11)C methionine positron emission tomography (PET) data—results of a pilot study in 32 surgical cases. *Acta Neurochir (Wien).* 2002;144(8):777–82; discussion 782.
9. Gross MW, Weber WA, Feldmann HJ, Bartenstein P, Schwaiger M, Molls M. The value of F-18-fluorodeoxyglucose PET for the 3-D radiation treatment planning of malignant gliomas. *Int J Radiat Oncol Biol Phys.* 1998;41(5):989–995.
10. Goldman S, Levivier M, Pirotte B, et al. Regional glucose metabolism and histopathology of gliomas. A study based on positron emission tomography-guided stereotactic biopsy. *Cancer.* 1996;78(5):1098–1106.
11. DiChiro G. Positron emission tomography using F-18 fluorodeoxyglucose in brain tumors. A powerful diagnostic and prognostic tool. *Invest Radiol.* 1986;22:360–371.
12. Alavi JB, Alavi A, Chawluk J, et al. Positron emission tomography in patients with glioma. A predictor of prognosis. *Cancer.* 1988;62(6):1074–1078.
13. Biersack HJ, Coenen HH, Stöcklin G, et al. Imaging of brain tumors with L-3-[123I]iodo-alpha-methyl tyrosine and SPECT. *J Nucl Med.* 1989;30(1):110–112.
14. Langen KJ, Coenen HH, Roosen N, et al. SPECT studies of brain tumors with L-3-[123I] iodo-alpha-methyl tyrosine: comparison with PET, 124IMT and first clinical results. *J Nucl Med.* 1990;31(3):281–286.
15. Langen KJ, Pauleit D, Coenen HH. 3-[(123)I]Iodo-alpha-methyl-L-tyrosine: uptake mechanisms and clinical applications. *Nucl Med Biol.* 2002;29(6):625–631.
16. Langen KJ, Roosen N, Coenen HH, et al. Brain and brain tumor uptake of L-3-[123I]iodo-alpha-methyl tyrosine: competition with natural L-amino acids. *J Nucl Med.* 1991;32(6):1225–1229.
17. Langen KJ, Ziemons K, Kiwit JC, et al. 3-[123I]iodo-alpha-methyltyrosine and [methyl-11C]-L-methionine uptake in cerebral gliomas: a comparative study using SPECT and PET. *J Nucl Med.* 1997;38(4):517–522.
18. Weber WA, Dick S, Reidl G, et al. Correlation between postoperative 3-[(123)I]iodo-L-alpha-methyltyrosine uptake and survival in patients with gliomas. *J Nucl Med.* 2001;42(8):1144–1150.
19. Weckesser M, Griessmeier M, Schmidt D, et al. Iodine-123 alpha-methyl tyrosine single-photon emission tomography of cerebral gliomas: standardised evaluation of tumour uptake and extent. *Eur J Nucl Med.* 1998;25(2):150–156.
20. Weckesser M, Matheja P, Rickert C, et al. Evaluation of the extension of cerebral gliomas by scintigraphy. *Strahlenther Onkol.* 2000;176(4):180–185.
21. Grosu AL, Feldmann H, Dick S, et al. Implications of IMT-SPECT for postoperative radiotherapy planning in patients with gliomas. *Int J Radiat Oncol Biol Phys.* 2002;54(3):842–854.
22. Grosu AL, Weber WA, Franz M, et al. Reirradiation of recurrent high-grade gliomas using amino acid PET (SPECT)/CT/MRI image fusion to determine gross tumor volume for stereotactic fractionated radiotherapy. *Int J Radiat Oncol Biol Phys.* 2005;63(2):511–519.
23. Pauleit D, Floeth F, Tellmann L, et al. Comparison of O-(2–18F-fluoroethyl)-L-tyrosine PET and 3–123I-iodo-alpha-methyl-L-tyrosine SPECT in brain tumors. *J Nucl Med.* 2004;45(3):374–381.
24. Weber WA, Wester HJ, Grosu AL, et al. O-(2-[18F]fluoroethyl)-L-tyrosine and L-[methyl-11C]methionine uptake in brain tumours: initial results of a comparative study. *Eur J Nucl Med.* 2000;27(5):542–549.
25. Grosu AL, Astner ST, Riedel E, et al. An interindividual comparison of O-(2-[18F]fluoroethyl)-L-tyrosine (FET)- and L-[methyl-11C]methionine (MET)-PET in patients with brain gliomas and metastases. *Int J Radiat Oncol Biol Phys.* 2011;81(4):1049–1058.
26. Riemann B, Könemann S, Pöpping D, et al. Early effects of irradiation on [(123)I]-IMT and [(18)F]-FDG uptake in rat C6 glioma cells. *Strahlenther Onkol.* 2004;180(7):434–441.
27. Schmidt D, Gottwald U, Langen KJ, et al. 3-[123I]Iodo-alpha-methyl-L-tyrosine uptake in cerebral gliomas: relationship to histological grading and prognosis. *Eur J Nucl Med.* 2001;28(7):855–861.
28. Langen KJ, Jarosch M, Mühlensiepen H, et al. Comparison of fluorotyrosines and methionine uptake in F98 rat gliomas. *Nucl Med Biol.* 2003;30(5):501–508.
29. Langen KJ, Bröer S. Molecular transport mechanisms of radiolabeled amino acids for PET and SPECT. *J Nucl Med.* 2004;45(9):1435–1436.

30. Herholz K, Hölzer T, Bauer B, et al. 11C-methionine PET for differential diagnosis of low-grade gliomas. *Neurology.* 1998;50(5):1316–1322.

31. Kaschten B, Stevenaert A, Sadzot B, et al. Preoperative evaluation of 54 gliomas by PET with fluorine-18-fluorodeoxyglucose and/or carbon-11-methionine. *J Nucl Med.* 1998;39(5):778–785.

32. Ribom D, Engler H, Blomquist E, Smits A. Potential significance of (11)C-methionine PET as a marker for the radiosensitivity of low-grade gliomas. *Eur J Nucl Med Mol Imaging.* 2002;29(5):632–640.

33. Kuwert T, Morgenroth C, Woesler B, et al. Uptake of iodine-123-alpha-methyl tyrosine by gliomas and non-neoplastic brain lesions. *Eur J Nucl Med.* 1996;23(10):1345–1353.

34. Woesler B, Kuwert T, Morgenroth C, et al. Non-invasive grading of primary brain tumours: results of a comparative study between SPET with 123I-alpha-methyl tyrosine and PET with 18F-deoxyglucose. *Eur J Nucl Med.* 1997;24(4):428–434.

35. Riemann B, Papke K, Hoess N, et al. Noninvasive grading of untreated gliomas: a comparative study of MR imaging and 3-(iodine 123)-L-alpha-methyltyrosine SPECT. *Radiology.* 2002;225(2):567–574.

36. Weber W, Bartenstein P, Gross MW, et al. Fluorine-18-FDG PET and iodine-123-IMT SPECT in the evaluation of brain tumors. *J Nucl Med.* 1997;38(5):802–808.

37. Voges J, Herholz K, Hölzer T, et al. 11C-methionine and 18F-2-fluorodeoxyglucose positron emission tomography: a tool for diagnosis of cerebral glioma and monitoring after brachytherapy with 125I seeds. *Stereotact Funct Neurosurg.* 1997;69(1–4 Pt 2):129–135.

38. Grosu AL, Weber WA. PET for radiation treatment planning of brain tumours. *Radiother Oncol.* 2010;96(3):325–327.

39. Rachinger W, Goetz C, Pöpperl G, et al. Positron emission tomography with O-(2-[18F]fluoroethyl)-l-tyrosine versus magnetic resonance imaging in the diagnosis of recurrent gliomas. *Neurosurgery.* 2005;57(3):505–11; discussion 505.

40. Tsuyuguchi N, Sunada I, Iwai Y, et al. Methionine positron emission tomography of recurrent metastatic brain tumor and radiation necrosis after stereotactic radiosurgery: is a differential diagnosis possible? *J Neurosurg.* 2003;98(5):1056–1064.

41. Samnick S, Bader JB, Hellwig D, et al. Clinical value of iodine-123-alpha-methyl-L-tyrosine single-photon emission tomography in the differential diagnosis of recurrent brain tumor in patients pretreated for glioma at follow-up. *J Clin Oncol.* 2002;20(2):396–404.

42. Grosu AL, Weber W, Feldmann HJ, et al. First experience with I-123-alpha-methyl-tyrosine spect in the 3-D radiation treatment planning of brain gliomas. *Int J Radiat Oncol Biol Phys.* 2000;47(2):517–526.

43. Pirotte B, Goldman S, Massager N, et al. Comparison of 18F-FDG and 11C-methionine for PET-guided stereotactic brain biopsy of gliomas. *J Nucl Med.* 2004;45(8):1293–1298.

44. Kracht LW, Miletic H, Busch S, et al. Delineation of brain tumor extent with [11C]L-methionine positron emission tomography: local comparison with stereotactic histopathology. *Clin Cancer Res.* 2004;10(21):7163–7170.

45. Pauleit D, Floeth F, Hamacher K, et al. O-(2-[18F]fluoroethyl)-L-tyrosine PET combined with MRI improves the diagnostic assessment of cerebral gliomas. *Brain.* 2005;128(Pt 3):678–687.

46. Grosu AL, Lachner R, Wiedenmann N, et al. Validation of a method for automatic image fusion (BrainLAB System) of CT data and 11C-methionine-PET data for stereotactic radiotherapy using a LINAC: first clinical experience. *Int J Radiat Oncol Biol Phys.* 2003;56(5):1450–1463.

47. Grosu AL, Weber WA, Riedel E, et al. L-(methyl-11C) methionine positron emission tomography for target delineation in resected high-grade gliomas before radiotherapy. *Int J Radiat Oncol Biol Phys.* 2005b;63(1):64–74.

48. Nuutinen J, Sonninen P, Lehikoinen P, et al. Radiotherapy treatment planning and long-term follow-up with [(11)C]-methionine PET in patients with low-grade astrocytoma. *Int J Radiat Oncol Biol Phys.* 2000;48:43–52.

49. Ullrich R, Backes H, Li H, et al. Glioma proliferation as assessed by 3'-fluoro-3'-deoxy-L-thymidine positron emission tomography in patients with newly diagnosed high-grade glioma. *Clin Cancer Res.* 2008 Apr 1;14(7):2049–2055.

50. Valk PE, Mathis CA, Prados MD, Gilbert JC, Budinger TF. Hypoxia in human gliomas: demonstration by PET with fluorine-18-fluoromisonidazole. *J Nucl Med.* 1992;33(12):2133–2137.

51. Beer AJ, Grosu AL, Carlsen J, et al. [18F]galacto-RGD positron emission tomography for imaging of alphavbeta3 expression on the neovasculature in patients with squamous cell carcinoma of the head and neck. *Clin Cancer Res.* 2007;13(22 Pt 1):6610–6616.

demos MEDICAL

RADIATION MEDICINE ROUNDS

Boron Neutron Capture Therapy as a Treatment Modality for High-Grade Gliomas

Rolf F. Barth,[1*] M. Graca H. Vicente,[2] Otto K. Harling,[3] Kent J. Riley,[4] Peter J. Binns,[5] W. S. Kiger III,[6] and Shinji Kawabata[7]

[1]*Department of Pathology, The Ohio State University, Columbus, OH*

[2]*Department of Chemistry, Louisiana State University, Baton Rouge, LA*

[3]*Department of Nuclear Science & Engineering, Massachusetts Institute of Technology, Cambridge, MA*

[4]*Department of Radiation Oncology, Massachusetts General Hospital, Boston, MA*

[5]*Department of Radiation Oncology, Mt. Auburn Hospital, Cambridge, MA*

[6]*Department of Radiation Oncology, Beth Israel Deaconess Medical Center, Harvard Medical School, Boston, MA*

[7]*Department of Neurosurgery, Osaka Medical College, Takatsuki City, Osaka, Japan*

■ ABSTRACT

Boron neutron capture therapy (BNCT) is based on the nuclear capture and fission reactions that occur when nonradioactive boron-10 is irradiated with low-energy thermal neutrons to yield high linear energy transfer alpha particles vand recoiling lithium-7 nuclei. Clinical interest in BNCT has focused primarily on the treatment of high-grade gliomas, head and neck cancer, and either primary or metastatic melanoma. Neutron sources for BNCT currently are limited to specially modified nuclear reactors and these are available in the United States, Japan, Argentina, several European countries, Taiwan, and China. Accelerators potentially also could be used to produce epithermal neutrons and these are being developed in a number of countries, including Japan, Russia, Belgium, and Argentina, but at this time none are being used for BNCT. The major challenge in the development of boron delivery agents has been the requirement for selective tumor targeting in order to achieve boron concentrations sufficient to deliver therapeutic doses of radiation to the tumor with minimal normal tissue toxicity. Two boron drugs have been used clinically, sodium borocaptate or "BSH" ($Na_2B_{12}H_{11}SH$) and a dihydroxyboryl derivative of phenylalanine referred to as boronophenylalanine or "BPA". In this chapter, we will provide an overview of other boron delivery agents that are under evaluation, neutron sources for BNCT, clinical dosimetry and treatment planning, and past and ongoing clinical studies. We will conclude with a summary of critical issues that must be addressed if BNCT is to move forward as a useful modality for the treatment of high-grade gliomas.

*Corresponding author, Department of Pathology, The Ohio State University, 165 Hamilton Hall, 1645 Neil Avenue, Columbus, OH 43210.

E-mail address: rolf.barth@osumc.edu

Radiation Medicine Rounds 3:2 (2012) 209–226.

DOI: 10.5003/2151–4208.3.2.209

■ INTRODUCTION

Boron neutron capture therapy (BNCT) in theory provides a way to selectively destroy malignant cells and spare normal cells. It is based on the nuclear capture and fission reactions that occur when boron-10, which is a nonradioactive constituent of natural elemental boron, is irradiated with low-energy thermal neutrons to yield high linear energy transfer (LET) alpha particles (^4He) and recoiling lithium-7 (^7Li) nuclei as shown below.

$$^{10}B + n_{th}\ (0.025\ eV) \rightarrow [^{11}B] \rightarrow {}^4He + {}^7Li + 2.79\ MeV\ (6\%)$$

$$[^{11}B] \rightarrow {}^4He + {}^7Li + 2.31\ MeV\ (94\%)$$

$$\downarrow$$

$$^7Li + \gamma + 0.48\ MeV$$

In order for BNCT to be successful, a sufficient amount of ^{10}B must be selectively delivered to the tumor (~20 μg/g weight or ~10^9 atoms/cell), and enough thermal neutrons must be absorbed by them to sustain lethal damage from the $^{10}B(n, \alpha)^7Li$ capture reaction. Since the high LET particles have limited path lengths in tissue (5–9 μm), the destructive effects of these high energy particles is limited to boron containing cells. Clinical interest in BNCT for the treatment of brain tumors has focused primarily on high-grade gliomas (1–3) and a subset of patients with meningiomas (4), who have failed surgery and conventional radiotherapy (RT). Since BNCT is primarily a biochemically rather than a physically targeted type of radiation treatment, the potential exists to destroy tumor cells dispersed in normal brain tissue, if sufficient amounts of ^{10}B and thermal neutrons are delivered to the target volume. In this chapter, we will provide an update on BNCT, specifically as it relates to the treatment of high-grade gliomas. Topics that will be covered will include boron delivery agents, neutron sources, clinical dosimetry, treatment planning techniques, and past and ongoing clinical trials in Japan, the United States, and Europe, and finally, critical issues that must be addressed if BNCT is to be successful. Readers interested in more in-depth coverage of these and other topics related to BNCT are referred to the Proceedings of 13th and 14th International Congresses on Neutron Capture Therapy (5,6).

■ BORON DELIVERY AGENTS

General Requirements

The development of boron delivery agents for BNCT began approximately 50 years ago and research in this area continues, although unfortunately progress has been slow. The most important requirements for a successful boron delivery agent are: (a) low systemic toxicity and normal tissue uptake with high-tumor uptake and concomitantly high tumor:brain (T:Br) and tumor:blood (T:Bl) concentration ratios (>3–4:1); (b) tumor concentrations of at least ~20 μg ^{10}B/g tumor; and (c) rapid clearance from blood and normal tissues and persistence in tumor during BNCT. At this time, there are only two clinically used boron delivery agents, the polyhedral boron anion, sodium mercaptoundecahydro-*closo*-dodecaborate ($Na_2B_{12}H_{11}SH$), commonly known as sodium borocaptate (BSH) (7), and the boron-containing amino acid (L)-4-dihydroxyborylphenylalanine known as boronophenylalanine (BPA). Neither of these fulfills all of the criteria indicated above. With the development of new chemical synthetic techniques and increased knowledge of the biological and biochemical requirements needed for effective agents and their modes of delivery, a number of new boron agents have emerged. The major challenge in their development has been the requirement for selective tumor targeting in order to achieve boron concentrations sufficient to deliver therapeutic doses of radiation to the tumor with minimal normal tissue toxicity. The selective destruction of glioblastoma (GBM) cells in the presence of normal cells represents an even greater challenge compared to malignancies at other anatomic sites, since high-grade gliomas are highly infiltrative of normal brain, histologically complex, and heterogeneous in their cellular composition.

Third-Generation Boron Delivery Agents

A compilation of third-generation low- and high-molecular weight boron delivery agents is summarized in Table 1. Interested readers are referred to a recent comprehensive review on this topic (8). Among the low-molecular weight BNCT delivery agents (8), boronated natural amino acids, such as BPA and derivatives of glycine, aspartic acid, tyrosine, cysteine, methionine, and serine, have been intensively investigated (9–11). Boron-containing unnatural amino acids, such as the boronated derivatives of 1-aminocyclobutane-1-carboxylic acid and 1-amino-3-boronocyclopentanecarboxylic acid (designated ABCPC), have shown promise as BNCT delivery agents due to their higher tumor selectivity and increased water solubility compared to BPA (10,11). Boronated linear and cyclic peptides have also been investigated and shown to have low toxicity and high-tumor selectivity (12). Of particular interest are those that are ligands for certain receptors that are over-expressed on tumor cells (e.g., epidermal growth

TABLE 1 Examples of new low- and high-molecular-weight boron delivery agents that are currently under evaluation

Boronated unnatural amino acids (9–11)	Carboranyl nucleosides (13–15)
Dodecaborate cluster lipids and cholesterol derivatives (13)	Boronated porphyrins (16–18)
Boronated EGF and anti-EGFR monoclonal antibodies MAbs (21–23)	
Boron-containing immunoliposomes (25) and liposomes (26–29)	Boron-containing nanoparticles (31,33,109)
Boronated DNA intercalators (19)	Carboranyl porphyrazines (112)
Transferrin–polyethylene glycol liposomes (30,119)	Boronated cyclic peptides (12)
Dodecahydro-closo-dodecaborate clusters (10,13)	Boron nitride nanotubes (32)

The numbers indicated in parentheses are cited in the reference section.

factor receptor [EGFR], vascular endothelial growth factor [VEGFR], and somatostatin receptors).

Boron-containing purines, pyrimidines, thymidines, nucleosides, and nucleotides have been investigated as boron delivery agents (13–15), especially 3-carboranyl thymidine analogues (3CTAs). For example, the 3-(dihydroxypropyl-carboranyl-pentyl) thymidine derivative designated N5–2OH has shown low toxicitiy, selective tumor uptake, and high rate of phosphorylation into the corresponding nucleotide (14). Furthermore, convection-enhanced delivery of N5–2OH was shown to be effective in selectively delivering therapeutic amounts of boron to rats bearing intracerebral implants of the RG2 glioma (15).

Several boron-containing porphyrin derivatives, including chlorin, bacteriochlorin, tetrabenzoporphyrin, corrole and phthalocyanine macrocycles, have been investigated as BNCT agents (16,17). Examples are BOPP (18), CuTCPH, and porphyrins of high-boron content such as H_2OCP. All of these porphyrins have been shown to deliver high amounts of boron to tumor-bearing mice with high tumor-to-blood and tumor-to-brain boron concentration ratios and long retention times in tumors. Boronated chlorins, bacteriochlorins, and phthalocyanines are promising agents for application as dual BNCT and photodynamic therapy photosensitizers. This is because of their strong absorptions of near-infrared light, which penetrates deeper into human tissues (16). In addition to these, other boronated DNA binding molecules, such as alkylating agents, intercalators, minor-groove binders, polyamines, and metal complexes, have been investigated (19), including derivatives of aziridines, acridines, phenanthridines, Pt(II) complexes, trimethoxyindoles, and carboranylpolyamines. These compounds usually show low-tumor selectivity and sometimes high toxicity due to their multiple cationic charges and ability for binding to DNA. Boronated carbohydrates, such as derivatives of glucose, mannose, ribose, galactose, maltose, and lactose, have also been investigated (8,20). These compounds usually display low toxicity and poor tumor uptake, perhaps as a result of their low hydrophobicity and fast clearance from tissues.

High-molecular BNCT agents include monoclonal antibodies (MAbs), liposomes, and nanoparticles. MAbs are a promising class of targeted delivery agents due to their very high specificity for the target, for example, EGF and VEGF receptors (21–24). Immunoliposomes have been shown to deliver small boronated molecules such as BSH into brain tumors via incorporation into their lipid bilayers (25,26). Liposomes have been used to transport large amounts of boronated molecules intracellularly, for example, polyethylene glycol [PEG]-based liposomes and these particles generally show increased tumor boron uptake (27). Extensive studies on liposomes as delivery agents of polyhedral boron anions have been carried out by Hawthorne and Feakes and their coworkers and their studies are summarized in a recent review on this topic (28). Sufficiently high-boron concentrations have been attained when these were encapsulated in tumor selective unilamellar liposomes. However, *in vivo* therapeutic efficacy has yet to be demonstrated. Boronated lipids bearing covalently bound boron also have been investigated. These particles avoid problems associated with leakage of encapsulated boronated compounds and were shown to deliver large amounts of boron to tumor-bearing mice with increased survival times following BNCT (29,30). Finally, other boron-containing nanoparticles have been proposed and investigated as delivery agents for BNCT (31,32) and interested readers are referred to a recent review on this topic (33).

■ NEUTRON SOURCES FOR BNCT

Nuclear Reactors

Clinical studies of BNCT originated at the Brookhaven National Laboratory (BNL) and the Massachusetts Institute of Technology (MIT) approximately 50 years ago (reviewed in (1,2)). The initial trials were carried out in patients with high-grade gliomas, the majority of which had GBMs, using fission reactors producing thermal neutron beams. The inadequate tissue-penetrating properties of these beams (3–4 cm) led the clinical team in the MIT-Harvard trials to introduce intraoperative, open cranium irradiations to increase neutron penetration. This approach subsequently was used by Hatanaka and Nakagawa and their coworkers (34–36) when they initiated clinical studies in Japan using BSH as the boron delivery agent (37). Based on the research of Mishima and his coworkers in Japan (38) and Coderre et al. at BNL (39), BPA has been used along with higher energy epithermal neutrons (~0.4 eV ≤ E ≤ 10 keV) in patients with GBM who were treated at BNL and MIT in the 1990s and early 2000s. A schematic diagram of the MIT research reactor (MITR) is shown in Figure 1. The use of epithermal neutrons obviated the need for intraoperative BNCT when treating brain tumors at depths greater than the useful penetration of thermal neutrons. Epithermal neutrons can reach tumors as deep as 8 cm with therapeutic ratios >1. They are now generally used for BNCT, although some intraoperative irradiations with thermal or mixed thermal and epithermal neutron beams have continued in Japan.

Desired Performance Characteristics

Based on recent clinical experience at Harvard-MIT, the suggested characteristics and performance of epithermal neutron irradiation facilities (40), which are suitable for high-throughput, routine clinical BNCT are summarized as follows:

1. Enough intensity to deliver an irradiation field in several minutes and during the time of optimum

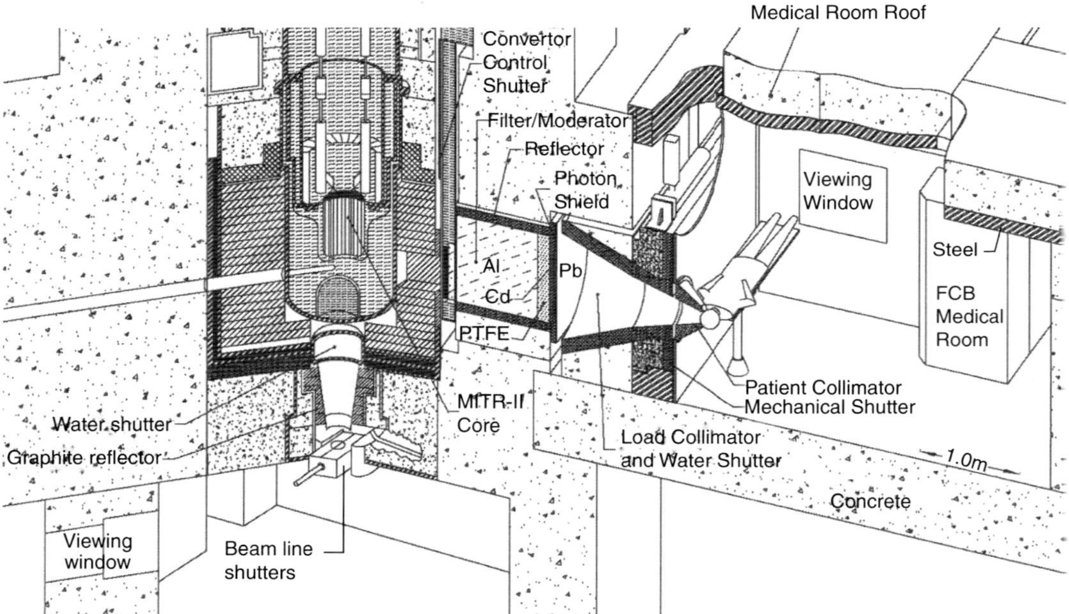

FIGURE 1 Schematic diagram of the Massachusetts Institute of Technology Reactor (MITR). The fission converter–based epithermal neutron irradiation (FCB) facility is housed in the experimental hall of the MITR and operates in parallel with other user applications. The FCB contains an array of 11 MITR-II fuel elements cooled by forced convection of heavy water coolant. The converter power is 120 kW at 6 MW reactor power. A shielded horizontal beam line contains an aluminum and Teflon® filter-moderator to tailor the neutron energy spectrum into the desired epithermal energy range. A patient collimator defines the beam aperture and extends into the shielded medical room to provide circular apertures ranging from 16 to 8 cm in diameter. The in-air epithermal flux is 6.2×10^9 n/cm^{2}s at the patient position with the 12 cm collimator. The measured specific absorbed doses are constant for all field sizes and are well below the inherent background of 2.8×10^{-12} Gy_w cm^2/n produced by epithermal neutrons in tissue. The dose distributions achieved with the FCB approach the theoretical optimum for boron neutron capture therapy (BNCT). Below the core of the reactor is located the initially constructed thermal neutron irradiation facility for NCT. This facilty is useful for clinical studies of superficial cancers and small animal studies.

boron distribution in both tumor (high) and brain around tumor (low) located within the neutron radiation field

2. Adequate neutron penetration to irradiate tumors at depth with a therapeutic ratio significantly >1.0
3. The specific fast neutron and photon dose rates should be less than the inherent background dose from the epithermal neutron beam, $<2.8\times10^{-12}$ $Gy_w\ cm^2/n$
4. Ease of patient setup to allow irradiation with multiple fields at all possible tumor sites
5. Easily variable beam collimation and size, neutron current/flux ratios $\gtrsim 0.75$ and beam aperture sizes, 0 to $\gtrsim 16$ cm
6. Accurate, reliable, and automated beam monitoring and control systems with ±1% accuracy in the delivered neutron fluence (n/cm^2)
7. A well-shielded irradiation room with audio and visual communication between patient and clinical staff and with quick access available to the patient at all times
8. Nearby patient care facilities for examinations, drug infusions, beam simulations, treatment setup, and planning

Approaches to Using Fission Reactor Sources for BNCT

The general design of reactor-based epithermal neutron irradiation facilities has been discussed in (40,41). Two approaches have been used for the design of epithermal neutron irradiation facilities at fission reactors. Direct use of the core neutrons as the source has been the predominant approach for modification or conversion of existing reactors for NCT. More than eight such facilities have been constructed for clinical use in the United States, Argentina, Europe, and Asia and several more are under construction. The performance of completed clinical NCT facilities has been summarized in a recent review by Harling and Riley (42).

An interesting new facility which makes direct use of core neutrons from a low power 30 kW reactor recently has been constructed in China. It was designed specifically for NCT and is located approximately 1 mile from a hospital in the outskirts of Beijing (43,44). The Chinese In-Hospital Neutron Irradiator (IHNI-1) uses core neutrons to feed a moderator from which a thermal beam is extracted on one side of the reactor and an epithermal neutron beam from a filter/moderator on the other side. This provides the capability of BNCT in small animals and clinical studies in patients with superficial tumors using the thermal neutron beam while the epithermal beam would be used for BNCT large animal studies or in clinical trials in patients. However, the initial beam intensity of this facility is much lower than is desirable for use in routine clinical BNCT. Therefore, increasing the reactor's power would be highly advantageous. The Beijing reactor is based upon an ultrasafe, "walk away safe," low cost, design suited for sites in populated areas.

While new special purpose reactors are a possible source of additional neutron irradiation facilities, it is unlikely that many will be constructed unless BNCT becomes more widely used radiotherapeutic modality. In the interim reactor, conversions and modifications are likely to be a primary source of new BNCT irradiation facilities. Another approach to using fission reactors is based upon the use of a fission converter that converts a reactor's thermal neutrons to higher energy fission neutrons. The fission neutrons are then moderated and filtered to produce epithermal neutron beams. This approach can be especially useful to modify existing multipurpose reactors. To date, one fission converter–based facility has been constructed at the MITR (45,46). The MIT fission converter beam (FCB) represents the current state of art for epithermal neutron irradiation facilities (Figure 1). Neutrons from the core of the MIT reactor are well thermalized in heavy water and graphite before they impinge upon the converter, which is composed of 11 standard MITR fuel elements. The sub-critical converter generates ~120 kW, at 6 MW reactor power, and is cooled with heavy water to reduce neutron moderation. Fission neutrons from the converter are moderated and filtered by aluminum, polytetrafluoroethylene (Teflon®), cadmium, and lead to produce a high-intensity and low-specific contamination epithermal neutron beam at the patient position. The design of the FCB, with three in-line beam shutters, allows it to operate essentially independent of all other reactor uses. This feature is important for multipurpose reactors. Converter-based epithermal neutron irradiation facilities can be useful for retrofitting some existing research and test reactors not originally designed for epithermal neutron BNCT. While the FCB is the first example of this design approach, other fission converter–based epithermal beams have been designed with excellent calculated beam performance (47). The MIT FCB meets all requirements for an epithermal neutron irradiation facility needed for routine high-throughput clinical NCT. An optimized treatment plan for brain tumors usually requires several irradiation fields from different directions. Figure 2 shows a patient setup for a lateral brain irradiation at the MIT FCB. For a compliant patient, strips of surgical tape or Velcro straps suffice to keep the patient positioned during

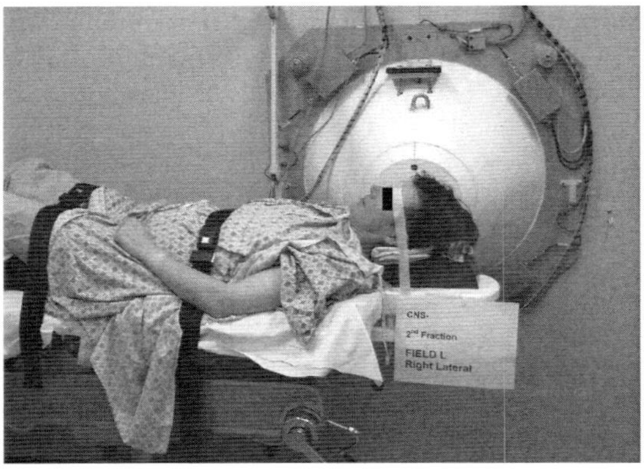

FIGURE 2 A typical patient setup for a lateral brain irradiation using the fission converter beam's (FCB's) epithermal neutron beam. A single strip of surgical tape is sufficient to immobilize the patient's head during the relatively short 5 to 15-minute treatment fields. The design of the patient collimator and the medical room allows positioning of the beam on any part of the patient.

the several minutes required for a typical irradiation field. The FCB's high intensity helps to assure that irradiations can occur during the optimum time in the boron delivery drug's biodistribution (i.e., high tumor and low blood and normal brain concentrations) and that the patient will be comfortable during the short irradiations.

Accelerator-Based Neutron Sources (ABNS)

To date, all BNCT clinical irradiations have been carried out at reactor neutron sources. However, accelerator-based neutron sources are being developed to provide neutron sources for use in hospital settings. Accelerator sources are expected to be much easier to license in a hospital setting than nuclear reactors. Proponents of accelerators also believe that they could be more compact and less expensive than comparable reactor sources. ABNS for BNCT have been reviewed (48,49), and a number of these (50–58) have been described at the recently held 14th International Congress on NCT. However, their low intensity, compared to reactors, has been a problem for existing accelerator sources. Increases in intensity by more than an order of magnitude would be necessary if accelerators are to be competitive with reactor sources for clinical BNCT. This would require that the accelerator current and target heat load also must be increased by more than an order of magnitude over that available with currently demonstrated technology. Managing heat loads of several tens of kWs, with neutron sources, which use low melting point lithium targets for the desirable (p,Li) reaction, is a major engineering challenge. The accelerator source designers have promising approaches for overcoming the limitations of current accelerator sources and it is hoped that this can be accomplished while containing costs and reducing their size. For example, operating with liquid metal targets is one approach to managing the low melting point of the lithium (50,51). Some accelerator neutron sources under development are based upon the (p,Be), (d,Be), or even the (d,t) reactions. These reactions eliminate the difficulty associated with the low melting temperature lithium targets, but the higher energy neutrons that are produced in these reactions require substantially more moderating materials to bring the neutrons into the desired energy range. Thicker moderators reduce neutron intensity. One such ABNS has been produced in Japan by Sumitomo Heavy Industries (52) and it is anticipated that a phase I clinical trial for patients with recurrent GBMs will be initiated in 2012. This will be followed by a trial in patients with recurrent head and neck cancer. If these trials result in improved survival data in the case of patients with GBMs and tumor control in patients with head and neck cancer, this should increase clinical interest in BNCT and ABNS.

■ CLINICAL DOSIMETRY AND TREATMENT PLANNING

Dosimetric Methods

The measurement of absorbed dose in an epithermal neutron beam is complicated because the incident radiation field, that consists primarily of neutrons in the energy range 0.5 eV to 10 keV, is accompanied by a small but non-negligible photon component, as well as fast neutrons, which have energies up to ~10 MeV for fission sources. Incident photons mainly include capture gammas created in the materials of the beam line. A significant photon source is also generated within the patient by the incident epithermal neutrons as they penetrate tissue and are moderated to thermal energies producing 2.2 MeV photons from subsequent neutron capture in hydrogen. The dosimetry of these neutron beams requires an assessment of the neutron and photon absorbed doses since each component possesses a markedly different relative biological effectiveness (RBE). In addition, the thermal flux must also be measured to determine the boron dose to normal tissue and tumor.

The twin ionization chamber technique (59) developed for fast neutron dosimetry (60) has been adopted as the method of choice for assessing the photon and neutron absorbed dose components (61,62). Pairs of detectors are employed with different sensitivities to the two radiation types such as A-150 tissue equivalent plastic- and graphite- (or magnesium-) walled ionization chambers. It is also necessary to separately determine the portion of the neutron dose arising from thermal neutron capture in boron, when present, and the elemental constituents of tissue (arising mainly from nitrogen) because the concentrations of these elements vary between tissues. These absorbed dose rates are determined from thermal neutron flux measurements obtained by neutron activation analysis of bare and cadmium-covered gold foils (61,63). Gamma rays emitted by the activated foils are counted using a gamma spectrometer incorporating either a high-purity germanium or sodium iodide detector. These, like their ionization chamber counterparts, have a calibration traceable to a national standards laboratory. The measured thermal flux is multiplied by the appropriate kerma coefficient for a given reaction and the weight fraction of nitrogen (or boron) in the tissue of interest.

Treatment Planning

Treatment planning for NCT differs markedly from treatment planning for external beam photons or electrons in conventional RT and, in some ways, is significantly more complex requiring specialized software for construction of the computational beam and patient geometry models needed for calculation and analysis of the absorbed doses (64–67). The computational models used for photon and electron dose calculations involve only a single low-LET dose component and do not apply to NCT, where the radiation field is a complex mixture of high- and low-LET dose components with varying biological effectiveness. The spatial distribution of each dose component is different and depends on the tissue composition as well as the neutron and photon energy spectra (Figure 3). Multiplicative weighting factors, which are generally RBE factors measured in animal models (68), are applied to the individual dose components to allow expression of their sum as

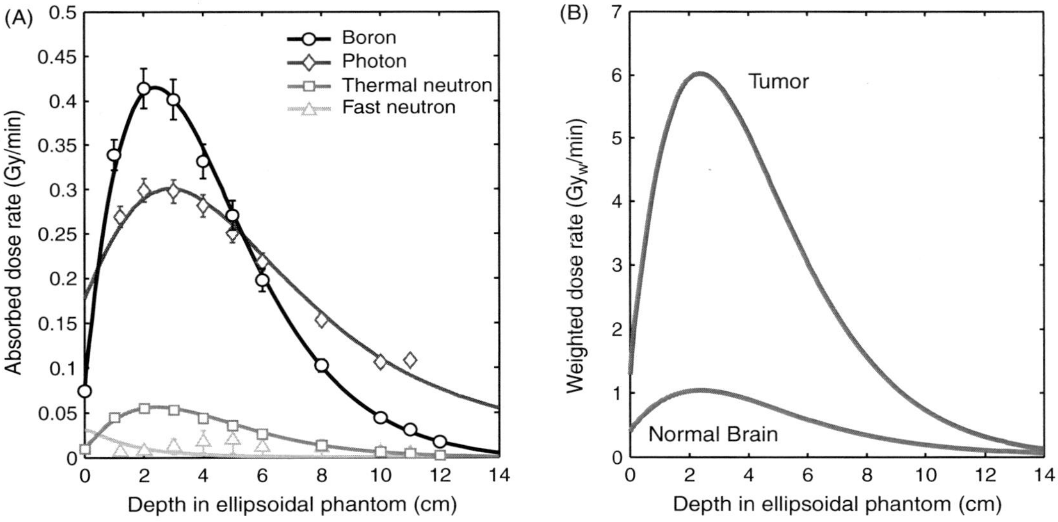

FIGURE 3 (A) Measured (points) and calculated (curves) absorbed dose rate profiles in brain as a function of depth along the central axis of an ellipsoidal water phantom for a 12 cm diameter beam at the fission converter–based epithermal neutron facility at Massachusetts Institute of Technology (MIT). (B) Biologically weighted dose profiles computed for boronophenylalanine (BPA)-based boron neutron capture therapy (BNCT) using the same neutron beam and phantom with boron concentrations of 15 μg/g for normal brain and 52.5 μg/g for tumor and biological weighting factors of 1.0, 3.2, 1.3, and 3.8 for photons, neutrons, boron in brain and boron in tumor, respectively. Error bars represent the absolute measurement uncertainties and the statistical uncertainty in the calculated curves is ≤0.6% of the maximum for each dose component. Adapted from measured data in Ref. (46) and Monte Carlo calculations in Ref. (69).

a single, total weighted dose (expressed as Gy_w) that is approximately equivalent in effect to the same dose of photon radiation.

Although generally regarded as the most accurate algorithms, direct solutions of the Boltzmann transport equation like Monte Carlo simulation or the discrete ordinates method are rarely used in photon RT because they are computationally expensive. NCT treatment planning systems, however, rely exclusively on Monte Carlo simulation for dose calculations because of the complex, scatter-dominated nature of the radiation transport processes involved. Monte Carlo calculations simulate transport of neutrons and photons through the patient's geometry and use track length density estimators of neutron and photon flux integrated against kerma coefficients to compute dose. Treatment planning systems require careful validation by evaluating agreement between dose calculations and in-phantom measurements, an example of which is shown in Figure 3 (69,70). Treatment plans are developed using individualized computational models with the geometry constructed from CT or MR images of the patient using combinations of manual and automated methods of image processing. While tissue (electron) density is the principal consideration for transport of megavoltage photon beams, the transport of neutrons is governed by nuclear interactions. The associated neutron cross sections can vary significantly for different elemental tissue composition so that dose calculations for NCT require modeling different tissue types in the region of interest.

Therapeutic advantage in BNCT is achieved principally through the tumor selectivity of the ^{10}B-containing delivery agent rather than by precise geometric targeting of multiple well-collimated radiation fields converging on the target volume. The low-energy neutron beams used in NCT are usually not highly collimated and any directionality is rapidly lost with depth in tissue due to neutron scattering and thermalization. Generally, only a small number of neutron fields are used to deliver treatment plans for brain tumors, typically not more than three. For superficially located target volumes, however, a single field may suffice. In such cases, an optimal plan often results by centering the beam on the target volume and aligning the field to minimize the depth of the deepest aspect of the target volume. Since dose declines with depth due to thermal neutron attenuation after its maximum at 2–3 cm depth, this field arrangement will maximize the minimum dose to the target volume. Proximity to dose-limiting tissues or organs at risk, however, must also be considered in the field arrangement. For deep-seated tumors, multiple fields, often directionally opposed, are generally necessary to achieve adequate dose coverage of the target at depth. Care must be taken to avoid overlap near the surface with multiple nonopposed fields. An example treatment plan using three fields is shown in Figure 4. As can be seen in the figure, the presentation of dose in BNCT treatment planning is somewhat unconventional. Typically, total weighted dose (expressed as Gy_w) for tumor and normal tissue(s) are calculated separately, each for the entire dose grid using different boron concentrations and weighting factors (RBEs) are assumed for each tissue. The rationale for this approach is that the exact boundary of the tumor is unknown and that microscopic deposits of tumor extend well beyond the enhancing volume detectable on imaging.

Absorbed Dose Profiles

The absolute uncertainties for individual BNCT dose components are given in Table 2 and although some are larger than the 3–5% recommended for RT (71), the boron and photon doses that comprise the principal components are known accurately enough notwithstanding the microscopic distribution of boron. Figure 3 shows depth-dose profiles for each dose component in an ellipsoidal water-filled phantom irradiated in an epithermal neutron beam (46). The boron, photon, and thermal neutron dose components exhibit a relatively low-entrance dose with a marked buildup occurring at shallow depths that peak between 20 and 30 mm in phantom. Conversely, the fast neutrons have a dose profile that is highest at the surface and rapidly attenuates with depth to very low levels. The fast neutron dose component is difficult to measure with acceptably low experimental uncertainty in the presence of the other dose components at depths beyond 40 mm in most beams. The photon and boron absorbed dose components dominate when using either BPA or BSH as the boron delivery agents with relatively little contribution from thermal and fast neutrons.

Dosimetric Intercomparisons

BNCT is still an experimental modality, and there are no standardized methods for either calibrating the mixed radiation fields employed or for calculating treatment plans that specify the prescription dose to the patient. This makes it difficult

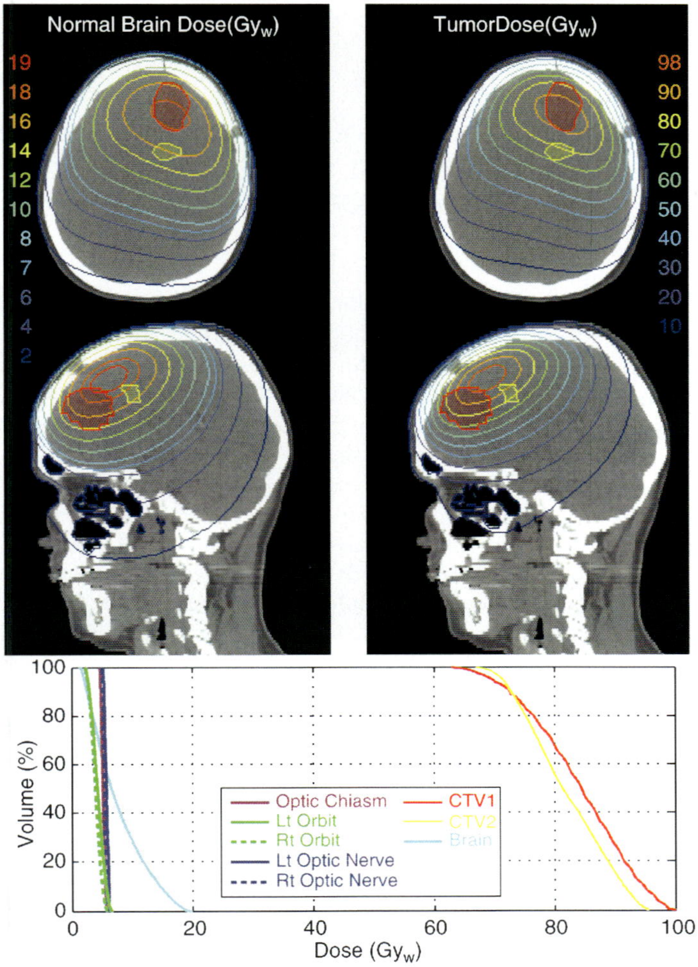

FIGURE 4 A three-field treatment plan for a brain tumor (GBM) patient calculated using the MiMMC treatment planning system. The prescription is a mean brain dose of 7.7 Gy$_w$. Isodose contours calculated for tumor and normal brain are shown on axial and sagittal slices through the target volumes. The integral dose volume histograms (DVHs) summarize dosimetry for structures of interest including target volumes and organs at risk.

TABLE 2 Summary of the absolute uncertainty for individual absorbed dose components measured in brain

Dose Component	Uncertainty (%)	Fraction of Total Dose at D_{max}	
		Absorbed Dose (Gy)	Weighted Dose (Gy$_w$)
Boron	4.0–6.5	0.52	0.48
Photon	4.4	0.37	0.27
Thermal neutron	4.0–6.5	0.07	0.16
Fast neutron	30	0.04	0.09

The right columns give the fraction of each dose component relative to the total dose in brain containing 15 μg/g of ^{10}B for both absorbed dose (unweighted) and weighted dose with radiobiological weighting factors of 1.3, 1.0, and 3.2 applied for boron, photons and neutrons (both thermal and fast) respectively.

to compare studies performed at different centers, and unfortunately precludes combining or sharing clinical data on safety and efficacy in any meaningful way because each group's specification of dose may not be the same. This absence in uniformity has been partly addressed by an extensive series of measurements and calculations performed between all clinical centers in the United States, Europe, and Argentina (72–76). This study established an empirical model relating the maximum weighted dose in brain specified by a particular center to an MIT-measured dose as a function of tissue boron concentration (Figure 5). In doing so, a first-order appraisal can be made by each participant of their own dose specification in relation to any other participant. Neglecting the uncertainties related to biological weighting factors, large variations between calculated and measured dose are apparent that depend upon the ^{10}B uptake in the tumor and normal tissues. If a boron concentration of 15 µg/g in normal tissue is assumed, for example, differences in the evaluated maximum dose to brain for the same nominal specification of 10 Gy_w at the different facilities range between 7.6 and 13.2 Gy_w in the trials using BPA. The magnitude of these variations cannot be fully explained by uncertainties or measurement errors, but may rather highlight inaccuracies in beam source definition (70) or inexact benchmarking of treatment planning systems (69,77). That was found to be the case at BNL where the source definition did not agree with measurements or fully account for beamline modifications implemented in 1996 (69,72,78,79).

Consequently, it is important to recognize that while individual centers achieve satisfactory consistency within their patient cohorts, dose specifications are different between centers and the various results of seemingly similar studies performed by different centers cannot then be directly compared. Although more comparisons of clinical outcomes, such as those recently published from the Swedish clinical trial (80–84), are needed to help advance BNCT, recognition of dosimetric disparities must be incorporated to limit the likelihood of erroneous conclusions.

■ CLINICAL STUDIES OF BNCT FOR BRAIN TUMORS

Early Studies in the United States and Japan

Although the clinical potential of BNCT first was recognized in the 1930s, it was not until the 1950s that the first clinical trials were initiated by Farr at the BNL in New York (85) and by Sweet and Brownell at the Massachusetts General Hospital (MGH) using the MITR (86) using several different low-molecular weight inorganic boron compounds as delivery agents. However, the results of these studies were disappointing in large part due to the nonselectivity of the low-molecular weight boron compounds that were used (87). No further clinical trials were carried out in the United States until the 1990s when BNCT was resumed at the Brookhaven National Laboratory Medical Research Reactor (88) and at Harvard-MIT using the MITR (89). BPA was used as the boron delivery agent and patients were irradiated with a collimated beam of higher energy epithermal neutrons, which had greater tissue-penetrating properties than thermal neutrons. This was well tolerated, but there were no significant differences in the median survival times of patients who had received BNCT compared to those who had received conventional therapy (89,90).

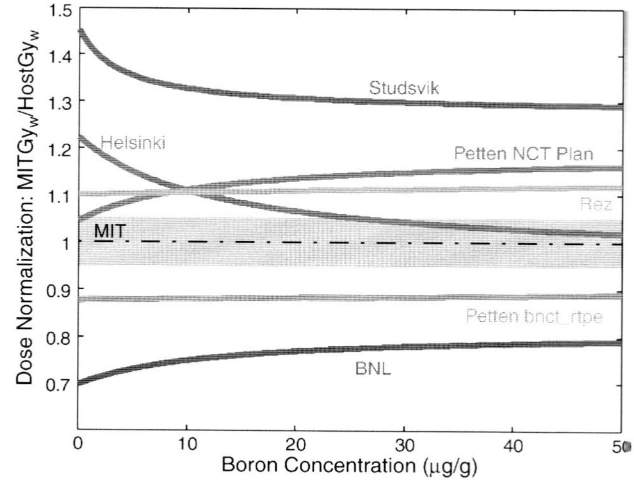

FIGURE 5 Graphical representation of a parameterized model converting the maximum weighted dose, calculated with the treatment planning systems from each center to a Massachusetts Institute of Technology (MIT) calibrated dose as a function of boron uptake in tissue (76). The plotted curves afford an easy and direct comparison of dose specification between participants.

Clinical Trials in Japan

Following a 2-year fellowship in Sweet's laboratory at the MGH, Hiroshi Hatanaka initiated clinical studies in Japan in 1967 using low-energy thermal neutron beams and BSH, which had been developed as a boron delivery agent by Soloway (37). In Hatanaka's procedure (34), which was based on that used by Sweet (86), as much of the tumor was surgically removed as possible ("debulking"), and at some time thereafter, BSH was administered by a slow intraarterial infusion (34) or, in later studies, intravenously (35,36). Twelve to fourteen hours following administration, BNCT was carried out at one or another of several different nuclear reactors. Since thermal neutrons have a limited depth of penetration in tissue, this necessitated reflecting the skin and raising the bone flap in order to directly irradiate the exposed brain. This eliminated radiation damage to the scalp and permitted treatment of more deep-seated residual tumors. A ping pong ball or silastic sphere was inserted into the resection cavity to create a void space in order to improve neutron penetration into deeper regions of the tumor bed and adjacent brain. This was a major difference between the intraoperative procedure carried out by Hatanaka and Nakagawa (36,91) and other Japanese neurosurgeons and the BNCT protocols that have been carried out in the United States, Europe, and in Japan (92–97). The latter have utilized epithermal neutron beams that have not required reflecting the scalp and raising the bone flap at the time of irradiation. This has made it difficult to directly compare Hatanaka's clinical results with those obtained elsewhere. The results using epithermal neutron beams are summarized in Table 3 and are described below.

Kawabata and Miyatake and their coworkers have carried out several clinical studies in which BPA alone or in combination with BSH were administered for treatment of patients with primary, surgically resected gliomas or those with recurrent GBMs who previously had received photon irradiation (92–94). In patients with newly diagnosed GBMs, favorable responses were seen using BNCT with BPA and BSH either with or without an x-ray boost especially in high-risk groups (93; Figure 7). The median survival time [MeST] of patients treated with this regimen was 23.5 months compared to 14.1 months for patients who had surgery followed by BNCT. For those patients who had surgery and BNCT alone (n = 21), the MeST was 15.6 months (95% confidence interval (CI): 12.2–23.9 months) after diagnosis. This was significantly longer than the 10.3 months MeST for the historical controls (n = 27) at Osaka Medical College who had undergone surgical resection followed by external beam photon irradiation and chemotherapy with nitrosourea (mainly ACNU in Japan (94)). Similarly, Nakai et al. have reported improved survival by combining BNCT with a photon boost (97). These clinical studies have validated the animal model data, reported by Barth and his coworkers (98), showing the efficacy of combining BNCT with an external beam photon irradiation. Fluorine-18 labeled BPA has been shown to be useful

TABLE 3 Boron neutron capture therapy (BNCT) clinical trials using epithermal neutron beams for BNCT of patients with gliomas

Facility[a]	No. of Patients & Duration of Trial	Delivery Agent	Median Survival Time (Months)	Reference No.
BMRR, United States	53 (1994–1999)	BPA 250–330 mg/kg	13–14	(88,90)
MITR M67 Beam, MIT, United States	20 (1996–1999)	BPA 250 or 350 mg/kg	13	(65,89)
MITR FCB, MIT, United States	6 (2002–2003)	BPA 14 g/m^2	Not indicated	(67)
KURRI, Japan	>43 (2002–present)	BPA 500 mg/kg	20.7	(91–94)
JRR4, JAEA, Japan	>100 (1998–2010)	BPA 250 mg/kg + BSH 5g	Not indicated	(95–97)
R2–0, Studsvik Medical AB, Sweden	29 (2001–2005)	BPA 900 mg/kg	17.7	(81–84)
FiR1, Finland	>50 (1999–present)	BPA 290–400 mg/kg	7 (recurrent patients)	(101)
HFR, Netherlands	26 (1997–2002)	BSH 100 mg/kg	13.2–15.0	(113,114)

MITR indicates Massachusetts Institute of Technology Reactor; FCB, fission converter beam; MIT, Massachusetts Institute of Technology; BPA, boronophenylalanine; BSH, sodium borocaptate.

in predicting the effectiveness of BNCT (99) and post treatment radiation effects (100). Representative radiographic changes in two patients, treated by Miyatake, Kawabata et al., who received BNCT, are shown in Figure 7 and PET imaging studies with fluorine-18 BPA are shown in Figure 8. As is well known in evaluating clinical trials, especially those involving BNCT, retrospective comparisons must be interpreted with caution (80). Nevertheless, the MeST from the date of diagnosis, calculated using the Kaplan–Meier method (Figure 6A, Figure 6B) for Protocol 2 (BNCT+XRT) was 23.5 months (95% CI: 10. 2 months to undetermined) after diagnosis (n = 11), compared to 10.3 months (95% CI: 7.4–13.2), log-rank test P = .0035) for historical controls. The MeST of patients in Protocol 1 (BNCT-XRT) was 14.1 months (95% CI: 9.9–18.5 months), which was not significantly different from historical controls. This study was compromised by low patient numbers since they had been subdivided into two protocols involving only 10 and 11 patients each. A future multicenter phase II Japanese clinical study will be carried out by Kawabata and Miyatake and their coworkers to evaluate BNCT in combination with temozolomide (Osaka-Tribrain 0902, NCT00974987).

Clinical Studies in Finland

The team of clinicians and physicists at the Helsinki University Central Hospital and VTT Technical Research Center of Finland recently have reported on 22 patients with GBMs who had undergone standard therapy, recurred, and subsequently received BNCT at the time of their recurrence using BPA as the boron delivery agent (101).The median time to progression was 3 month, and the overall MST was 7 months. It is difficult to compare these results with other reported results in patients with recurrent GBMs, but they are a starting point for future studies using BNCT as salvage therapy in patients with recurrent tumors.

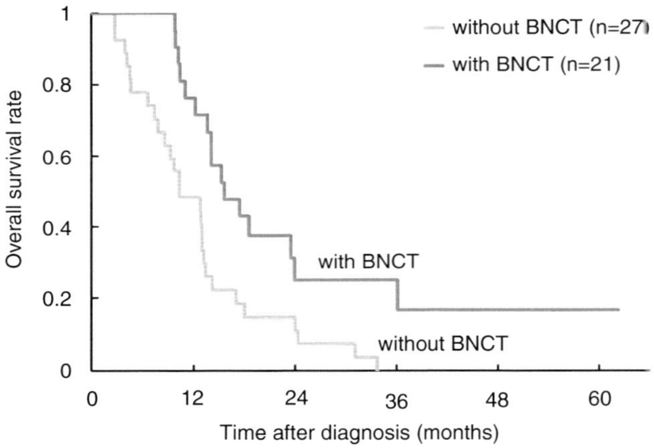

FIGURE 6A Kaplan–Meier estimates of overall survival for all newly diagnosed glioblastoma (WHO grade 4, n = 21). The continuous line was recent historical control treated by external beam x-ray irradiation. The median survival time of the BNCT group was 15.6 months. There was statistical significance between both groups in Log-rank test (P = .0035).

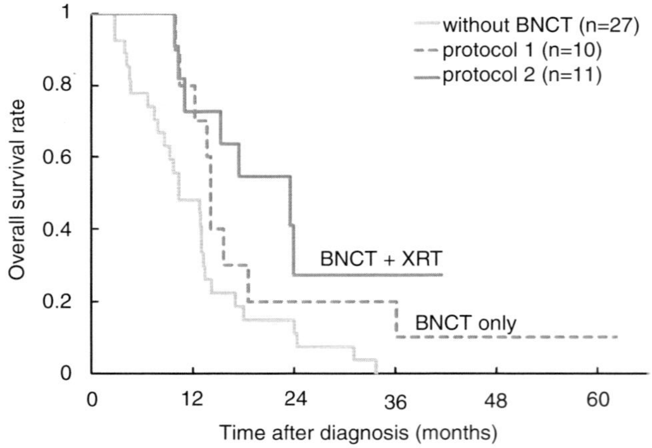

FIGURE 6B Kaplan–Meier estimates of overall survival for all newly diagnosed glioblastoma patients (protocol 1 and 2). External beam x-ray irradiation (XRT) boost after BNCT (protocol 2, continuous line) was for the latter 11 cases. This improved the median survival time to 23.5 months (14.1 months for BNCT only protocol 1, dotted line).

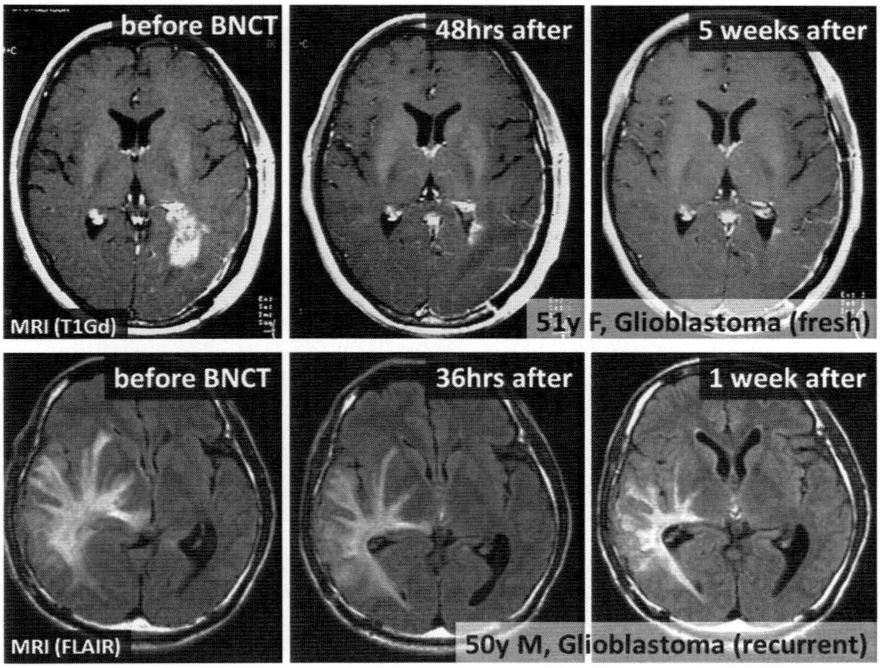

FIGURE 7 Radiographic changes following boron neutron capture therapy (BNCT) in two representative patients with glioblastoma (GBM). In both, there was a reduction in both mass and peritumoral edema without the administration of corticosteroids or mannitol within a few days. This is also shown in the FLAIR image of Case #12.

Clinical Studies in Sweden

Finally, to conclude this section, the following is a summary of a clinical trial that was carried out in Sweden using BPA and an epithermal neutron beam, which had greater tissue penetration properties than the thermal beams originally used in Japan. This study differed significantly from all previous clinical trials in that the total amount of BPA administered was increased to 900 mg/kg b.w., and it was infused intravenously over 6 hours (80). This regimen was based on animal studies in F98 glioma bearing rats that showed that boron concentrations in invading tumor cells increased from 37% to 71% of that in the main tumor if the infusion time was increased from 2 hours to 6 hours (102). The longer infusion time of the drug was well tolerated by the 29 patients who were enrolled in this study (80–84). All were treated with two fields, and the mean weighted whole brain dose was 3.2 to 6.1 Gy_w and the minimum dose to the tumor ranged from 15.4 to 54.3 Gy_w. There has been some disagreement among the Swedish investigators who carried out this study in terms of evaluation of the results. One group reported survival data that was compiled before all the patients had succumbed to their tumors (81). Based on complete survival data, the other group (82–84) reported that the MeST was 17.7 months compared to 15.5 months, which has been reported for patients who received standard therapy of surgery, followed by RT and temozolomide (103,104). Furthermore, the frequency of adverse events was less after BNCT (14%) than after RT alone (21%) and both of these were less than those seen following RT in combination with temozolomide. If this improved survival data, obtained using the higher dose of BPA and a 6-hour infusion time can be confirmed by others, preferably in a randomized clinical trial, it could represent a significant step forward in BNCT of brain tumors especially if combined with a photon boost.

■ CONCLUSIONS

What then is the future of BNCT? It probably lies in filling a niche for those malignancies, whether primary or recurrent, for which there is no effective therapy. What are some of the advantages of BNCT?

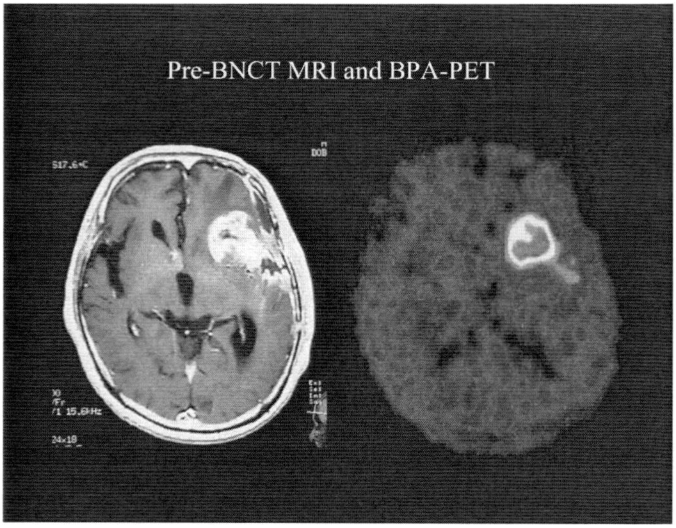

FIGURE 8 Contrast-enhanced T1-weighted MRI of representative glioblastoma patient and ^{18}F-labeled BPA-PET image after initial debulking surgery. The patients received ^{18}F-BPA-PET to assess the distribution of boronophenylalanine (BPA) and to estimate the boron concentration in tumors before boron neutron capture therapy (BNCT) without direct determination of boron concentration in the tumor. The lesion to normal brain (L/N) ratio of the enhanced tumor was 7.8 in this case. Note that even the periphery of the main mass, that is, the infiltrative portion of the tumor, showed BPA uptake. The L/N ratio of BPA uptake can be estimated from this study and dose planning was done according to this L/N ratio, and if the L/N ratio was more than 2.5, then BNCT was initiated. ^{18}F-BPA-PET accurate BPA provided an accurate estimate of the accumulation and distribution of BPA as previously reported (99,100).

First, it has the ability to selectively deliver a high-radiation dose to the tumor with a much lower dose to surrounding normal tissues. This is an important feature that makes BNCT particularly attractive for salvage therapy of patients who have been treated to tolerance with photon irradiation. *Second*, it has the ability to more effectively target multicentric deposits of tumor than is possible with stereotactic radiosurgery of primary and metastatic brain tumors. *Third*, although it may be only palliative, it can produce striking clinical responses, as evidenced by the experience of several groups treating patients with recurrent, therapeutically refractory head and neck cancer (105–109).

Critical issues that must be addressed include: (a) development of new low- and high-molecular weight boron agents and optimization of their delivery; (b) obtaining approval for the clinical use of these new agents from regulatory agencies and carrying out biodistribution studies in glioma patients prior to resection of their primary tumors; (c) improvement of methods for determining the boron dose delivered to the residual tumor volume on both macroscopic and microscopic levels to enable more accurate tumor dose specifications; (d) development of neutron sources that can be easily sited in hospitals; (e) initiate randomized clinical trials; and (f) be prepared to compete with or complement new therapeutic approaches. In this chapter, we have summarized the current status of BNCT as a treatment for high-grade gliomas and outlined the problems that we believe are important to solve in order to move forward with BNCT as a treatment modality. It is up to investigators, both in basic and clinical research, to come up with solutions to these problems.

■ ACKNOWLEDGMENTS

This paper is dedicated to Professor Emeritus Albert H. Soloway in celebration of his 87th birthday. Dr. Barth thanks Mrs. Heidi Bosworth for expert secretarial assistance in the preparation of this manuscript. Research of Drs. Barth, Binns, Harling, Kiger, Riley, and Vicente has been supported by numerous grants from the United States Department of Energy and the National Institutes of Health. Dr. Kawabata's clinical studies have been supported by grants from the Ministry of Health, Labor and Welfare from the government of Japan.

REFERENCES

1. Barth RF, Coderre JA, Vicente MG, Blue TE. Boron neutron capture therapy of cancer: current status and future prospects. *Clin Cancer Res.* 2005;11(11):3987–4002.
2. Slatkin DN. A history of boron neutron capture therapy of brain tumours. Postulation of a brain radiation dose tolerance limit. *Brain.* 1991;114:1609–1629.
3. Barth RF. Boron neutron capture therapy: a critical assessment. *J Neurooncol.* 2003;62:1–210.
4. Miyatake S, Kawabata S, Nonoguchi N, et al. Pseudoprogression in boron neutron capture therapy for malignant gliomas and meningiomas. *Neuro-oncology.* 2009;11(4):430–436.
5. Altieri S, Bortolussi S, Barth RF, Roveda L, Zonta A (eds.). Thirteenth International Congress on Neutron Capture Therapy. *Appl Radiat Isot.* 2009;67(7–8 Suppl):S1–S379.
6. Kreiner A (ed.). 14th International Congress on Neutron Capture Therapy. *Appl Radiat Isot.* 2011;69:1631–1939.
7. Soloway AH, Tjarks W, Barnum BA, et al. The Chemistry of Neutron Capture Therapy. *Chem Rev.* 1998;98(4):1515–1562.
8. Sibrian-Vazquez M, Vicente MGH. Boron tumor-delivery for BNCT: Recent developments and perspectives. In: Hosmane NS, ed. *Boron Science: New Technologies & Applications*: CRC Press; 2011:203–32.
9. Semioshkin A NE, Godovikov I, et al.. Reactions of oxonium derivatives of $[B^{12}H^{12}]^{2-}$ with amines: Synthesis and structure of novel B_{12}-based ammonium salts and amino acids. *V. J. Organomet. Chem.* 2007;692:4020–8.
10. Kabalka GW, Wu Z, Yao M-L. Synthesis of a series of boronated unnatural cyclic amino acids as potential boron capture therapy agents. *Appl. Organomet. Chem.* 2008;22:516–22.
11. Kabalka GW, Yao ML, Marepally SR, Chandra S. Biological evaluation of boronated unnatural amino acids as new boron carriers. *Appl Radiat Isot.* 2009;67(7–8 Suppl):S374–S379.
12. Mier W, Gabel, D, Haberkorn, U. Conjugation of the closo-borane mereaptoundeca-hydrododecaborate (BSH) to a tumor selective peptide. *Anorg. Allg. Chem.* 2004;630:1258–62.
13. Bregadze V, Sivaev I. Polyhedral Boron Compounds for BNCT. In: Hosmane N, ed. *Boron Science: New Technologies and Applications*: CRC Press; 2012:181–208.
14. Al-Madhoun AS, Johnsamuel J, Barth RF, et al. Evaluation of human thymidine kinase 1 substrates as new candidates for boron neutron capture therapy. *Cancer Res.* 2004;64(17):6280–6286.
15. Barth RF, Yang W, Wu G, et al. Thymidine kinase 1 as a molecular target for boron neutron capture therapy of brain tumors. *Proc Natl Acad Sci USA.* 2008;105(45):17493–17497.
16. Renner MW, Miura M, Easson MW, Vicente MG. Recent progress in the syntheses and biological evaluation of boronated porphyrins for boron neutron-capture therapy. *Anticancer Agents Med Chem.* 2006;6(2):145–157.
17. Ol'shevskaya V, Zaytsev A, Savchenko A, et al. Boronated porphyrins and chlorins as potential anticancer drugs. *Bull. Korean Chem. Soc.* 2007;28:1910–6.
18. Kahl S, Koo M. Synthesis and properties of tebrakis-carborane-carboxylate esters of 2;4-bis (-dehydroryethyl) dereteroporphyrin IX. In: Allen B, Moore D, Harrington B, eds. *Progress Neutron Capture Therapy.* New York: Plenium Press; 1992:223–6.
19. Crossley EL, Ziolkowski EJ, Coderre JA, Rendina LM. Boronated DNA-binding compounds as potential agents for boron neutron capture therapy. *Mini Rev Med Chem.* 2007;7(3):303–313.
20. Orlova A, Kononov, LO, Kimel, BG, et al. Conjugates of polyhedral boron compounds with carbohydrates. 4. Hydrolytic stability of carborane-lactose conjugates depends on the structure of a spacer between the carborane cage and sugar moiety. *Appl. Organometal. Chem.* 2006;20:416–20.
21. Capala J, Barth RF, Bendayan M, et al. Boronated epidermal growth factor as a potential targeting agent for boron neutron capture therapy of brain tumors. *Bioconjug Chem.* 1996;7(1):7–15.
22. Wu G, Yang W, Barth RF, et al. Molecular targeting and treatment of an epidermal growth factor receptor-positive glioma using boronated cetuximab. *Clin Cancer Res.* 2007;13(4):1260–1268.
23. Yang W, Wu G, Barth RF, et al. Molecular targeting and treatment of composite EGFR and EGFRvIII-positive gliomas using boronated monoclonal antibodies. *Clin Cancer Res.* 2008;14(3):883–891.
24. Backer MV, Gaynutdinov TI, Patel V, et al. Vascular endothelial growth factor selectively targets boronated dendrimers to tumor vasculature. *Mol Cancer Ther.* 2005;4(9):1423–1429.
25. Pan X, Wu G, Yang W, et al. Synthesis of cetuximab-immunoliposomes via a cholesterol-based membrane anchor for targeting of EGFR. *Bioconjug Chem.* 2007; 18(1):101–108.
26. Nakamura H. Liposomal boron delivery system for neutron capture therapy of cancer. In: Hosmane N, ed. *Boron Science: New Technologies and Applications*: CRC Press; 2012:165–79.
27. Altieri S, Balzi M, Bortolussi S, et al. Carborane derivatives loaded into liposomes as efficient delivery systems for boron neutron capture therapy. *J Med Chem.* 2009;52(23):7829–7835.
28. Feakes DA. Design and development of polyhedral borane anions for liposomal delivery. In: Hosmane NS, ed. *Boron Science: New Technologies and Applications*: CRC Press; 2011:277–92.

29. Li T, Hamdi J, Hawthorne MF. Unilamellar liposomes with enhanced boron content. *Bioconjug Chem.* 2006;17(1):15–20.

30. Doi A, Kawabata S, Iida K, et al. Tumor-specific targeting of sodium borocaptate (BSH) to malignant glioma by transferrin-PEG liposomes: a modality for boron neutron capture therapy. *J Neurooncol.* 2008;87(3):287–294.

31. Zhu Y, Yan K, Maguire J, et al. Recent developments in boron neutron capture therapy (BNCT) driven by nanotechnology. *Curr. Chem. Biol.* 2007;1:141–9.

32. Menichetti L, De Marchi D, Calucci L, et al. Boron nitride nanotubes for boron neutron capture therapy as contrast agents in magnetic resonance imaging at 3 T. *Appl Radiat Isot.* 2011;69(12):1725–1727.

33. Yinghuai Z, Cheng Yan K, Maguire JA. Recent developments in boron neutron capture therapy driven by nanotechnology. In: Hosmane NS, ed. *Boron Science: New Technologies and Applications*: CRC Press; 2007:147–63.

34. Hatanaka H. Boron neutron capture therapy for brain tumors. In: Karim A, Laws E, eds. *Glioma*: Berlin, Springer-Verlag; 1991: 233–49.

35. Hatanaka H, Nakagawa Y. Clinical results of long-surviving brain tumor patients who underwent boron neutron capture therapy. *Int J Radiat Oncol Biol Phys.* 1994;28(5):1061–1066.

36. Nakagawa Y, Hatanaka H. Boron neutron capture therapy. Clinical brain tumor studies. *J Neurooncol.* 1997;33(1–2):105–115.

37. Soloway AH, Hatanaka H, Davis MA. Penetration of brain and brain tumor. VII. Tumor-binding sulfhydryl boron compounds. *J Med Chem.* 1967;10(4):714–717.

38. Mishima Y. Selective thermal neutron capture therapy of cancer cells using their specific metabolic activities - melanoma as prototype. In: Mishima Y, ed. *Cancer Neutron Capture Therapy.* New York: Plenum Press; 1996:1–26.

39. Coderre JA, Glass JD, Fairchild RG, et al. Selective delivery of boron by the melanin precursor analogue p-boronophenylalanine to tumors other than melanoma. *Cancer Res.* 1990;50(1):138–141.

40. Harling OK. Fission reactor based epithermal neutron irradiation facilities for routine clinical application in BNCT–Hatanaka memorial lecture. *Appl Radiat Isot.* 2009;67(7–8 Suppl):S7–11.

41. Moss RL, Aizawa O, Beynon D, et al. The requirements and development of neutron beams for neutron capture therapy of brain cancer. *J Neurooncol.* 1997;33(1–2):27–40.

42. Harling OK, Riley KJ. Fission reactor neutron sources for neutron capture therapy–a critical review. *J Neurooncol.* 2003;62(1–2):7–17.

43. Guotu K, Ziyong, S., Feng, S. . The study of physics and thermal characteristics for in hospital neutron irradiator (IHNI). *Appl. Radiat. Isotop.* 2009;67:S234-S7.

44. Yiguo L, Pu, X, Wang, X, et al. Start-up of the first in-hospital Neutron Irradiator (IHNI1) & presentation of the BNCT development status in China. In: Proc. 14th Int'l. Cong. on Neutron Capture Therapy Buenos Aires, Argentina; 2010. p. 371–4.

45. Harling OK, Riley KJ, Newton TH, et al. The fission converter based epithermal neutron ir-radiation facility at the Massachusetts Institute of Technology Reactor. *Nucl. Sci. and Eng.* 2002;140:223–40.

46. Riley KJ, Binns PJ, Harling OK. Performance characteristics of the MIT fission converter based epithermal neutron beam. *Phys Med Biol.* 2003;48(7):943–958.

47. Liu HB, Razvi, J., Rucker, R., et al. TRIGA fuel based converter assembly design for a dual-mode neutron beam system at the McClellan Nuclear Radiation Center. In: Hawthorne MF, Shelly, K., Wiersema, R.J., ed. *Frontiers in Neutron Capture Therapy.* New York: Kluwer Academic/Plenum Publishers; 2001:295–300.

48. Blue TE, Yanch JC. Accelerator-based epithermal neutron sources for boron neutron capture therapy of brain tumors. *J Neurooncol.* 2003;62(1–2):19–31.

49. Nigg DW. Neutron sources and applications in radiotherapy- A brief history and current trends. In: Proc. 12th Intl. Cong. Neutron Capture Therapy. Takamatsu, Japan; 2006.

50. Halfon S, Paul M, Arenshtam A, et al. High-power liquid-lithium target prototype for accelerator-based boron neutron capture therapy. *Appl Radiat Isot.* 2011;69(12):1654–1656.

51. Kononov V, Bokhovko, K., Kononov, O. High-power liquid lithium neutron production target design for accelerator based intensive neutron source. In: Proc. 14th Intl. Cong. Neutron Capture Therapy. Beunos Aires, Argentina; 2010. p. 466–7.

52. Tanaka H, Sakurai Y, Suzuki M, et al. Experimental verification of beam characteristics for cyclotron-based epithermal neutron source (C-BENS). *Appl Radiat Isot* 2011;69(12):1642–1645.

53. Kandiev Y, Kashaeva E, Malyshkin G, et al. Optimization of the target of an accelerator-driven neutron source through Monte Carlo numerical simulation of neutron and gamma transport by the PRIZMA code. *Appl Radiat. Isot.* 2011;69(12):1632–1634.

54. Aleynik V, Burdakov A, Davydenko V, et al. BINP accelerator based epithermal neutron source. *Appl Radiat Isot.* 2011;69(12):1635–1638.

55. Imoto M, Tanaka H, Fujita K, et al. Evaluation for activities of component of Cyclotron-Based Epithermal Neutron Source (C-BENS) and the surface of concrete wall in irradiation room. *Appl Radiat Isot.* 2011;69(12):1646–1648.

56. Vento VT, Bergueiro J, Cartelli D, et al. Electrostatic design and beam transport for a folded tandem electrostatic quadrupole accelerator facility for accelerator-based boron neutron capture therapy. *Appl Radiat Isot.* 2011;69(12):1649–1653.

57. Kreiner AJ, Castell W, Di Paolo H, et al. Development of a Tandem-Electrostatic-Quadrupole facility for Accelerator-Based Boron Neutron Capture Therapy. *Appl Radiat Isot.* 2011;69:1672–5.

58. Ceballos C, Esposito J, Agosteo S, et al. Towards the final BSA modeling for the accelerator-driven BNCT facility at INFN LNL. *Appl Radiat Isot.* 2011;69(12):1660–1663.

59. Attix FH. Introduction to Radiological Physics and Radiation Dosimetry. New York: Wiley; 1986:475–501.

60. International Commission on Radiation Units and Measurements. Clinical Neutron Dosimetry, Part 1: Determination of Absorbed Dose in a Patient Treated by External Beams of Fast Neutrons. Bethesda, MD; ICRU Report 45, 1989.

61. Rogus RD, Harling OK, Yanch JC. Mixed field dosimetry of epithermal neutron beams for boron neutron capture therapy at the MITR-II research reactor. *Med Phys.* 1994;21(10):1611–1625.

62. Raaijmakers CP, Konijnenberg MW, Verhagen HW, Mijnheer BJ. Determination of dose components in phantoms irradiated with an epithermal neutron beam for boron neutron capture therapy. *Med Phys.* 1995;22(3):321–329.

63. American Society for Testing and Materials. Standard test method for determining thermal neutron reaction and fluence rates by radioactivation techniques. West Conshohocken, PA; ASTM E262–97, 1997.

64. Zamenhof R, Redmond E 2nd, Solares G, et al. Monte Carlo-based treatment planning for boron neutron capture therapy using custom designed models automatically generated from CT data. *Int J Radiat Oncol Biol Phys.* 1996;35(2):383–397.

65. Palmer MR, Goorley JT, Kiger WS, et al. Treatment planning and dosimetry for the Harvard-MIT Phase I clinical trial of cranial neutron capture therapy. *Int J Radiat Oncol Biol Phys.* 2002;53(5):1361–1379.

66. Nigg DW. Computational dosimetry and treatment planning considerations for neutron capture therapy. *J Neurooncol.* 2003;62(1–2):75–86.

67. Kiger WS 3rd, Lu XQ, Harling OK, et al. Preliminary treatment planning and dosimetry for a clinical trial of neutron capture therapy using a fission converter epithermal neutron beam. *Appl Radiat Isot.* 2004;61(5):1075–1081.

68. Coderre JA, Morris GM. The radiation biology of boron neutron capture therapy. *Radiat Res.* 1999;151(1):1–18.

69. Albritton JR. Computational aspects of treatment planning for neutron capture therapy. Thesis]. Cambridge, MA: Massachusetts Institute of Technology; 2009.

70. Albritton JR, Kiger III WS. Neutron beam source definition techniques for NCT treatment planning. In: Zonta A, Altieri S, Roveda L, Barth RF, Eds. Proceedings of the 13th International Congress on Neutron Capture Therapy: A New Option Against Cancer. Rome: ENEA; 2008. p. 571–4.

71. Mijnheer BJ, Battermann JJ, Wambersie A. What degree of accuracy is required and can be achieved in photon and neutron therapy? *Radiother Oncol.* 1987;8(3):237–252.

72. Riley KJ, Binns PJ, Greenberg DD, Harling OK. A physical dosimetry intercomparison for BNCT. *Med Phys.* 2002;29(5):898–904.

73. Binns PJ, Riley KJ, Harling OK, et al. Progress with the NCT international dosimetry exchange. *Appl Radiat Isot.* 2004;61(5):865–868.

74. Binns PJ, Riley KJ, Harling OK, et al. An international dosimetry exchange for boron neutron capture therapy. Part I: Absorbed dose measurements. *Med Phys.* 2005;32(12):3729–3736.

75. Riley KJ, Binns PJ, Harling OK, et al. Unifying dose specification between clinical BNCT centers in the Americas. *Med Phys.* 2008;35(4):1295–1298.

76. Riley KJ, Binns PJ, Harling OK, et al. An international dosimetry exchange for BNCT part II: computational dosimetry normalizations. *Med Phys.* 2008;35(12):5419–5425.

77. Albritton JR, Kiger III WS. Development of Reference Problems for Neutron Capture Therapy Treatment Planning Systems. In: Nakagawa Y, Kobayashi T, Fukuda H, eds. *Advances in Neutron Capture Therapy 2006.* Takamatsu, Japan: International Society for Neutron Capture Therapy; 2006:496–9.

78. Albritton JR, Binns PJ, Riley KJ, et al. Comparison of Doses Delivered in Clinical Trials of Neutron Capture Therapy in the USA. In: Nakagawa Y, Kobayashi T, Fukuda H, eds. *Advances in Neutron Capture Therapy 2006.* Takamatsu, Japan: International Society for Neutron Capture Therapy; 2006:56–9.

79. Liu HB, Greenberg DD, Capala J, Wheeler FJ. An improved neutron collimator for brain tumor irradiations in clinical boron neutron capture therapy. *Med Phys.* 1996;23(12):2051–2060.

80. Capala J, Stenstam BH, Sköld K, et al. Boron neutron capture therapy for glioblastoma multiforme: clinical studies in Sweden. *J Neurooncol.* 2003;62(1–2):135–144.

81. Henriksson R, Capala J, Michanek A, et al.; Swedish Brain Tumour Study Group. Boron neutron capture therapy (BNCT) for glioblastoma multiforme: a phase II study evaluating a prolonged high-dose of boronophenylalanine (BPA). *Radiother Oncol.* 2008;88(2):183–191.

82. Sköld K, H-Stenstam B, Diaz AZ, et al. Boron Neutron Capture Therapy for glioblastoma multiforme: advantage of prolonged infusion of BPA-f. *Acta Neurol Scand.* 2010;122(1):58–62.

83. Sköld K, Gorlia T, Pellettieri L, et al. Boron neutron capture therapy for newly diagnosed glioblastoma multiforme: an assessment of clinical potential. *Br J Radiol.* 2010;83(991):596–603.

84. Hopewell JW, Gorlia T, Pellettieri L, et al. Boron neutron capture therapy for newly diagnosed glioblastoma multiforme: an assessment of clinical potential. *Appl Radiat Isot.* 2011;69(12):1737–1740.

85. Farr LE, Sweet WH, Robertson JS, et al. Neutron capture therapy with boron in the treatment of glioblastoma multiforme. *Am J Roentgenol Radium Ther Nucl Med.* 1954;71(2):279–293.

86. Sweet WH. Practical problems in the past in the use of boron-slow neutron capture therapy in the treatment of glioblastoma multiforme. In: Proceedings of the First

International Symposium on Neutron Capture Therapy. 1983. p. 376–8.

87. Asbury AK, Ojemann RG, Nielsen SL, Sweet WH. Neuropathologic study of fourteen cases of malignant brain tumor treated by boron-10 slow neutron capture radiation. *J Neuropathol Exp Neurol.* 1972;31(2):278–303.

88. Chanana AD, Capala J, Chadha M, et al. Boron neutron capture therapy for glioblastoma multiforme: interim results from the phase I/II dose-escalation studies. *Neurosurgery.* 1999;44(6):1182–92; discussion 1192.

89. Busse PM, Harling OK, Palmer MR, et al. A critical examination of the results from the Harvard-MIT NCT program phase I clinical trial of neutron capture therapy for intracranial disease. *J Neurooncol.* 2003;62(1–2):111–121.

90. Diaz AZ. Assessment of the results from the phase I/II boron neutron capture therapy trials at the Brookhaven National Laboratory from a clinician's point of view. *J Neurooncol.* 2003;62(1–2):101–109.

91. Nakagawa Y, Pooh K, Kobayashi T, et al. Clinical review of the Japanese experience with boron neutron capture therapy and a proposed strategy using epithermal neutron beams. *J Neurooncol.* 2003;62(1–2):87–99.

92. Miyatake S, Kawabata S, Yokoyama K, et al. Survival benefit of Boron neutron capture therapy for recurrent malignant gliomas. *J Neurooncol.* 2009;91(2):199–206.

93. Kawabata S, Miyatake S, Kuroiwa T, et al. Boron neutron capture therapy for newly diagnosed glioblastoma. *J Radiat Res.* 2009;50(1):51–60.

94. Kawabata S, Miyatake S, Hiramatsu R, et al. Phase II clinical study of boron neutron capture therapy combined with X-ray radiotherapy/temozolomide in patients with newly diagnosed glioblastoma multiforme–study design and current status report. *Appl Radiat Isot.* 2011;69(12):1796–1799.

95. Yamamoto T, Nakai K, Nariai T, et al. The status of Tsukuba BNCT trial: BPA-based boron neutron capture therapy combined with X-ray irradiation. *Appl Radiat Isot.* 2011;69(12):1817–1818.

96. Aiyama H, Nakai K, Yamamoto T, et al. A clinical trial protocol for second line treatment of malignant brain tumors with BNCT at University of Tsukuba. *Appl Radiat Isot.* 2011;69(12):1819–1822.

97. Nakai K, Yamamoto T, Aiyama H, et al. Boron neutron capture therapy combined with fractionated photon irradiation for glioblastoma: a recursive partitioning analysis of BNCT patients. *Appl Radiat Isot.* 2011;69(12):1790–1792.

98. Barth RF, Grecula JC, Yang W, et al. Combination of boron neutron capture therapy and external beam radiotherapy for brain tumors. *Int J Radiat Oncol Biol Phys.* 2004;58(1):267–277.

99. Imahori Y, Ueda S, Ohmori Y, et al. Fluorine-18-labeled fluoroboronophenylalanine PET in patients with glioma. *J Nucl Med.* 1998;39(2):325–333.

100. Miyashita M, Miyatake S, Imahori Y, et al. Evaluation of fluoride-labeled boronophenylalanine-PET imaging for the study of radiation effects in patients with glioblastomas. *J Neurooncol.* 2008;89(2):239–246.

101. Kankaanranta L, Seppälä T, Koivunoro H, et al. L-boronophenylalanine-mediated boron neutron capture therapy for malignant glioma progressing after external beam radiation therapy: a Phase I study. *Int J Radiat Oncol Biol Phys.* 2011;80(2):369–376.

102. Smith DR, Chandra S, Barth RF, et al. Quantitative imaging and microlocalization of boron-10 in brain tumors and infiltrating tumor cells by SIMS ion microscopy: relevance to neutron capture therapy. *Cancer Res.* 2001;61(22):8179–8187.

103. Stupp R, Hegi ME, Mason WP, et al. Radiotherapy plus concomitant and adjuvant temozolomide for glioblastoma. *N Engl J Med.* 2005;352:987–996.

104. Stupp R, Hegi ME, Mason WP, et al. Effects of radiotherapy with concomitant and adjuvant temozolomide versus radiotherapy alone on survival in glioblastoma in a randomised phase III study: 5-year analysis of the EORTC-NCIC trial. *Lancet Oncol.* 2009;10:459–466.

105. Aihara T, Hiratsuka J, Morita N, et al. First clinical case of boron neutron capture therapy for head and neck malignancies using ^{18}F-BPA PET. *Head Neck.* 2006;28(9):850–855.

106. Kato I, Ono K, Sakurai Y, et al. Effectiveness of BNCT for recurrent head and neck malignancies. *Appl Radiat Isot.* 2004;61(5):1069–1073.

107. Kato I, Fujita Y, Maruhashi A, et al. Effectiveness of boron neutron capture therapy for recurrent head and neck malignancies. *Appl Radiat Isot.* 2009;67(7–8 Suppl):S37–S42.

108. Kankaanranta L, Seppälä T, Koivunoro H, et al. Boron neutron capture therapy in the treatment of locally recurred head-and-neck cancer: final analysis of a phase I/II trial. *Int J Radiat Oncol Biol Phys.* 2012;82(1):e67–e75.

109. Wang LW, Wang SJ, Chu PY, et al. BNCT for locally recurrent head and neck cancer: preliminary clinical experience from a phase I/II trial at Tsing Hua Open-Pool Reactor. *Appl Radiat Isot.* 2011;69(12):1803–1806.

110. Bregadze VI, Sivaev IB, Lobanova IA, et al. Conjugates of boron clusters with derivatives of natural chlorin and bacteriochlorin. *Appl Radiat Isot.* 2009;67(7–8 Suppl):S101–S104.

111. Ito Y, Kimura Y, Shimahara T, et al. Disposition of TF-PEG-Liposome-BSH in tumor-bearing mice. *Appl Radiat Isot.* 2009;67(7–8 Suppl):S109–S110.

112. Pietrangeli D, Ricciardi G. Neutral and polyanionic carboranylporphyrazines: synthesis and physico-chemical properties. *Appl Radiat Isot.* 2009;67(7–8 Suppl):S97–S100.

113. Vos MJ, Turowski B, Zanella FE, et al. Radiologic findings in patients treated with boron neutron capture therapy for glioblastoma multiforme within EORTC trial 11961. *Int J Radiat Oncol Biol Phys.* 2005;61(2):392–399.

114. Wittig A, Hideghety K, Paquis P, et al. Current Clinical Results of the EORTC-Study 11961. In: Sauerwein W, Moss R, Wittig A, eds. *Research and Development in Neutron Capture Therapy.* Bologna: Monduzzi Editore - International Proceedings Division; 2002:1117–22.

demos MEDICAL

RADIATION MEDICINE ROUNDS

Molecular Classification of Malignant Gliomas

Aditya Raghunathan and Kenneth D. Aldape*

Department of Pathology, University of Texas MD Anderson Cancer Center, Houston, TX

■ ABSTRACT

Diffuse gliomas, consisting of diffuse astrocytoma and oligodendroglioma, are the most prevalent form of primary brain tumors. Traditionally, histologic features have been used to grade gliomas, in an attempt to help predict tumor behavior and patient outcome. However, these existing classification schemes do not entirely explain the differences in clinical behavior of tumors, even within the same histologic grade. Emerging understanding of molecular alterations at work in these tumors indicates extensive diversity within these tumor grades. In this chapter, we review major molecular features identified in diffuse gliomas, including isocitrate dehydrogenase (IDH) mutations, codeletion of 1p and 19q chromosomal arms, O^6-methylguanine-DNA methyltransferase (*MGMT*) promoter hypermethylation, *TP53* mutations, selected receptor tyrosine kinase alterations, glioma CpG island methylator phenotype (G-CIMP), and the proneural/mesenchymal glioblastoma multiforme (GBM) subtypes that have emerged from integrated genomic analysis. These alterations appear to play a role in determining patient prognosis, predicting response to therapy, as well as providing targets for individualized therapy regimens. Although the development of molecular-based grading schemes is still a work in progress, incorporating these molecular features into the existing histologic grading may help refine the future grading schemes.

Keywords: IDH-1, G-CIMP, MGMT, p53, molecular, classification, gliomas

■ INTRODUCTION

Histology-Based Classification of Diffuse Gliomas

Histological grading of neoplasia is based on identifying morphologic features that have been associated with clinical behavior and patient outcomes, and helps guide the choice of therapy within a cancer type. Although different grading schemes have been proposed for grading brain tumors, the World Health Organization (WHO) Classification of Tumors of the Central Nervous System (CNS) is the most widely accepted set of guidelines for the grading of gliomas (1). A major goal of a grading scheme is to classify tumors according to their expected clinical behavior. In other words, lower grade tumors are generally associated with more indolent behavior than those with higher grades. Standardized application of such a grading scheme helps ensure clear communication among health care providers regarding the potential behavior of a tumor.

Diffuse gliomas, which include infiltrating astrocytomas and oligodendrogliomas, are primary brain tumors that are characterized by their ability to infiltrate the brain parenchyma (1). Distinguishing astrocytoma from oligodendroglioma is based on determination of characteristic

*Corresponding author, Department of Pathology, University of Texas MD Anderson Cancer Center, 1515 Holcombe Boulevard, Unit 85, Houston, TX 77030.

E-mail address: Kaldape@mdanderson.org

Radiation Medicine Rounds 3:2 (2012) 227–240.

DOI: 10.5003/2151–4208.3.2.227

cellular morphologic features. Diffuse astrocytoma is identified by pleomorphic, irregular, oval-to-elongated nuclei, and ranges from WHO grades II to IV. A grade II diffuse astrocytoma shows atypical nuclei, cellularity that is slightly to moderately higher than normal white matter, but with inconspicuous mitoses. In contrast, WHO grade III astrocytoma shows higher cellularity, increased nuclear atypia and exhibits brisk mitotic activity. GBM is considered a WHO grade IV diffuse astrocytoma, and is diagnosed by the presence of a highly cellular, mitotically active glioma with the additional features of tumor necrosis and microvascular proliferation. Two clinically distinct types of GBM have long been identified based on the initial presentation of the patient. "Secondary" (progressive) GBM arises in the setting of a previously diagnosed lower grade diffuse astrocytoma, whereas "primary" GBM presents *de novo*, without prior history of glioma.

Oligodendrogliomas have more uniform, round-to-oval nuclei and are generally more monomorphic than astrocytomas. The nuclei are characteristically surrounded by perinuclear halos and a network of delicate, branching blood vessels is usually identified within the tumor. The WHO categorizes oligodendroglioma into grades II and III based on cellularity, cytologic atypia, mitotic activity, microvascular proliferation, and necrosis, the presence of which elevate the tumor to grade III. It is important to note that while morphologic criteria can be used to distinguish "textbook" examples of astrocytoma from oligodendroglioma, many cases are encountered in daily practice that are difficult to classify as one or the other with certainty. Perhaps to emphasize this difficulty, the WHO recognizes oligoastrocytoma as a diffusely infiltrating glioma that exhibits intermediate/indeterminate features in the continuum between classic astrocytoma on one end and classic oligodendroglioma on the other.

The cells of origin of astrocytoma and oligodendroglioma, and whether they derive from one or two different cell types, are not known. The fact that both astrocytoma and oligodendroglioma exhibit *IDH* mutations, whereas other neuroepithelial tumors do not, provides some evidence for a single cell of origin. Although GBM has traditionally been considered an astrocytic tumor, the latest iteration of the WHO classification highlights this uncertainty by including "Glioblastoma with oligodendroglioma component," a morphological variant of GBM that contains foci that resemble oligodendroglioma.

The Utility of Proliferation Markers

In general, all categories of diffuse glioma behave more aggressively with increasing proliferative activity, as histologically identified by mitoses. However the identification and scoring of mitoses is subject to inaccuracies due to variation in tumor cellularity, as well as technical artifacts. Indeed, the current WHO guidelines do not establish cut-off values for mitoses to distinguish grade II and grade III gliomas.

Ki-67 is a labile, nonhistone nuclear protein that is a marker of cell proliferation. It is expressed in the G1 thru M phases of the cell cycle, being is rapidly degraded at the end of M phase and not detectable in resting/G0 and early in the G1 phases MIB-1 is a monoclonal antibody directed against the Ki-67 protein that can be used in formalin-fixed paraffin-embedded tissue. Proliferating cells show strong nuclear staining for Ki-67/MIB-1, and widespread Ki-67/ MIB-1 labeling among tumor cells is indicative of a rapidly proliferating neoplasm. The Ki-67/ MIB-1 labeling index has been shown to be significantly correlated with proliferative activity among grades II and III diffuse gliomas, as well as to patient outcomes (2–5). Other studies, however, have failed to find a similar correlation with survival on multivariate analysis, after taking into account clinical parameters known to be associated with patient survival (6,7). Although proliferation index is widely used in lower grade (grade II and III) gliomas, it has not shown clinical utility in GBM.

The histone H3 protein is one of five histone proteins involved in the structure of chromatin in eukaryotic cells. In mitosis, histone H3 is specifically phosphorylated at the serine 10 residue during chromatin condensation (8). The antibody to serine 10-phosphorylated histone H3 (***pHH3***) is a reliable and robust marker of mitoses and allows for the additional morphologic validation of mitotic figures that are stained (9,10). Among diffuse gliomas, the pHH3 staining has been shown to correlate well with the Ki-67/ MIB-1 labeling index as well as other markers of proliferation (4,5). However, the correlation of MIB-1 proliferation index with mitotic activity can occasionally be challenging due to artifactual tissue distortion and the resultant difficulty in morphologically identifying stained mitotic figures (4).

An elevated pHH3 labeling index as well as an elevated Ki-67/MIB-1 labeling index have been associated with a significantly shorter survival among non-GBM diffuse astrocytomas (4,5). The uniform application of such immunohistochemistry (IHC)-based markers, therefore, may help accurately assess the proliferative activity and potential for biological aggressiveness among diffuse gliomas. However, due to the variability in staining and counting techniques between laboratories, establishing standardized cut-off values for the purpose of reproducible grading remains a challenge (11). With that said, the use of pHH3 has an advantage, at least in theory, as compared to MIB-1 as a proliferation marker. Staining conditions and antibody concentrations differ among laboratories, and can result in systematic differences in MIB-1 counting. Since pHH3 relies on both positive staining as well as morphological features of mitosis, the pHH3 index may be less sensitive to interlaboratory technical considerations.

■ COMMON MOLECULAR ABNORMALITIES IN DIFFUSE GLIOMAS

IDH Mutations

The nicotinamide adenine dinucleotide phosphate (NADP)-dependent isocitrate dehydrogenase 1, 2, and 3 (IDH1, IDH2, and IDH3) enzymes catalyze the oxidative decarboxylation of isocitrate to alpha-ketoglutarate in the citric acid cycle. The IDH1 enzyme is found in the cytoplasm and peroxisomes, and the IDH2 enzyme is found in mitochondria (12). The *IDH1* gene is located at 2q33.3 (13), whereas the *IDH2* gene is located on 15q26.1 (14). Mutations of these genes were initially observed among a small percentage of GBMs (15). Subsequently, *IDH1*/*IDH2* mutations have been observed in a large proportion of WHO grade II and III diffuse gliomas and secondary GBMs (16–19). Mutations in *IDH3* have not been described. In gliomas, these are almost exclusively point mutations, resulting in substitution of arginine at residue 132 of IDH1 (R132), or at residue 172 of IDH2 (R172) (17,20). The *IDH* mutation status of diffuse gliomas is conserved before the development of other aberrations during tumor progression from a lower to a higher grade, suggesting that this is an early event during glioma genesis (18,21,22). Although mutations involving *IDH1* are more common than those involving *IDH2* overall (20), *IDH2* mutations are more frequently present in oligodendroglioma than diffuse astrocytoma (17,23–25). Thus far, the vast majority of diffuse gliomas with combined deletion of chromosomal arms 1p and 19q also show mutations in either IDH1 or IDH2 (23,24). *IDH1*/*IDH2* mutations are not seen in primary GBM and in practice, *IDH* mutation status can be viewed as a defining lesion that distinguishes primary from secondary/progressive GBM (Figure 1). *IDH* mutations are not seen in other types of common CNS tumors (16–19), and may be of value in helping to identify diffuse gliomas from other CNS tumors and nonneoplastic mimics in limited biopsy specimens (19,26–29). *IDH* mutations have also recently been shown to repress lineage-specific cell differentiation by impairing histone demethylation, particularly of histone H3, via increased 2-hydroxyglutarate, supporting the role of these mutations as tumor-initiating events (30). Although *IDH* mutations are associated with a younger age at presentation (17,20,31) and have been identified among diffuse gliomas in adolescents (32), these mutations are rarely identified in pediatric gliomas, the suggesting that an alternative pathway may be involved in the evolution of diffuse gliomas in pediatric patients (33). Recent whole exome sequencing of pediatric GBMs revealed recurrent mutations in regulatory proteins participating in chromatin remodeling—*H3F3A* (which encodes the replication-independent histone variant H3.3), *ATRX*, and *DAXX* (34). The *H3F3A-ATRX-DAXX* mutations appear to be more prevalent in GBMs from pediatric, adolescent, and young adult patients, and have not yet been identified in adult GBMs. Further, mutations in these genes and *IDH1* mutations appear to be mutually exclusive. The identification of these mutations further supports the pathogenesis of pediatric GBMs as being distinct from adult GBMs.

In addition to aiding diagnosis of diffuse gliomas, *IDH* mutations have also been shown to be associated with clinical outcome. Within each WHO grade, diffuse gliomas that harbor *IDH* mutations appear to have significantly longer overall survival than those without *IDH* mutations (35–39). Further, anaplastic astrocytomas that do not harbor *IDH1* mutations appear to have worse prognosis than GBM with mutant *IDH1* (31). Although this finding requires further validation, the implication is that a tumor with lower grade histologic features may have consistently worse outcome than a higher grade tumor, based on the absence or presence of *IDH*, or other as yet unidentified, mutations. The effect of *IDH* mutation status on the response to chemotherapy has yet to be fully established, however, with reports suggesting favorable response among low-grade diffuse gliomas and secondary GBMs (40,41) being contradicted by reports of prognostic but not predictive significance of *IDH*-mutations (25,42).

The most common *IDH* mutation involves *IDH1*, with the exchange of guanine for adenine (G395A) resulting in the replacement of arginine by histidine at position 132 (R132H). IHC utilizing a

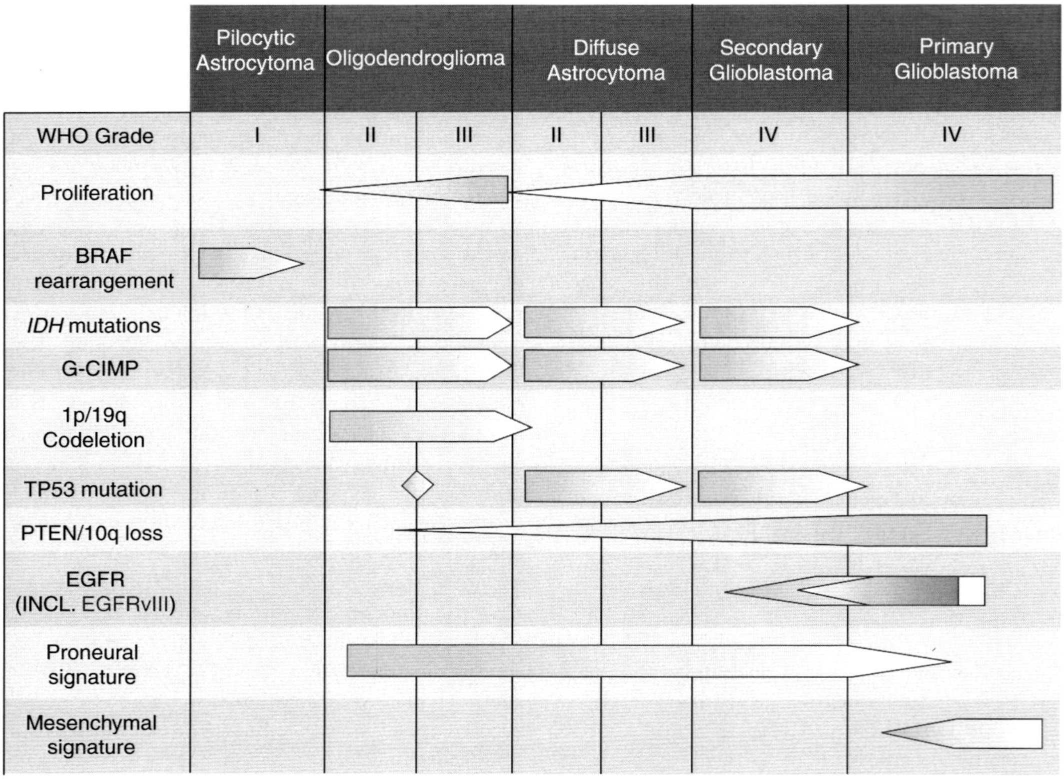

FIGURE 1 A simplified schematic diagram illustrating the prevalence of common genetic/molecular alterations in diffuse gliomas.

mutation-specific mouse monoclonal antibody has been demonstrated to have high specificity and sensitivity for detecting the IDH1R132H mutant protein in histological sections from formalin-fixed, paraffin-embedded tissue (43–45). We find this antibody to be extremely useful in daily practice, not only as a prognostic marker, but also as a diagnostic marker. In addition, since the IDH1 – R132H mutation is tumor specific, the use of the IHC stain provides the ability to identify tumor cells in a background of nonneoplastic neuropil, providing, for example, visual representations of glioma infiltration.

The CpG Island Methylator Phenotype

A CpG island methylator phenotype (CIMP) was first identified as a cancer-specific CpG island hypermethylation in a subset of patients with colorectal carcinoma (46). Colorectal CIMP was found in tumors involving the proximal colon and was found to be associated with *BRAF* mutations and microsatellite instability caused by MLH1 promoter hypermethylation and transcriptional silencing (47). Cancer-specific promoter CpG island hypermethylation generally results in transcriptional silencing of the associated gene (48). Such promoter-associated CpG island hypermethylation has been reported in GBMs, as well as other glioma subtypes (49–53). Secondary GBMs appear to have a higher frequency of promoter methylation than primary GBMs (48,54,55).

Recently, the Cancer Genome Atlas (TCGA) project has identified a distinct subset of gliomas that displays concerted hypermethylation at a large number of loci, suggestive of a glioma-CIMP (G-CIMP) phenotype (56). The presence of G-CIMP has been found to be significantly more prevalent among lower grade gliomas than GBM. Among these lower grade gliomas, G-CIMP positivity is twice more common among oligodendroglioma than astrocytoma (56,57), and appears to be a better predictor of survival than O^6-methylguanine-DNA methyltransferase (*MGMT*) methylation status (58). G-CIMP positive status also appears to be correlated with improved patient outcome within each WHO grade. Patients with G-CIMP positive tumors have been found to be younger at the time of diagnosis, with significantly improved outcomes. G-CIMP status, positive or negative, appears to be retained at recurrence, indicating stability of the G-CIMP phenotype over time, and providing some evidence that it is critical for tumor formation and maintenance (56). Among GBMs, G-CIMP-positive tumors appear to be strongly associated with *IDH* mutations (56,57,59). Further, it has recently been shown that the *IDH1* mutation may be the molecular basis for gliomas acquiring a G-CIMP phenotype (60). A small proportion of G-CIMP-positive but *IDH1* wild-type GBMs also appear to have prolonged overall survival, suggesting that the G-CIMP-positive status may be an indicator of good prognosis independent of the *IDH1* status (56). Indeed, G-CIMP positive tumors appear to have a significantly better survival on multivariate analysis, after adjusting for patient age, recurrence, and primary/secondary GBM status.

1p/19q Codeletion

Since their initial identification (61), combined deletions of the short arm of chromosome 1 (1p) and the long arm of chromosome 19 (19q) have been found in a majority of oligodendroglioma (62,63). The combined 1p/19q loss is strongly correlated with longer progression-free survival (64–67) and is an independent predictor of response to chemotherapy (68–72). This combined loss has been strongly associated with "classic" oligodendroglioma histology across grades (66,73–75), and with the presence of *IDH* mutations (23,24,76). Although tightly correlated with oligodendroglial histology, concurrent loss of the entire 1p and 19q may occasionally be identified among diffuse gliomas that lack characteristic features of oligodendroglioma (77). In contrast, partial deletions involving 1p or 19q may be identified in diffuse astrocytoma and GBM, but do not appear to be associated with improved overall survival (77,78). Complete hemizygous losses of 1p have been shown to be tightly associated with 19q loss, classic oligodendroglioma morphology, and longer overall and progression-free survival. In contrast, partial 1p deletions are not associated with 19q loss, are mainly observed in tumors with astrocytoma morphology, and have a negative prognostic value (79). Evaluation of widespread 1p and 19q loss with the use of fluorescence in situ hybridization probes or multiple PCR-based markers along the chromosomal arms is therefore required to appreciate the real clinical significance of 1p loss in gliomas. With respect to molecular pathogenesis, 1p/19q codeletion probably occurs after *IDH* mutation, since practically all 1p/19q codeleted tumors exhibit *IDH* mutations, but the converse is not true. Among GBMs in which an oligodendroglioma-like component is identified on histology, 1p/19q codeletions appear to be rare (80,81). However, the prognostic significance of finding such oligodendroglioma-like areas on histologic examination needs further clarification (80,81).

The losses of chromosomal arms 1p and 19q have been associated with an unbalanced pericentromeric translocation that produces the derivative chromosome der (1,19) (q10; p10) (67,82). The other derivative chromosome may not be formed or may be unstable, leading to a net loss of the 1p and 19q chromosomal arms. A recent deep sequencing study of oligodendroglioma revealed inactivating mutations of the *CIC* gene (homolog of the *Drosophila* gene *capicua*) on 19q and *FUBP1* gene (encoding far upstream element (FUSE) binding protein) on 1p in a significant proportion of tumors (83). In particular, *CIC* mutations appear strongly correlated with classic oligodendroglioma morphology, 1p/19q codeletion and *IDH1*/*IDH2* mutations, and are rare in tumors that lack the codeletion (76). Further exploration of the role of *CIC* mutations may help better understand the role of 1p/19q codeletions in gliomagenesis.

TP53 Mutations

The p53 protein is a tumor suppressor involved cell cycle arrest in G1 phase and initiation of apoptosis. Mutations of the *TP53* gene result in nonfunctional p53 protein, and have been identified in lower grade astrocytomas and in the secondary GBMs that evolve from these (84–87). Mutated forms of the p53 protein may be more stable, and so can be detected by IHC staining (88). However, mutations of the *TP53* gene and the expression of the p53 protein have not been definitely correlated with prognosis or with response to therapy (86,89–91). On integrating genomic findings across their respective regulatory pathways, the *p53* pathway appears to be disrupted in a majority of GBMs (92), either directly or through alterations in mdm2 and IN4A/ARF (93–95). Recent data also suggests that p53 overexpression may be significantly associated with improved progression-free survival among patients treated with prolonged therapy with adjuvant temozolomide (96), and may warrant further exploration in prospective clinical trials.

MGMT Promoter Hypermethylation

In diffuse gliomas, the DNA repair enzyme MGMT has been the subject of investigation due to its association with response to alkylating chemotherapeutic agents (97). The *MGMT* gene is located on chromosome 10q26, and its promoter region contains 97 CG-dinucleotide (CpG)-rich sites. In normal tissue, these CpG sites are unmethylated. In tumors, the cytosine in these CpG-rich sites may be methylated, leading to binding of proteins to the DNA, alteration of the chromatin structure, preventing the binding of transcription factors and leading to the silencing of *MGMT* expression relative to normal tissue (48,98). *MGMT* promoter methylation status appears to be a more reliable predictor of susceptibility to adjuvant therapy and prognosis of GBM than MGMT protein or gene expression levels (99). The epigenetic silencing of *MGMT* expression has been associated with response to radiation therapy (100), as well as to alkylating chemotherapeutic agents that damage DNA by methylating the O-6 position of the guanine (101,102). It appears that *MGMT* silencing helps identify a subset of patients with high-grade gliomas and GBM in whom adjuvant chemotherapy may significantly prolong overall survival, at initial diagnosis (103,104) as well as at recurrence (105). The strong correlation of *MGMT* promoter hypermethylation status with *IDH* mutation status raises the possibility that this may be early events in the evolution of diffuse gliomas (21,106–108). Reports demonstrating stability of the methylation status in recurrent tumors (107) are at odds with prior reports of change in the status in recurrent tumors following treatment (109). However, the initial promoter methylation of *MGMT*, in conjunction with temozolomide treatment, may result in selective pressure to lose mismatch repair function, resulting in aggressive recurrent tumors with a hypermethylator phenotype (92,101,110). These conflicting results may be due to differences in testing methodologies (111–113), and the optimal technique to reliably identify the methylation status needs to be defined in order to reduce variability in the results from different laboratories. Recently, a classification scheme based more comprehensive analysis of the methylation status of all the CpG sites in the *MGMT* promoter using a novel methylation-specific multiplex ligation-dependent probe amplification (MS-MLPA) test has been proposed as being significantly predictive of progression-free survival in GBM (114).

Overall, *MGMT* promoter methylation status appears to be a marker of good prognosis in high-grade astrocytoma and GBM, and was found to be associated with better prognosis and overall survival on meta-analysis (103), whereas its role in lower grade (grades II and III) gliomas is less clear. It may also be, at least in part, a predictive marker. On meta-analysis, MGMT silencing was found to be a predictor of improved outcome in patients who received chemotherapy as compared to patients who did not receive chemotherapy. However, it also showed, to a lesser extent, a prognostic effect in patients who received adjuvant radiation therapy, as compared to no adjuvant therapy. MGMT is probably best thought of as a partially predictive marker. In turn, adjuvant chemotherapy may provide a benefit, albeit smaller, in patients whose tumors are MGMT unmethylated. This finding, coupled with the fact that alternative therapies have not been identified for MGMT unmethylated tumors, has resulted in the use of adjuvant chemoradiation as the standard of care in both MGMT-methylated and MGMT unmethylated tumors (103). However, it may help to identify patients who may have better outcome and who may benefit from radiation therapy and alkylating chemotherapy (99–105), and may also be useful as a marker to predict pseudoprogression and distinguish this from true tumor progression (115). However, the MGMT promoter methylation phenotype does not perfectly correlate with the response to therapy, suggesting the presence of other prognostic and predictive genetic mechanisms in GBMs (94,106,116,117).

Receptor Tyrosine Kinase Alterations

Several diffuse gliomas show alterations in receptor tyrosine kinases and their downstream pathways. Amplification of the epidermal growth factor receptor (EGFR), located on chromosome 7p12, is the most prevalent receptor tyrosine kinase abnormality in GBMs (87,92). High-level amplification of *EGFR* appears to be a late event during the tumorigenesis of GBMs (118). Frequently, this amplification is associated with a truncated mutant variant—EGFRvIII—which is characterized by deletion of exons 2 to 7 (119). The EGFRvIII variant and other less frequently identified missense mutations (120) lead to ligand-independent constitutive activation of EGFR and result in persistent activation of the downstream phosphatidylinositol 3′-kinase (PI3K) signaling pathway. Activation of the EGFR-mediated signaling pathway has been observed in a small percentage of lower grade diffuse gliomas as well, although the presence of EGFR amplification can practically be viewed as indicative of GBM in a high-grade glioma sample that otherwise lacks the necessary histologic requirements for this diagnosis. Accordingly, EGFR overexpression and the presence of EGFRvIII have been reported as indicators of poor prognosis in anaplastic astrocytoma and GBM (121–123), and as indicators of poor response to radiation therapy (124). However, the association of EGFR aberrations with patient outcomes in GBM remains to be further clarified.

Somatic mutations of the downstream ***PI3K complex*** have also been identified in a small but significant subset of GBMs. These mutations most frequently involve the *PIK3CA* gene that encodes the catalytically active p110α protein and, less frequently, the *PIK3R1* gene that encodes the regulatory p85α protein (92,125–127), and appear to be mutually exclusive (92). Phosphorylation and activation of Akt (p-Akt) and the mitogen-activated protein kinase (MAPK) pathway also appear to be activated in high-grade astrocytoma and GBM, and may be involved in the proliferation and invasion of GBM cells (128–130). Activation of this pathway has also been associated with resistance to radiotherapy (131–133).

The mammalian target of rapamycin (mTOR) is both, a downstream target of the PI3K-Akt pathway, as well as an upstream activator of Akt. The phosphatase and tensin homologue (*PTEN*) is a tumor-suppressor gene located on the long arm of chromosome 10 (10q), and is a negative regulator of the PI3K-Akt-mTOR and MAPK pathways. It is frequently mutated in GBMs (92), most commonly associated with loss of 10q (134). Loss of heterozygosity of 10q has frequently been identified in high-grade gliomas. However, the 10q deletion is rarely seen in tumors harboring classical oligodendroglioma morphology and true codeletion of 1p/19q chromosomal arms (135,136). Overall, the interactions between EGFR and downstream signaling pathways, including PI3K-Akt-mTOR and PTEN, are complex (137–140) and appear to play a central role in the regulation of glioma growth, invasion, angiogenesis, and apoptosis.

Among other receptor tyrosine kinase systems, the platelet-derived growth factor (***PDGF***) system also shows receptor amplification, phosphorylation, mutation, or ligand overexpression in diffuse astrocytomas and GBMs, as well as in oligodendrogliomas (141,142).

The MAPK pathway also includes Ras/Raf/MEK (MAP2K mitogen-activated protein kinase/extracellular signal-regulated kinase [ERK])/ERK signaling cascade. ERK has one of the largest range of effectors described for a kinase, and affects a multitude of diverse fundamental cellular programs (143). Activation of the MAPK pathway has been identified in low-grade astrocytomas, particularly in pilocytic astrocytoma, a WHO grade I tumor (144,145). The tandem duplication of the ***BRAF*** locus at 7q34, leading to fusion between *KIAA1549* and *BRAF*, has been identified in a high proportion (500%) of pilocytic astrocytomas (145–149). The *KIAA1549*: *BRAF* fusion incorporates the *BRAF* kinase domain without the autoinhibitory domain, leading to its constitutive activation (146,149). This *KIAA1549*: *BRAF* fusion product has been identified in pilocytic astrocytomas occurring at all ages and at various locations, but appears to be particularly frequent among pediatric cases and in the cerebellum (147,150–152). This novel fusion product appears to be rare in diffuse astrocytoma and so may be of value in helping to distinguish these two categories of tumors in small biopsy samples (153,154). On the other hand, *BRAF* activation by point mutation involving the hotspot at residue 600 (BRAF V600E) has also been identified in pediatric diffuse astrocytoma, pleomorphic xanthoastrocytoma (WHO grade II), ganglioglioma (WHO grade I), and a small proportion of extracerebellar pilocytic astrocytomas (155,156). Alternate mechanisms of MAPK pathway activation, such as the 3p25 tandem duplication leading to a *SRGAP3*:*RAF1* fusion gene, have also rarely been reported in pilocytic astrocytoma (147,148,157). Although frequently identified in pilocytic astrocytomas, the prognostic significance of the *KIAA1549*: *BRAF* fusion is yet to be determined (150).

A small percentage of GBMs also appears to show intermingled cell subpopulations that have amplifications of different receptor tyrosine kinase genes, including *EGFR*, *MET*, and *PDGFRA* (158,159). The effect of such genetic heterogeneity on the response of such tumors to different targeted therapeutic agents and different treatment regimens requires further evaluation as therapies targeting various RTK pathways become increasingly available.

Transcriptional Signature-Based GBM Subtypes

Differences in the gene expression profiles between GBMs and lower grade diffuse gliomas have been well established, leading to findings that markers such as VEGF (142,160), IGFBP2 (160), and CHI3L1 (50,161) being associated with poor outcome and/or higher glioma grade. The idea of utilizing gene expression patterns to determine prognosis among diffuse gliomas has been explored in the past, with two to four major subtypes based on the gene expression profiles being proposed (50,160–166). These subtypes have been linked to variations in patterns of DNA methylation, in chromosomal copy-numbers, in the DNA sequence alterations, and in proteomic markers of signaling pathways (56,161,163,165–167). These findings have also been examined in the TCGA dataset, wherein these genetic changes correlated with patient information, including mutations involving *TP53*, *PTEN*, *EGFR*, *RB1*, *NF1*, *ERBB2*, *PIK3CA*, and *PIK3R1* (92). This was complemented by the identification of novel somatic mutations in *IDH1* in a subset of GBMs that predominantly consisted of young patients and patients with secondary GBM, and were, as expected, associated with an increase in overall survival (15).

In 2006, three high-grade astrocytoma groups were defined based on the differential expression of prognostic markers, and were termed proneural, proliferative, and mesenchymal based on the predominant profiles of the molecular signatures identified within each group (167). The proneural group was characterized by markers associated with neurogenesis, the proliferative group demonstrated markers of cellular proliferation, and the mesenchymal group expressed markers found in tissues of mesenchymal origin. Among these three, the proneural group was associated with the most favorable outcome, whereas the proliferative and mesenchymal groups were both associated with poor outcome. GBMs in the proliferative group had elevated Ki-67/ MIB-1 indices, whereas those in the mesenchymal group demonstrated increased angiogenesis.

Similarly, integrated genomic analysis of the TCGA dataset revealed four GBM expression subtypes: proneural, neural, mesenchymal, and classic (165). The proneural subtype was strongly associated with *IDH1* mutations and/or *PDGFRA* amplification, the classical subtype was associated with *EGFR* amplification and/or mutations, and the mesenchymal subtype was associated with loss and/or mutation of *NF1*. On DNA methylation profiling performed on the TCGA dataset, majority of G-CIMP tumors were found to belong to the proneural subgroup (56). Within the proneural subgroup, G-CIMP positive patients had longer survival than G-CIMP negative patients, and the G-CIMP status. Although the subgroups and the G-CIMP status were not perfectly concordant, among the proneural subgroup, G-CIMP-negative tumors were found to be similar to GBMs in the mesenchymal subgroup, whereas G-CIMP-positive tumors were distinct from this subgroup.

A meta-analysis compiling and comparing the results of these two studies found a strong agreement in the assignment of samples to the proneural and mesenchymal subgroups, indicating robust reproducibility in subcategorizing diffuse gliomas in this manner (168). The proneural signature was more frequently identified in lower grade gliomas and secondary GBMs, whereas the Mesenchymal signature was strongly associated with primary GBMs. Although there is no uniform agreement on the type and number of expression-based glioma subtypes, the proneural/mesenchymal phenotypes appear to show some consensus among a variety of investigators.

Determining the independent prognostic and predictive value of gene expression-based subtyping is complicated by the extent of overlap with the status of other prognostic molecular signatures, such as *IDH* mutation, 1p/19q codeletion, MGMT promoter methylation, and G-CIMP. Indeed, this may be a reflection of the multiple mechanisms that are independently and/or interactively responsible for heterogeneity in the clinical behavior of diffuse gliomas.

■ SUMMARY AND CONCLUSIONS

The aim of diffuse glioma classification remains to help predict tumor behavior and to guide appropriate therapy. Although morphology-based classification provides some information regarding the clinical behavior of glioma, it is imprecise and subject to interobserver variability. The use of molecular alterations provides an opportunity to refine a purely morphology-based classification system by identifying subtypes which may differ in their natural history and/or responsiveness to specific therapeutics. For example, the IDH mutation/G-CIMP subclass in diffuse gliomas is clinically distinct from the IDH wild-type/G-CIMP-negative tumors. Given the relative ease of detecting the mutant IDH1 R132H protein by IHC (in ~90% of cases), we speculate that IDH status will become integral to the standard classification of diffuse gliomas in the near future. It is likely that future standard-of-care treatment regimens will be based on the molecular status of the tumor, as well as the histologic subclass and grade. As a diagnostic tool, molecular signatures can provide objective data which may reduce the subjectivity inherent in morphology-based classification. At present, the understanding of various molecular alterations and their impact on patient outcomes and response to therapy is a field in evolution. As our knowledge and understanding of these improve, we believe future diffuse glioma classification schemes will necessarily be a "hybrid," incorporating the status of various clinically relevant molecular biomarkers into the well-established, morphology-based classification.

■ REFERENCES

1. Louis DN, Ohgaki H, Wiestler OD, Cavenee WK, eds. WHO classification of tumours of the central nervous

system. 4th ed. Lyon: International Agency for Research on Cancer; 2007:13–67.

2. Giannini C, Scheithauer BW, Burger PC, et al. Cellular proliferation in pilocytic and diffuse astrocytomas. *J Neuropathol Exp Neurol.* 1999;58(1):46–53.
3. McKeever PE, Strawderman MS, Yamini B, Mikhail AA, Blaivas M. MIB-1 proliferation index predicts survival among patients with grade II astrocytoma. *J Neuropathol Exp Neurol.* 1998;57(10):931–936.
4. Habberstad AH, Gulati S, Torp SH. Evaluation of the proliferation markers Ki-67/MIB-1, mitosin, survivin, pHH3, and DNA topoisomerase IIa in human anaplastic astrocytomas—an immunohistochemical study. *Diagn Pathol.* 2011;6:43.
5. Colman H, Giannini C, Huang L, et al. Assessment and prognostic significance of mitotic index using the mitosis marker phospho-histone H3 in low and intermediate-grade infiltrating astrocytomas. *Am J Surg Pathol.* 2006;30(5):657–664.
6. Rodríguez-Pereira C, Suárez-Peñaranda JM, Vázquez-Salvado M, et al. Value of MIB-1 labelling index (LI) in gliomas and its correlation with other prognostic factors. A clinicopathologic study. *J Neurosurg Sci.* 2000;44(4):203–9; discussion 209.
7. Moskowitz SI, Jin T, Prayson RA. Role of MIB1 in predicting survival in patients with glioblastomas. *J Neurooncol.* 2006;76(2):193–200.
8. Hendzel MJ, Wei Y, Mancini MA, et al. Mitosis-specific phosphorylation of histone H3 initiates primarily within pericentromeric heterochromatin during G2 and spreads in an ordered fashion coincident with mitotic chromosome condensation. *Chromosoma.* 1997;106(6):348–360.
9. Ribalta T, McCutcheon IE, Aldape KD, Bruner JM, Fuller GN. The mitosis-specific antibody anti-phospho-histone-H3 (PHH3) facilitates rapid reliable grading of meningiomas according to WHO 2000 criteria. *Am J Surg Pathol.* 2004;28(11):1532–1536.
10. Tapia C, Kutzner H, Mentzel T, Savic S, Baumhoer D, Glatz K. Two mitosis-specific antibodies, MPM-2 and phospho-histone H3 (Ser28), allow rapid and precise determination of mitotic activity. *Am J Surg Pathol.* 2006;30(1):83–89.
11. Hsu CY, Ho DM, Yang CF, Chiang H. Interobserver reproducibility of MIB-1 labeling index in astrocytic tumors using different counting methods. *Mod Pathol.* 2003;16(9):951–957.
12. Rakheja D, Mitui M, Boriack RL, DeBerardinis RJ. Isocitrate dehydrogenase ½ mutational analyses and 2-hydroxyglutarate measurements in Wilms tumors. *Pediatr Blood Cancer.* 2011;56(3):379–383.
13. Narahara K, Kimura S, Kikkawa K, et al. Probable assignment of soluble isocitrate dehydrogenase (IDH1) to 2q33.3. *Hum Genet.* 1985;71(1):37–40.
14. Oh IU, Inazawa J, Kim YO, Song BJ, Huh TL. Assignment of the human mitochondrial NADP(+)-specific isocitrate dehydrogenase (IDH2) gene to 15q26.1 by in situ hybridization. *Genomics.* 1996;38(1):104–106.
15. Parsons DW, Jones S, Zhang X, et al. An integrated genomic analysis of human glioblastoma multiforme. *Science.* 2008;321(5897):1807–1812.
16. Bleeker FE, Lamba S, Leenstra S, et al. IDH1 mutations at residue p.R132 (IDH1(R132)) occur frequently in high-grade gliomas but not in other solid tumors. *Hum Mutat.* 2009;30(1):7–11.
17. Hartmann C, Meyer J, Balss J, et al. Type and frequency of IDH1 and IDH2 mutations are related to astrocytic and oligodendroglial differentiation and age: a study of 1,010 diffuse gliomas. *Acta Neuropathol.* 2009;118(4):469–474.
18. Ichimura K, Pearson DM, Kocialkowski S, et al. IDH1 mutations are present in the majority of common adult gliomas but rare in primary glioblastomas. *Neuro-oncology.* 2009;11(4):341–347.
19. Capper D, Reuss D, Schittenhelm J, et al. Mutation-specific IDH1 antibody differentiates oligodendrogliomas and oligoastrocytomas from other brain tumors with oligodendroglioma-like morphology. *Acta Neuropathol.* 2011;121(2):241–252.
20. Yan H, Parsons DW, Jin G, et al. IDH1 and IDH2 mutations in gliomas. *N Engl J Med.* 2009;360(8):765–773.
21. Watanabe T, Nobusawa S, Kleihues P, Ohgaki H. IDH1 mutations are early events in the development of astrocytomas and oligodendrogliomas. *Am J Pathol.* 2009;174(4):1149–1153.
22. Lai A, Kharbanda S, Pope WB, et al. Evidence for sequenced molecular evolution of IDH1 mutant glioblastoma from a distinct cell of origin. *J Clin Oncol.* 2011;29(34):4482–4490.
23. Labussière M, Idbaih A, Wang XW, et al. All the 1p19q codeleted gliomas are mutated on IDH1 or IDH2. *Neurology.* 2010;74(23):1886–1890.
24. Mukasa A, Takayanagi S, Saito K, et al. Significance of IDH mutations varies with tumor histology, grade, and genetics in Japanese glioma patients. *Cancer Sci.* 2011.
25. Dubbink HJ, Taal W, van Marion R, et al. IDH1 mutations in low-grade astrocytomas predict survival but not response to temozolomide. *Neurology.* 2009;73(21):1792–1795.
26. Camelo-Piragua S, Jansen M, Ganguly A, Kim JC, Louis DN, Nutt CL. Mutant IDH1-specific immunohistochemistry distinguishes diffuse astrocytoma from astrocytosis. *Acta Neuropathol.* 2010;119(4):509–511.
27. Capper D, Sahm F, Hartmann C, Meyermann R, von Deimling A, Schittenhelm J. Application of mutant IDH1 antibody to differentiate diffuse glioma from nonneoplastic central nervous system lesions and therapy-induced changes. *Am J Surg Pathol.* 2010;34(8):1199–1204.
28. Horbinski C, Kofler J, Kelly LM, Murdoch GH, Nikiforova MN. Diagnostic use of IDH1/2 mutation analysis in routine clinical testing of formalin-fixed, paraffin-embedded glioma tissues. *J Neuropathol Exp Neurol.* 2009;68(12):1319–1325.
29. Camelo-Piragua S, Jansen M, Ganguly A, et al. A sensitive and specific diagnostic panel to distinguish diffuse astrocytoma from astrocytosis: chromosome 7 gain with

mutant isocitrate dehydrogenase 1 and p53. *J Neuropathol Exp Neurol.* 2011;70(2):110–115.

30. Lu C, Ward PS, Kapoor GS, et al. IDH mutation impairs histone demethylation and results in a block to cell differentiation. *Nature.* 2012;483(7390):474–478.

31. Hartmann C, Hentschel B, Wick W, et al. Patients with IDH1 wild type anaplastic astrocytomas exhibit worse prognosis than IDH1-mutated glioblastomas, and IDH1 mutation status accounts for the unfavorable prognostic effect of higher age: implications for classification of gliomas. *Acta Neuropathol.* 2010;120(6):707–718.

32. Pollack IF, Hamilton RL, Sobol RW, et al.; Children's Oncology Group. IDH1 mutations are common in malignant gliomas arising in adolescents: a report from the Children's Oncology Group. *Childs Nerv Syst.* 2011;27(1):87–94.

33. Antonelli M, Buttarelli FR, Arcella A, et al. Prognostic significance of histological grading, p53 status, YKL-40 expression, and IDH1 mutations in pediatric high-grade gliomas. *J Neurooncol.* 2010;99(2):209–215.

34. Schwartzentruber J, Korshunov A, Liu XY, et al. Driver mutations in histone H3.3 and chromatin remodelling genes in paediatric glioblastoma. *Nature.* 2012;482(7384):226–231.

35. Sanson M, Marie Y, Paris S, et al. Isocitrate dehydrogenase 1 codon 132 mutation is an important prognostic biomarker in gliomas. *J Clin Oncol.* 2009;27(25):4150–4154.

36. Bujko M, Kober P, Matyja E, et al. Prognostic value of IDH1 mutations identified with PCR-RFLP assay in glioblastoma patients. *Mol Diagn Ther.* 2010;14(3):163–169.

37. Nobusawa S, Watanabe T, Kleihues P, Ohgaki H. IDH1 mutations as molecular signature and predictive factor of secondary glioblastomas. *Clin Cancer Res.* 2009;15(19):6002–6007.

38. Metellus P, Coulibaly B, Colin C, et al. Absence of IDH mutation identifies a novel radiologic and molecular subtype of WHO grade II gliomas with dismal prognosis. *Acta Neuropathol.* 2010;120(6):719–729.

39. Thon N, Eigenbrod S, Kreth S, et al. IDH1 mutations in grade II astrocytomas are associated with unfavorable progression-free survival and prolonged postrecurrence survival. *Cancer.* 2012;118(2):452–460.

40. Houillier C, Wang X, Kaloshi G, et al. IDH1 or IDH2 mutations predict longer survival and response to temozolomide in low-grade gliomas. *Neurology.* 2010;75(17):1560–1566.

41. SongTao Q, Lei Y, Si G, et al. IDH mutations predict longer survival and response to temozolomide in secondary glioblastoma. *Cancer Sci.* 2012;103(2):269–273.

42. van den Bent MJ, Dubbink HJ, Marie Y, et al. IDH1 and IDH2 mutations are prognostic but not predictive for outcome in anaplastic oligodendroglial tumors: a report of the European Organization for Research and Treatment of Cancer Brain Tumor Group. *Clin Cancer Res.* 2010;16(5):1597–1604.

43. Capper D, Zentgraf H, Balss J, Hartmann C, von Deimling A. Monoclonal antibody specific for IDH1 R132H mutation. *Acta Neuropathol.* 2009;118(5):599–601.

44. Preusser M, Wöhrer A, Stary S, Höftberger R, Streubel B, Hainfellner JA. Value and limitations of immunohistochemistry and gene sequencing for detection of the IDH1-R132H mutation in diffuse glioma biopsy specimens. *J Neuropathol Exp Neurol.* 2011;70(8):715–723.

45. Mellai M, Piazzi A, Caldera V, et al. IDH1 and IDH2 mutations, immunohistochemistry and associations in a series of brain tumors. *J Neurooncol.* 2011;105(2):345–357.

46. Toyota M, Ahuja N, Ohe-Toyota M, Herman JG, Baylin SB, Issa JP. CpG island methylator phenotype in colorectal cancer. *Proc Natl Acad Sci USA.* 1999;96(15):8681–8686.

47. Weisenberger DJ, Siegmund KD, Campan M, et al. CpG island methylator phenotype underlies sporadic microsatellite instability and is tightly associated with BRAF mutation in colorectal cancer. *Nat Genet.* 2006;38(7):787–793.

48. Nakagawachi T, Soejima H, Urano T, et al. Silencing effect of CpG island hypermethylation and histone modifications on O6-methylguanine-DNA methyltransferase (MGMT) gene expression in human cancer. *Oncogene.* 2003;22(55):8835–8844.

49. Dong SM, Pang JC, Poon WS, et al. Concurrent hypermethylation of multiple genes is associated with grade of oligodendroglial tumors. *J Neuropathol Exp Neurol.* 2001;60(8):808–816.

50. Liang Y, Diehn M, Watson N, et al. Gene expression profiling reveals molecularly and clinically distinct subtypes of glioblastoma multiforme. *Proc Natl Acad Sci USA.* 2005;102(16):5814–5819.

51. Kim TY, Zhong S, Fields CR, Kim JH, Robertson KD. Epigenomic profiling reveals novel and frequent targets of aberrant DNA methylation-mediated silencing in malignant glioma. *Cancer Res.* 2006;66(15):7490–7501.

52. Martinez R, Martin-Subero JI, Rohde V, et al. A microarray-based DNA methylation study of glioblastoma multiforme. *Epigenetics.* 2009;4(4):255–264.

53. Uhlmann K, Rohde K, Zeller C, et al. Distinct methylation profiles of glioma subtypes. *Int J Cancer.* 2003;106(1):52–59.

54. Nakamura M, Watanabe T, Yonekawa Y, Kleihues P, Ohgaki H. Promoter methylation of the DNA repair gene MGMT in astrocytomas is frequently associated with G:C –> A:T mutations of the TP53 tumor suppressor gene. *Carcinogenesis.* 2001;22(10):1715–1719.

55. Ohgaki H, Kleihues P. Genetic pathways to primary and secondary glioblastoma. *Am J Pathol.* 2007;170(5):1445–1453.

56. Noushmehr H, Weisenberger DJ, Diefes K, et al.; Cancer Genome Atlas Research Network. Identification of a CpG island methylator phenotype that defines a distinct subgroup of glioma. *Cancer Cell.* 2010;17(5):510–522.

57. Laffaire J, Everhard S, Idbaih A, et al. Methylation profiling identifies 2 groups of gliomas according to their tumorigenesis. *Neuro-oncology.* 2011;13(1):84–98.

58. van den Bent MJ, Gravendeel LA, Gorlia T, et al. A hypermethylated phenotype is a better predictor of survival than MGMT methylation in anaplastic oligodendroglial brain tumors: a report from EORTC study 26951. *Clin Cancer Res.* 2011;17(22):7148–7155.

59. Christensen BC, Smith AA, Zheng S, et al. DNA methylation, isocitrate dehydrogenase mutation, and survival in glioma. *J Natl Cancer Inst.* 2011;103(2):143–153.

60. Turcan S, Rohle D, Goenka A, et al. IDH1 mutation is sufficient to establish the glioma hypermethylator phenotype. *Nature.* 2012;483(7390):479–483.

61. Jenkins RB, Curran W, Scott CB, Cairncross G. Pilot evaluation of 1p and 19q deletions in anaplastic oligodendrogliomas collected by a national cooperative cancer treatment group. *Am J Clin Oncol.* 2001;24(5):506–508.

62. Reifenberger J, Reifenberger G, Liu L, James CD, Wechsler W, Collins VP. Molecular genetic analysis of oligodendroglial tumors shows preferential allelic deletions on 19q and 1p. *Am J Pathol.* 1994;145(5):1175–1190.

63. Bello MJ, Vaquero J, de Campos JM, et al. Molecular analysis of chromosome 1 abnormalities in human gliomas reveals frequent loss of 1p in oligodendroglial tumors. *Int J Cancer.* 1994;57(2):172–175.

64. Thiessen B, Maguire JA, McNeil K, Huntsman D, Martin MA, Horsman D. Loss of heterozygosity for loci on chromosome arms 1p and 10q in oligodendroglial tumors: relationship to outcome and chemosensitivity. *J Neurooncol.* 2003;64(3):271–278.

65. van den Bent MJ, Looijenga LH, Langenberg K, et al. Chromosomal anomalies in oligodendroglial tumors are correlated with clinical features. *Cancer.* 2003;97(5):1276–1284.

66. Kim SH, Kim H, Kim TS. Clinical, histological, and immunohistochemical features predicting 1p/19q loss of heterozygosity in oligodendroglial tumors. *Acta Neuropathol.* 2005;110(1):27–38.

67. Jenkins RB, Blair H, Ballman KV, et al. A t(1;19)(q10;p10) mediates the combined deletions of 1p and 19q and predicts a better prognosis of patients with oligodendroglioma. *Cancer Res.* 2006;66(20):9852–9861.

68. Streffer J, Schabet M, Bamberg M, et al. A role for preirradiation PCV chemotherapy for oligodendroglial brain tumors. *J Neurol.* 2000;247(4):297–302.

69. van den Bent MJ, Taphoorn MJ, Brandes AA, et al.; European Organization for Research and Treatment of Cancer Brain Tumor Group. Phase II study of first-line chemotherapy with temozolomide in recurrent oligodendroglial tumors: the European Organization for Research and Treatment of Cancer Brain Tumor Group Study 26971. *J Clin Oncol.* 2003;21(13):2525–2528.

70. Mikkelsen T, Doyle T, Anderson J, et al. Temozolomide single-agent chemotherapy for newly diagnosed anaplastic oligodendroglioma. *J Neurooncol.* 2009;92(1):57–63.

71. Cairncross G, Berkey B, Shaw E, et al.; Intergroup Radiation Therapy Oncology Group Trial 9402. Phase III trial of chemotherapy plus radiotherapy compared with radiotherapy alone for pure and mixed anaplastic oligodendroglioma: Intergroup Radiation Therapy Oncology Group Trial 9402. *J Clin Oncol.* 2006;24(18):2707–2714.

72. Cairncross G, Macdonald D, Ludwin S, et al. Chemotherapy for anaplastic oligodendroglioma. National Cancer Institute of Canada Clinical Trials Group. *J Clin Oncol.* 1994;12(10):2013–2021.

73. Giannini C, Burger PC, Berkey BA, et al. Anaplastic oligodendroglial tumors: refining the correlation among histopathology, 1p 19q deletion and clinical outcome in Intergroup Radiation Therapy Oncology Group Trial 9402. *Brain Pathol.* 2008;18(3):360–369.

74. Scheie D, Cvancarova M, Mørk S, et al. Can morphology predict 1p/19q loss in oligodendroglial tumours? *Histopathology.* 2008;53(5):578–587.

75. McDonald JM, See SJ, Tremont IW, et al. The prognostic impact of histology and 1p/19q status in anaplastic oligodendroglial tumors. *Cancer.* 2005;104(7):1468–1477.

76. Yip S, Butterfield YS, Morozova O, et al. Concurrent CIC mutations, IDH mutations, and 1p/19q loss distinguish oligodendrogliomas from other cancers. *J Pathol.* 2012;226(1):7–16.

77. Vogazianou AP, Chan R, Bäcklund LM, et al. Distinct patterns of 1p and 19q alterations identify subtypes of human gliomas that have different prognoses. *Neuro-oncology.* 2010;12(7):664–678.

78. Kaneshiro D, Kobayashi T, Chao ST, Suh J, Prayson RA. Chromosome 1p and 19q deletions in glioblastoma multiforme. *Appl Immunohistochem Mol Morphol.* 2009;17(6):512–516.

79. Idbaih A, Marie Y, Pierron G, et al. Two types of chromosome 1p losses with opposite significance in gliomas. *Ann Neurol.* 2005;58(3):483–487.

80. Hegi ME, Janzer RC, Lambiv WL, et al.; European Organisation for Research and Treatment of Cancer Brain Tumour and Radiation Oncology Groups; National Cancer Institute of Canada Clinical Trials Group. Presence of an oligodendroglioma-like component in newly diagnosed glioblastoma identifies a pathogenetically heterogeneous subgroup and lacks prognostic value: central pathology review of the EORTC_26981/NCIC_CE.3 trial. *Acta Neuropathol.* 2012;123(6):841–852.

81. Wang Y, Li S, Chen L, et al. Glioblastoma with an oligodendroglioma component: distinct clinical behavior, genetic alterations, and outcome. *Neuro Oncol.* 2012.

82. Griffin CA, Burger P, Morsberger L, et al. Identification of der(1;19)(q10;p10) in five oligodendrogliomas suggests mechanism of concurrent 1p and 19q loss. *J Neuropathol Exp Neurol.* 2006;65(10):988–994.

83. Bettegowda C, Agrawal N, Jiao Y, et al. Mutations in CIC and FUBP1 contribute to human oligodendroglioma. *Science.* 2011;333(6048):1453–1455.

84. von Deimling A, Eibl RH, Ohgaki H, et al. p53 mutations are associated with 17p allelic loss in grade II and grade III astrocytoma. *Cancer Res.* 1992;52(10):2987–2990.

85. Louis DN, von Deimling A, Chung RY, et al. Comparative study of p53 gene and protein alterations in human astrocytic tumors. *J Neuropathol Exp Neurol.* 1993;52(1):31–38.

86. Kraus JA, Wenghoefer M, Glesmann N, et al. TP53 gene mutations, nuclear p53 accumulation, expression of Waf/p21, Bcl-2, and CD95 (APO-1/Fas) proteins are not prognostic factors in de novo glioblastoma multiforme. *J Neurooncol.* 2001;52(3):263–272.

87. Ohgaki H, Dessen P, Jourde B, et al. Genetic pathways to glioblastoma: a population-based study. *Cancer Res.* 2004;64(19):6892–6899.
88. Lotfi M, Afsharnezhad S, Raziee HR, et al. Immunohistochemical assessment of MGMT expression and p53 mutation in glioblastoma multiforme. *Tumori.* 2011;97(1):104–108.
89. Stark AM, Witzel P, Strege RJ, Hugo HH, Mehdorn HM. p53, mdm2, EGFR, and msh2 expression in paired initial and recurrent glioblastoma multiforme. *J Neurol Neurosurg Psychiatr.* 2003;74(6):779–783.
90. Ruano Y, Ribalta T, de Lope AR, et al. Worse outcome in primary glioblastoma multiforme with concurrent epidermal growth factor receptor and p53 alteration. *Am J Clin Pathol.* 2009;131(2):257–263.
91. Blough MD, Beauchamp DC, Westgate MR, Kelly JJ, Cairncross JG. Effect of aberrant p53 function on temozolomide sensitivity of glioma cell lines and brain tumor initiating cells from glioblastoma. *J Neurooncol.* 2011;102(1):1–7.
92. Comprehensive genomic characterization defines human glioblastoma genes and core pathways. *Nature.* 2008;455(7216):1061–1068.
93. Hede SM, Nazarenko I, Nistér M, Lindström MS. Novel Perspectives on p53 Function in Neural Stem Cells and Brain Tumors. *J Oncol.* 2011;2011:852970.
94. Sato A, Sunayama J, Matsuda K, et al. MEK-ERK signaling dictates DNA-repair gene MGMT expression and temozolomide resistance of stem-like glioblastoma cells via the MDM2-p53 axis. *Stem Cells.* 2011;29(12):1942–1951.
95. Kumar M, Lu Z, Takwi AA, et al. Negative regulation of the tumor suppressor p53 gene by microRNAs. *Oncogene.* 2011;30(7):843–853.
96. Malkoun N, Chargari C, Forest F, et al. Prolonged temozolomide for treatment of glioblastoma: preliminary clinical results and prognostic value of p53 overexpression. *J Neurooncol.* 2012;106(1):127–133.
97. Thon N, Eigenbrod S, Grasbon-Frodl EM, et al. Predominant influence of MGMT methylation in non-resectable glioblastoma after radiotherapy plus temozolomide. *J Neurol Neurosurg Psychiatr.* 2011;82(4):441–446.
98. Esteller M, Garcia-Foncillas J, Andion E, et al. Inactivation of the DNA-repair gene MGMT and the clinical response of gliomas to alkylating agents. *N Engl J Med.* 2000;343(19):1350–1354.
99. Uno M, Oba-Shinjo SM, Camargo AA, et al. Correlation of MGMT promoter methylation status with gene and protein expression levels in glioblastoma. *Clinics (Sao Paulo).* 2011;66(10):1747–1755.
100. Rivera AL, Pelloski CE, Gilbert MR, et al. MGMT promoter methylation is predictive of response to radiotherapy and prognostic in the absence of adjuvant alkylating chemotherapy for glioblastoma. *Neuro-oncology.* 2010;12(2):116–121.
101. Hegi ME, Diserens AC, Gorlia T, et al. MGMT gene silencing and benefit from temozolomide in glioblastoma. *N Engl J Med.* 2005;352(10):997–1003.
102. Ishii D, Natsume A, Wakabayashi T, et al. Efficacy of temozolomide is correlated with 1p loss and methylation of the deoxyribonucleic acid repair gene MGMT in malignant gliomas. *Neurol Med Chir (Tokyo).* 2007;47(8):341–9; discussion 350.
103. Olson RA, Brastianos PK, Palma DA. Prognostic and predictive value of epigenetic silencing of MGMT in patients with high grade gliomas: a systematic review and meta-analysis. *J Neurooncol.* 2011;105(2):325–335.
104. Mellai M, Monzeglio O, Piazzi A, et al. MGMT promoter hypermethylation and its associations with genetic alterations in a series of 350 brain tumors. *J Neurooncol.* 2012;107(3):617–631.
105. Sadones J, Michotte A, Veld P, et al. MGMT promoter hypermethylation correlates with a survival benefit from temozolomide in patients with recurrent anaplastic astrocytoma but not glioblastoma. *Eur J Cancer.* 2009;45(1):146–153.
106. Gömöri E, Pál J, Kovács B, Dóczi T. Concurrent hypermethylation of DNMT1, MGMT and EGFR genes in progression of gliomas. *Diagn Pathol.* 2012;7:8.
107. Mulholland S, Pearson DM, Hamoudi RA, et al. MGMT CpG island is invariably methylated in adult astrocytic and oligodendroglial tumors with IDH1 or IDH2 mutations. *Int J Cancer.* 2011.
108. Ohka F, Natsume A, Motomura K, et al. The global DNA methylation surrogate LINE-1 methylation is correlated with MGMT promoter methylation and is a better prognostic factor for glioma. *PLoS ONE.* 2011;6(8):e23332.
109. Jung TY, Jung S, Moon KS, et al. Changes of the O6-methylguanine-DNA methyltransferase promoter methylation and MGMT protein expression after adjuvant treatment in glioblastoma. *Oncol Rep.* 2010;23(5):1269–1276.
110. Cahill DP, Levine KK, Betensky RA, et al. Loss of the mismatch repair protein MSH6 in human glioblastomas is associated with tumor progression during temozolomide treatment. *Clin Cancer Res.* 2007;13(7):2038–2045.
111. Preusser M, Elezi L, Hainfellner JA. Reliability and reproducibility of PCR-based testing of O6-methylguanine-DNA methyltransferase gene (MGMT) promoter methylation status in formalin-fixed and paraffin-embedded neurosurgical biopsy specimens. *Clin Neuropathol.* 2008;27(6):388–390.
112. Preusser M. MGMT analysis at DNA, RNA and protein levels in glioblastoma tissue. *Histol Histopathol.* 2009;24(4):511–518.
113. Kreth S, Thon N, Eigenbrod S, et al. O-methylguanine-DNA methyltransferase (MGMT) mRNA expression predicts outcome in malignant glioma independent of MGMT promoter methylation. *PLoS ONE.* 2011;6(2):e17156.
114. Shah N, Lin B, Sibenaller Z, et al. Comprehensive analysis of MGMT promoter methylation: correlation with MGMT expression and clinical response in GBM. *PLoS ONE.* 2011;6(1):e16146.
115. Brandes AA, Franceschi E, Tosoni A, et al. MGMT promoter methylation status can predict the incidence

and outcome of pseudoprogression after concomitant radiochemotherapy in newly diagnosed glioblastoma patients. *J Clin Oncol.* 2008;26(13):2192–2197.

116. Shibahara I, Sonoda Y, Kanamori M, et al. IDH1/2 gene status defines the prognosis and molecular profiles in patients with grade III gliomas. *Int J Clin Oncol.* 2011.

117. Li S, Zhang W, Chen B, Jiang T, Wang Z. Prognostic and predictive value of p53 in low MGMT expressing glioblastoma treated with surgery, radiation and adjuvant temozolomide chemotherapy. *Neurol Res.* 2010;32(7):690–694.

118. Attolini CS, Cheng YK, Beroukhim R, et al. A mathematical framework to determine the temporal sequence of somatic genetic events in cancer. *Proc Natl Acad Sci USA.* 2010;107(41):17604–17609.

119. Sugawa N, Ekstrand AJ, James CD, Collins VP. Identical splicing of aberrant epidermal growth factor receptor transcripts from amplified rearranged genes in human glioblastomas. *Proc Natl Acad Sci USA.* 1990;87(21):8602–8606.

120. Lee JC, Vivanco I, Beroukhim R, et al. Epidermal growth factor receptor activation in glioblastoma through novel missense mutations in the extracellular domain. *PLoS Med.* 2006;3(12):e485.

121. Quaranta M, Divella R, Daniele A, et al. Epidermal growth factor receptor serum levels and prognostic value in malignant gliomas. *Tumori.* 2007;93(3):275–280.

122. Heimberger AB, Hlatky R, Suki D, et al. Prognostic effect of epidermal growth factor receptor and EGFRvIII in glioblastoma multiforme patients. *Clin Cancer Res.* 2005;11(4):1462–1466.

123. Quan AL, Barnett GH, Lee SY, et al. Epidermal growth factor receptor amplification does not have prognostic significance in patients with glioblastoma multiforme. *Int J Radiat Oncol Biol Phys.* 2005;63(3):695–703.

124. Martinou M, Giannopoulou E, Malatara G, Argyriou AA, Kalofonos HP, Kardamakis D. Ionizing radiation affects epidermal growth factor receptor signalling and metalloproteinase secretion in glioma cells. *Cancer Genomics Proteomics.* 2011;8(1):33–38.

125. Gallia GL, Rand V, Siu IM, et al. PIK3CA gene mutations in pediatric and adult glioblastoma multiforme. *Mol Cancer Res.* 2006;4(10):709–714.

126. Mueller W, Mizoguchi M, Silen E, D'Amore K, Nutt CL, Louis DN. Mutations of the PIK3CA gene are rare in human glioblastoma. *Acta Neuropathol.* 2005;109(6):654–655.

127. Hartmann C, Bartels G, Gehlhaar C, Holtkamp N, von Deimling A. PIK3CA mutations in glioblastoma multiforme. *Acta Neuropathol.* 2005;109(6):639–642.

128. Weber GL, Parat MO, Binder ZA, Gallia GL, Riggins GJ. Abrogation of PIK3CA or PIK3R1 reduces proliferation, migration, and invasion in glioblastoma multiforme cells. *Oncotarget.* 2011;2(11):833–849.

129. Kwiatkowska A, Kijewska M, Lipko M, Hibner U, Kaminska B. Downregulation of Akt and FAK phosphorylation reduces invasion of glioblastoma cells by impairment of MT1-MMP shuttling to lamellipodia and downregulates MMPs expression. *Biochim Biophys Acta.* 2011;1813(5):655–667.

130. Molina JR, Hayashi Y, Stephens C, Georgescu MM. Invasive glioblastoma cells acquire stemness and increased Akt activation. *Neoplasia.* 2010;12(6):453–463.

131. Pelloski CE, Lin E, Zhang L, et al. Prognostic associations of activated mitogen-activated protein kinase and Akt pathways in glioblastoma. *Clin Cancer Res.* 2006;12(13):3935–3941.

132. Li HF, Kim JS, Waldman T. Radiation-induced Akt activation modulates radioresistance in human glioblastoma cells. *Radiat Oncol.* 2009;4:43.

133. Kao GD, Jiang Z, Fernandes AM, Gupta AK, Maity A. Inhibition of phosphatidylinositol-3-OH kinase/Akt signaling impairs DNA repair in glioblastoma cells following ionizing radiation. *J Biol Chem.* 2007;282(29):21206–21212.

134. Jeuken JW, Nelen MR, Vermeer H, et al. PTEN mutation analysis in two genetic subtypes of high-grade oligodendroglial tumors. PTEN is only occasionally mutated in one of the two genetic subtypes. *Cancer Genet Cytogenet.* 2000;119(1):42–47.

135. Horbinski C, Nikiforova MN, Hobbs J, et al. The importance of 10q status in an outcomes-based comparison between 1p/19q fluorescence in situ hybridization and polymerase chain reaction-based microsatellite loss of heterozygosity analysis of oligodendrogliomas. *J Neuropathol Exp Neurol.* 2012;71(1):73–82.

136. Fallon KB, Palmer CA, Roth KA, et al. Prognostic value of 1p, 19q, 9p, 10q, and EGFR-FISH analyses in recurrent oligodendrogliomas. *J Neuropathol Exp Neurol.* 2004;63(4):314–322.

137. Zhang X, Wu A, Fan Y, Wang Y. Increased transforming growth factor-ß2 in epidermal growth factor receptor variant III-positive glioblastoma. *J Clin Neurosci.* 2011;18(6):821–826.

138. Magnus N, Garnier D, Rak J. Oncogenic epidermal growth factor receptor up-regulates multiple elements of the tissue factor signaling pathway in human glioma cells. *Blood.* 2010;116(5):815–818.

139. Liu M, Yang Y, Wang C, et al. The effect of epidermal growth factor receptor variant III on glioma cell migration by stimulating ERK phosphorylation through the focal adhesion kinase signaling pathway. *Arch Biochem Biophys.* 2010;502(2):89–95.

140. Rong Y, Belozerov VE, Tucker-Burden C, et al. Epidermal growth factor receptor and PTEN modulate tissue factor expression in glioblastoma through JunD/activator protein-1 transcriptional activity. *Cancer Res.* 2009;69(6):2540–2549.

141. Westermark B, Heldin CH, Nistér M. Platelet-derived growth factor in human glioma. *Glia.* 1995;15(3):257–263.

142. Karcher S, Steiner HH, Ahmadi R, et al. Different angiogenic phenotypes in primary and secondary glioblastomas. *Int J Cancer.* 2006;118(9):2182–2189.

143. Niault TS, Baccarini M. Targets of Raf in tumorigenesis. *Carcinogenesis.* 2010;31(7):1165–1174.

144. Bar EE, Lin A, Tihan T, Burger PC, Eberhart CG. Frequent gains at chromosome 7q34 involving BRAF in pilocytic astrocytoma. *J Neuropathol Exp Neurol.* 2008;67(9):878–887.

145. Pfister S, Janzarik WG, Remke M, et al. BRAF gene duplication constitutes a mechanism of MAPK pathway activation in low-grade astrocytomas. *J Clin Invest.* 2008;118(5):1739–1749.

146. Jones DT, Kocialkowski S, Liu L, et al. Tandem duplication producing a novel oncogenic BRAF fusion gene defines the majority of pilocytic astrocytomas. *Cancer Res.* 2008;68(21):8673–8677.

147. Forshew T, Tatevossian RG, Lawson AR, et al. Activation of the ERK/MAPK pathway: a signature genetic defect in posterior fossa pilocytic astrocytomas. *J Pathol.* 2009;218(2):172–181.

148. Jones DT, Kocialkowski S, Liu L, Pearson DM, Ichimura K, Collins VP. Oncogenic RAF1 rearrangement and a novel BRAF mutation as alternatives to KIAA1549:BRAF fusion in activating the MAPK pathway in pilocytic astrocytoma. *Oncogene.* 2009;28(20):2119–2123.

149. Sievert AJ, Jackson EM, Gai X, et al. Duplication of 7q34 in pediatric low-grade astrocytomas detected by high-density single-nucleotide polymorphism-based genotype arrays results in a novel BRAF fusion gene. *Brain Pathol.* 2009;19(3):449–458.

150. Horbinski C, Hamilton RL, Nikiforov Y, Pollack IF. Association of molecular alterations, including BRAF, with biology and outcome in pilocytic astrocytomas. *Acta Neuropathol.* 2010;119(5):641–649.

151. Hasselblatt M, Riesmeier B, Lechtape B, et al. BRAF-KIAA1549 fusion transcripts are less frequent in pilocytic astrocytomas diagnosed in adults. *Neuropathol Appl Neurobiol.* 2011;37(7):803–806.

152. Tihan T, Ersen A, Qaddoumi I, et al. Pathologic characteristics of pediatric intracranial pilocytic astrocytomas and their impact on outcome in 3 countries: a multi-institutional study. *Am J Surg Pathol.* 2012;36(1):43–55.

153. Korshunov A, Meyer J, Capper D, et al. Combined molecular analysis of BRAF and IDH1 distinguishes pilocytic astrocytoma from diffuse astrocytoma. *Acta Neuropathol.* 2009;118(3):401–405.

154. Jacob K, Albrecht S, Sollier C, et al. Duplication of 7q34 is specific to juvenile pilocytic astrocytomas and a hallmark of cerebellar and optic pathway tumours. *Br J Cancer.* 2009;101(4):722–733.

155. Schiffman JD, Hodgson JG, VandenBerg SR, et al. Oncogenic BRAF mutation with CDKN2A inactivation is characteristic of a subset of pediatric malignant astrocytomas. *Cancer Res.* 2010;70(2):512–519.

156. Schindler G, Capper D, Meyer J, et al. Analysis of BRAF V600E mutation in 1,320 nervous system tumors reveals high mutation frequencies in pleomorphic xanthoastrocytoma, ganglioglioma and extra-cerebellar pilocytic astrocytoma. *Acta Neuropathol.* 2011;121(3):397–405.

157. Cin H, Meyer C, Herr R, et al. Oncogenic FAM131B-BRAF fusion resulting from 7q34 deletion comprises an alternative mechanism of MAPK pathway activation in pilocytic astrocytoma. *Acta Neuropathol.* 2011;121(6):763–774.

158. Snuderl M, Fazlollahi L, Le LP, et al. Mosaic amplification of multiple receptor tyrosine kinase genes in glioblastoma. *Cancer Cell.* 2011;20(6):810–817.

159. Szerlip NJ, Pedraza A, Chakravarty D, et al. Intratumoral heterogeneity of receptor tyrosine kinases EGFR and PDGFRA amplification in glioblastoma defines subpopulations with distinct growth factor response. *Proc Natl Acad Sci USA.* 2012;109(8):3041–3046.

160. Sallinen SL, Sallinen PK, Haapasalo HK, et al. Identification of differentially expressed genes in human gliomas by DNA microarray and tissue chip techniques. *Cancer Res.* 2000;60(23):6617–6622.

161. Nigro JM, Misra A, Zhang L, et al. Integrated array-comparative genomic hybridization and expression array profiles identify clinically relevant molecular subtypes of glioblastoma. *Cancer Res.* 2005;65(5):1678–1686.

162. Freije WA, Castro-Vargas FE, Fang Z, et al. Gene expression profiling of gliomas strongly predicts survival. *Cancer Res.* 2004;64(18):6503–6510.

163. Maher EA, Brennan C, Wen PY, et al. Marked genomic differences characterize primary and secondary glioblastoma subtypes and identify two distinct molecular and clinical secondary glioblastoma entities. *Cancer Res.* 2006;66(23):11502–11513.

164. Idbaih A, Marie Y, Lucchesi C, et al. BAC array CGH distinguishes mutually exclusive alterations that define clinicogenetic subtypes of gliomas. *Int J Cancer.* 2008;122(8):1778–1786.

165. Verhaak RG, Hoadley KA, Purdom E, et al.; Cancer Genome Atlas Research Network. Integrated genomic analysis identifies clinically relevant subtypes of glioblastoma characterized by abnormalities in PDGFRA, IDH1, EGFR, and NF1. *Cancer Cell.* 2010;17(1):98–110.

166. Brennan C, Momota H, Hambardzumyan D, et al. Glioblastoma subclasses can be defined by activity among signal transduction pathways and associated genomic alterations. *PLoS ONE.* 2009;4(11):e7752.

167. Phillips HS, Kharbanda S, Chen R, et al. Molecular subclasses of high-grade glioma predict prognosis, delineate a pattern of disease progression, and resemble stages in neurogenesis. *Cancer Cell.* 2006;9(3):157–173.

168. Huse JT, Phillips HS, Brennan CW. Molecular subclassification of diffuse gliomas: seeing order in the chaos. *Glia.* 2011;59(8):1190–1199.

demos MEDICAL

RADIATION MEDICINE ROUNDS

Antiangiogenesis Therapies for Malignant Gliomas

Phyllis Wachsberger,[1*] Wenyin Shi,[1] and Adam P. Dicker[2]

[1]*Assistant Professor, Department of Radiation Oncology, Thomas Jefferson University, Philadelphia, PA;*

[2]*Professor and Chair, Department of Radiation Oncology, Professor of Pharmacology and Experimental Therapeutics, and Director of Christine Baxter Research Laboratory for Experimental Cancer Therapeutics, Jefferson Medical College of Thomas Jefferson University, Philadelphia, PA*

ABSTRACT

The approval by the United States Food and Drug Administration (FDA) of bevacizumab for use in recurrent glioblastoma multiforme (GBM) has made antiangiogenic therapy a valid strategy for further development in the treatment of malignant gliomas. Approval of bevacizumab has triggered significant interest in additional antiangiogenic agents and therapeutic strategies for patients with both recurrent and newly diagnosed GBM. Many clinical trials are currently ongoing combining new antiangiogenic agents with chemotherapy and/or radiation. To date, however, the survival benefits of antiangiogenic treatments have been relatively modest. Among the major challenges in the application of antiangiogenic therapy for GBM are identifying better targets, overcoming resistance to existing antiangiogenic agents, determining optimal scheduling, timing, and dosing of these agents with cytotoxic therapies and identifying clinically useful biomarkers for predicting efficacy of these agents. A better understanding of the biology of tumor angiogenesis will aid in overcoming these existing challenges.

Keywords: glioblastoma multiforme, angiogenesis, chemoradioresistance, VEGF-targeted therapies, hypoxia

INTRODUCTION

Glioblastoma multiforme (GBM) is the most common and the most lethal astrocytic primary malignant glioma in adults and accounts for nearly 40% of all malignant gliomas. The standard of care for newly diagnosed GBM is maximal surgical resection followed by radiotherapy (RT) and concurrent and adjuvant chemotherapy with the alkylating agent, temozolomide (TMZ), producing a median survival of only 14.6 months (1,2). The vast majority of GBM patients experience recurrent disease with a median time to recurrence of 7 months (3). A variety of factors contribute to poor treatment response, including (a) restricted delivery of chemotherapy because of the blood–brain barrier; (b) restricted efficacy of RT because of restricted delivery of oxygen to tumor resulting from abnormal vascular network produced by tumor angiogenesis; (c) high tumoral interstitial fluid pressure (IFP), which is largely the result of high levels of expression of the permeability factor, vascular endothelial growth factor (VEGF) (4), which contributes to vascular cerebral edema, and short survival in patients with GBM (5); (d) intrinsic

*Corresponding author, Department of Radiation Oncology, Thomas Jefferson University, 111 S. 11th Street, Philadelphia, PA 19107.

E-mail address: Phyllis.wachsberger@jeffersonhospital.org

Radiation Medicine Rounds 3:2 (2012) 241–260.

DOI: 10.5003/2151–4208.3.2.241

resistance to radiation and chemotherapy (6); (e) acquired resistance to chemotherapy (i.e., TMZ resistance develops during adjuvant therapy in over 30% of patients, contributing to recurrent disease); highly infiltrative nature of GBM resulting in tumor cells migrating extensively throughout the brain making it difficult to eliminate all tumor foci. In addition, the existence of marked genetic heterogeneities within GBMs gives rise to redundant and overlapping cellular signaling pathways driving tumor cell proliferation, survival, and angiogenesis that cannot be targeted by any single agent. Recent data also suggest that glioma cell subpopulations, either as cancer stem cells or through clonal selection, may be important in the development of resistance to therapy (7).

Over the past 15 years, developments in the field of tumor angiogenesis have given rise to the concept that targeting tumor vasculature is a viable strategy for overcoming resistance to standard treatment interventions. This concept has been validated by the approval of angiogenesis inhibitors for clinical use in lung, colon, breast, kidney, hepatocellular carcinomas, and GBM. These agents include sorafenib, sunitinib, and bevacizumab. In particular, bevacizumab, a humanized antibody directed against VEGF, was granted accelerated approval by the United States Food and Drug Administration (FDA) in 2009 for its use in the treatment of recurrent GBM. Currently, bevacizumab is undergoing clinical trials as a single agent and in combination with chemotherapy for newly diagnosed GBM. Approval of bevacizumab has triggered significant interest in additional antiangiogenic agents and therapeutic strategies for patients with both recurrent and newly diagnosed GBM. This chapter focuses on recent advances in antiangiogenic therapies for GBMs, clinical experience with these agents, current limitations of antiangiogenesis as a treatment strategy, and future directions for optimizing antiangiogenic treatment for both newly diagnosed and recurrent GBM.

■ ANGIOGENESIS AS A RELEVANT TARGET FOR GBM THERAPY

The importance of targeting tumor vasculature development and function first became apparent through the seminal studies of Judah Folkman who in 1971 formulated the angiogenic hypothesis (8). It is now well established that the growth of solid tumors is dependent upon a highly integrated ecosystem containing tumor cells, stromal elements, and endothelial cells; further progression of solid tumors requires a competent and expanding vascular supply since cells in solid tumors, like normal tissue, must receive oxygen and other nutrients to survive and grow (9). GBMs make good candidates for antiangiogenic therapy because they are among the most highly vascularized of human tumors and, therefore, dependent on angiogenesis for development and progression. They often express high levels of proangiogenic factors such as VEGF, basic fibroblast growth factor (bFGF), platelet-derived growth factor (PDGF), and interleukin-8 (IL-8) (10).

■ ROLE OF VEGF AND HYPOXIA IN ANGIOGENESIS IN GBM

VEGF has been the best studied angiogenic factor and is known to be central to initiating and maintaining tumor angiogenesis throughout the disease process (11). Studies evaluating VEGF levels in plasma and tumor fluid from patients show that GBMs express relatively high levels of VEGF (12). There is a direct correlation between VEGF overexpression and poor prognosis (13). VEGF is a potent stimulator of new blood vessel growth, inducing endothelial cell proliferation, migration, and survival, via activation of VEGFR-2 on the surface of endothelial cells. VEGF stimulates the budding of new capillaries and their growth toward tumor cells to form new vascular tubes and loops. VEGF is also a major vascular permeability factor (4); its overexpression causes excessive vascular permeability that facilitates leakage of proangiogenic proteins into the tumor microenvironment, thereby intensifying the angiogenic process.

There is a close relationship between VEGF production and hypoxia in GBM, which is related to the unique microvascular features of this tumor. GBMs are characterized by extensive hypoxia/necrotic areas which are typically surrounded by hypercellular zones referred to as pseudopalisades. Pseudopalisades give rise to regions of microvascular hyperplasia known as glomeruloid bodies and are associated with intense nuclear staining with antihypoxia-inducible factor-1 (HIF-1) antibodies (10). Pseudopalisading cells also secrete high levels of proangiogenic molecules such as VEGF because of increased transcriptional activity of HIF-1. Secretion of VEGF, in turn, causes vascular hyperplasia, including glomeruloid vascular proliferation, one of the pathological features of GBM (14). HIF-1-induced VEGF secretion can also be stimulated through regulation of hypoxia-independent growth factor–induced VEGF expression. In this regard, GBMs commonly exhibit overactivation of the epidermal growth factor receptor (EGFR) and the loss of the tumor suppressor PTEN, both of which can affect HIF expression. Activation of EGFR by ligand binding or gene amplification or constitutive activity of the mutant EGFRvIII results in activation of the PI3K pathway which increases HIF activity. PTEN loss of function results in dysregulation of the PI3K/AKT pathway and is associated with increased HIF-1 expression and increased vascularization in gliomas15.

INTERACTIONS OF ANGIOGENESIS INHIBITORS WITH CYTOTOXIC THERAPIES

Preclinical and clinical studies indicate that antiangiogenic agents enhance the cytotoxic effects of RT and/or chemotherapy (16,17) and actually work best in combination with other cancer therapies (18). In gliomas, a number of studies have indicated a benefit (see review) (3). The molecular mechanisms of interaction of antiangiogenic agents with cytotoxic therapies are potentially multifold. It is essential to gain a better understanding of these mechanisms in order to optimize incorporation of this class of agents into standard of care regimens with the goal of reducing chemoradioresistance and improving overall response. The following section and Figure 1 lists potential interactions with radiation and chemotherapy that could lead to enhanced tumor response:

Blockade of Radiation-Induced Angiogenesis, Thereby Preventing Tumor Regrowth

Radiation, acting as a cytotoxic stress, can induce angiogenesis and prosurvival signaling mechanisms, leading to subsequent tumor radioresistance. In particular, radiation is known to stimulate the production of proangiogenic molecules such as VEGF through Hif-1α induction (19,20). The administration of antiangiogenic agents with RT may counteract VEGF-mediated radioresistance, thereby sensitizing tumors and associated vasculature to the ionizing effects of radiation.

Increase in Tumor Oxygenation and Radiosensitization

Oxygen is a potent radiosensitizer and tumor reoxygenation will significantly increase tumor response to radiation. Antiangiogenic agents can theoretically improve tumor oxygenation by three mechanisms: (a) a reduction in oxygen-consuming tumor cell and endothelial cell population, (b) a reduction in small immature blood vessels, and (c) an increase in perfusion of so-called normalized vessels (21). A reduction in cell population will decrease the number of oxygen-consuming cells and reduce vascular resistance, whereas a reduction

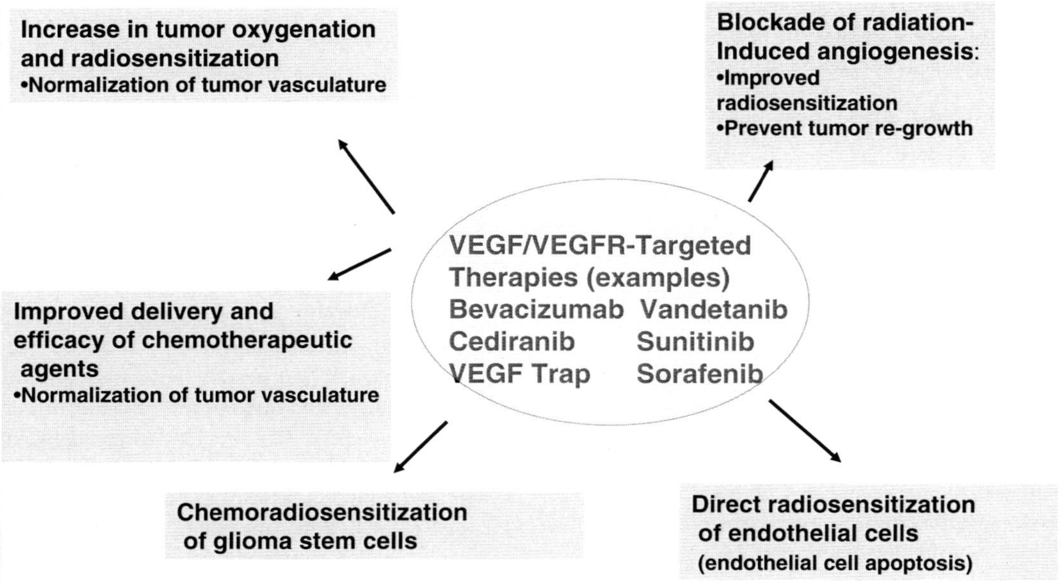

FIGURE 1 Rationale for combining antiangiogenic agents with cytotoxic therapies to improve therapeutic outcome for GBM.

of small, leaky vessels will reduce IFP and increase tumor perfusion and oxygen delivery.

Improved Delivery and Efficacy of Chemotherapeutic Agents

It has been shown both preclinically (22) and clinically (23) that VEGF blockade can result in a window of "normalized vasculature" characterized by less leaky, dilated and tortuous vessels with a more normal basement membrane and greater coverage by pericytes. It was consequently hypothesized that during this period, addition of radiation therapy and chemotherapy should give the best outcome because of improved tumor oxygenation. and improved delivery of chemotherapy. This concept was validated in the clinic when cediranib (AZD2171), a VEGFR inhibitor, was shown to temporarily induce a "normalization" time window' in tumor vessels in patients with recurrent GBM (23). This normalization led to a reduction in microvessel density and diminished permeability.

Direct Radiosensitization of Endothelial Cells (Endothelial Cell Apoptosis)

The tumor response to radiation is determined not only by tumor cell phenotype but also by endothelial cell sensitivity (24). By inducing HIF-1α mediated expression of VEGF in tumor cells, radiation also promotes endothelial cell survival, thereby minimizing vascular damage and radiation sensitivity (19). Therefore inhibitors of HIF-1α should overcome endothelial cell radioresistance following radiation.

Chemoradiosensitization of Glioma Stem Cells

Antiangiogenic agents have been shown to target glioma stem-like cells, a subpopulation of self-renewing tumor cells that contribute to treatment resistance (25,26). These glioma stem cells are associated with perivascular niches within the tumor from which high levels of VEGF are secreted, and exhibit chemoradioresistance compared with tumors derived from a low fraction of stem cells. Tumors derived from glioma stem cells are more angiogenic than those derived from nonglioma stem cells (25), exhibiting increased microvessel density, perfusion, recruitment of endothelial progenitor cells and high levels of VEGF and stromal-derived factor-1 (25,26). Antiangiogenic agents may disrupt the perivascular niche, thereby sensitizing gliomas to cytotoxic agents.

■ CURRENT ANTIANGIOGENIC STRATEGIES IN MALIGNANT GLIOMAS

A variety of antiangiogenic strategies are currently being employed in preclinical and clinical trials that have the potential to overcome resistance to standard cytotoxic therapies by mechanisms as outlined above (see Figure 2 for overview). Virtually all of the approved and investigational antiangiogenic agents target VEGF or its receptors. The three primary categories of antiangiogenic drugs are anti-VEGF monoclonal antibodies, soluble decoy receptors created from the VEGFR-1 receptor which selectively inhibit VEGF (27,28) and oral tyrosine kinase inhibitors (TKIs). Agents that target the VEGF ligand include bevacizumab, a recombinant humanized monoclonal antibody, approved for recurrent GBM that binds all isoforms of VEGF with high affinity and specificity (11) and VEGF Trap (aflibercept), a soluble, recombinant, decoy receptor, composed of the second Ig domain of VEGFR-1 and the third Ig domain of VEGFR-2 bound to the hinge region of the Fc portion of human IgG1 that sequesters all isoforms of VEGF-A and placental growth factor (PlGF) (28). Aflibercept was shown preclinically to enhance radiation therapy (29) and is currently in phase I and phase II clinical trials for initial and recurrent GBM (30). TKIs inhibit VEGFR kinase activity, and often other receptor and cytoplasmic kinases, of endothelial cells as well as in malignant and stromal cells. A number of TKIs are currently undergoing clinical evaluation (see section below). Among these are vatalinib, cediranib, pazopanib and vandetanib (30). XL184, currently in phase II trials for recurrent GBM, inhibits VEGFR-2, MET and RET kinases, and has the potential to inhibit both angiogenesis and invasiveness of GBM tumors. Agents that target alternate circulating angiogenic factors, such as PlGF, angiopoietin 1, 2 (Ang 1–2), bFGF, and endoglin, as well as additional receptors for VEGF, including neuropilins 1 and 2 (NRP-1, NRP-2)1, are in development. Examples of such agents are AMG 386, which targets the Ang-2 (31) and is currently in phase II study for recurrent GBM. In addition, integrin signaling which is associated

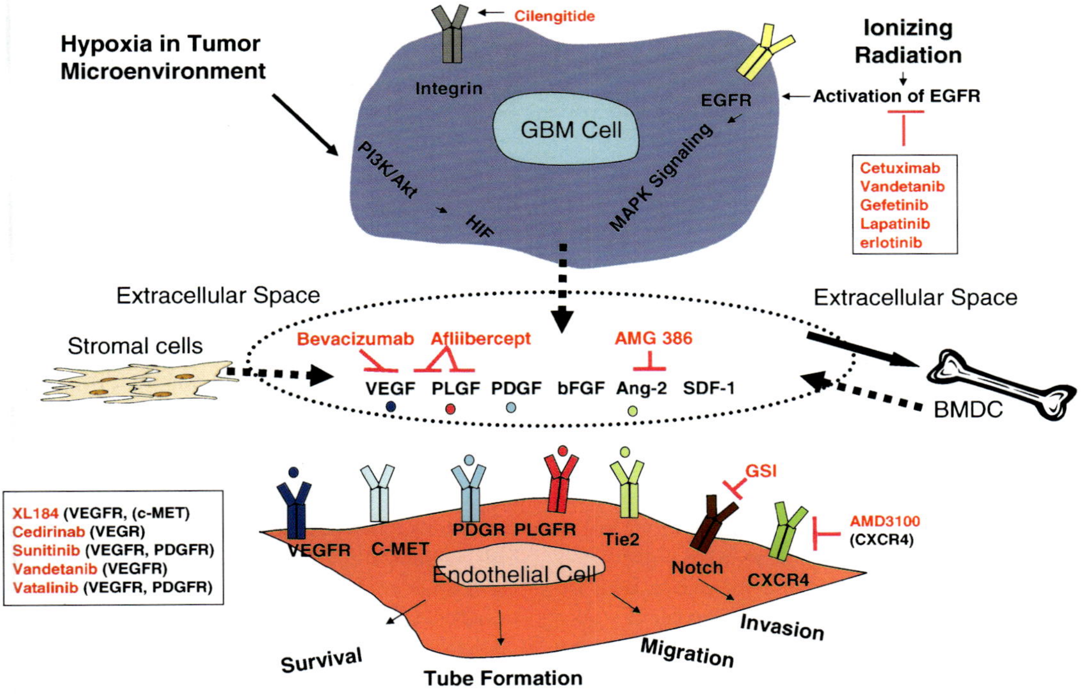

FIGURE 2 Current antiangiogenic strategies. The diagram depicts angiogenic targets on the GBM tumor cell, such as integrin and epidermal growth factor receptor, activated by factors in the tumor microenvironment (i.e., hypoxia, ionizing radiation), signaling to key intracellular pathways (i.e., PI3K/Akt, MAPK), leading to secretion of proangiogenic molecules into the extracellular space surrounding GBM cells (i.e., VEGF, PlGF, PDGR, bFGF, Ang-2, SDF-1). The extracellular space contains host stromal cells, which can also secrete proangiogenic molecules. In addition, proangiogenic molecules such as VEGF can mobilize bone marrow–derived cells (BMDCs depicted by solid arrow) to the tumor microenvironment to secrete additional angiogenic factors. The endothelial cell expresses a variety of cell surface receptors (i.e., VEGFR, cMET, PDGFR, PlGFR, Tie-2, Notch, CXCR4), which can bind the secreted proangiogenic molecules to stimulate angiogeneisis-related processes such as endothelial cell survival, tube formation, migration, and invasion. Drugs that target secreted angiogenic molecules and their receptors are depicted in red. Arrows: Dashed arrows depict secretion of angiogenic molecules. bFGF = basic fibroblast growth factor; PlGF = placental growth factor; PDGF = platelet-derived growth factor; VEGF = vascular endothelial growth factor.

with endothelial cell migration and invasion, is being targeted by cilengitide, a selective blocker of αvβ3 (which correlates with glioma tumor grade) (32) and αvβ5 integrins (33). The relative benefits of these different strategies have yet to be determined clinically (see following section below).

In addition to direct inhibitors of tumor angiogenesis, targeted drug therapies for GBM that are currently in clinical trials also include receptor TKIs (RTKIs) that indirectly inhibit tumor angiogenesis by targeting growth factor receptor–induced angiogenesis and their downstream signaling molecules. Examples of these agents include inhibitors of EGFR, such as gefetinib, lapatinib, erlotinib, and cetuximab (30).

■ CLINICAL EXPERIENCE WITH ANTIANGIOGENIC AGENTS IN GBM

VEGF-Targeted Therapy: Bevacizumab

Bevacizumab (Avastin) was the first antiangiogenesis agent to be approved by the FDA in 2004. It was initially approved for use in metastatic colorectal cancer. Its clinical use was subsequently extended to other cancers, including lung, breast, renal cell, and recently GBM (34).

The majority of clinical trials with bevacizumab for GBM patients are aimed at recurrent disease. In the initial trial, bevacizumab was evaluated in combination with concomitant irinotecan (35,36). This combination was supported by the activity of bevacizumab and irinotecan containing regimens in patients with metastatic colorectal cancer (37). In the first prospective phase II study, patients with recurrent GBM received bevacizumab and irinotecan in one of two treatment cohorts. The first cohort of 23 patients received bevacizumab 10 mg/kg every 2 weeks with irinotecan in a 6-week cycle. In the second cohort of 12 patients, patients received bevacizumab 15 mg/kg every 3 weeks with irinotecan in a 6-week cycle (35,36). The 6-month progression-free survival (PFS) was 46%, and 6-month overall survival (OS) was 77%. Recently, the 4-year survival rate was also reported to be 11% (38). The follow-up phase II trials further evaluated the role of bevacizumab alone in recurrent GBM patients. In the first single-arm phase II study, 48 patients with recurrent GBM received bevacizumab 10 mg/kg every 2 weeks. After tumor progression, patients were immediately treated with bevacizumab in combination with irinotecan 340 mg/m^2 or 125 mg/m^2 every 2 weeks, depending on concurrent use of enzyme-inducing antiepileptic drugs (39). The 6-month PFS was 29%. The 6-month OS was 57%. Median OS was 31 weeks. The second trial randomized 167 patients at first or second recurrence to either bevacizumab alone, or bevacizumab with irinotecan (40). In the bevacizumab-alone and the bevacizumab-plus-irinotecan groups, estimated 6-month PFS rates were 42.6% and 50.3%, respectively. Of the patients treated with bevacizumab alone or bevacizumab-plus-irinotecan, 46.4% and 65.8%, respectively, experienced grade ≥3 adverse events, the most common of which were hypertension (8.3%) and convulsion (6.0%) in the bevacizumab-alone group and convulsion (13.9%), neutropenia (8.9%), and fatigue (8.9%) in the bevacizumab-plus-irinotecan group. Intracranial hemorrhage was noted in two patients (2.4%) in the bevacizumab-alone group (grade I) and in three patients (3.8%) in the bevacizumab-plus-irinotecan group (grades I, II, and IV, respectively) (40). The authors concluded that bevacizumab, alone or in combination with irinotecan, was well tolerated and active in recurrent GBM. The outcome for patients treated with bevacizumab alone appears similar to patients who received bevacizumab and irinotecan. Based on these studies, FDA granted accelerated approval of single-agent bevacizumab for recurrent GBM in May 2009. The basis for the FDA's accelerated approval was a clinical and meaningful and durable objective tumor response rate determined by independent radiographic review. On the other hand, the European Medicines Agency did not approve bevacizumab, primarily because there was no bevacizumab control arm in these studies (41,42).

Subsequent studies have focused on evaluating a variety of bevacizumab regimens for recurrent GBM patients. Table 1 (modified from [42]) lists currently published trials of bevacizumab in recurrent glioma. In the bevacizumab monotherapy studies, 15 mg every 3 weeks appears to have similar outcome compared to bevacizumab 10 mg every 2 weeks (43). A variety of small molecular targeted agents and chemotherapy agents have also been studied in combination with bevacizumab. However, there is no clear

TABLE 1 Currently published trials of bevacizumab in adult patients with recurrent glioblastoma

Study	Design	Patient Number	PFS-6 (%)	OS (week)	Ref
Bev alone	Phase II	85	42	37	40
Bev alone	Phase II	48	29	31	39
Bev alone	Phase II	50	25	26	43
Bev + Etoposide	Phase II	27	45	46	150
Bev + Irinotecan	Phase II	23	30	40	36
Bev + Irinotecan	Phase II	35	46	42	35
Bev + Irinotecan	Phase II	82	50	35	40
Bev + Irinotecan + cetuximab	Phase II	43	30	29	151
Bev + Erlotinib	Phase II	25	29	45	152
Bev + Carboplatin + Irinotecan	Phase II	40	46.5	33	153
Bev + Temozolomide	Phase II	32	18.8	37	154

Abbreviations: BEV = bevacizumab; OS = overall survival; PFS = progression-free survival.

evidence that the combination approach is superior to bevacizumab alone. Over 50 clinical trials are currently open evaluating regimens containing bevacizumab in patients with recurrent glioma (www.clinicaltrial.gov).

Another attractive strategy is to combine bevacizumab with reirradiation for recurrent GBM patients. Retrospective studies have demonstrated that bevacizumab combined with fractionated reirradiation is safe and effective (44,45). The 6-month PFS rates are in the range of 55% to 65%, although these data are from limited studies (44,45). The safety and efficacy of stereotactic radiosurgery (SRS) and adjuvant bevacizumab have also been studied (46). Median PFS is 5.2 months, and 1-year OS is 50%. Prospective trials are in active development (NCT00595322, NCT01478321, NCT01017250, NCT01086345, RTOG 1109).

The greatest challenge for treatment of recurrent GBM patients receiving bevacizumab is what therapy to offer patients after disease progression on bevacizumab. Although additional agents after bevacizumab have been tried, disease prognosis is extremely poor, with a median survival of 37.5 days and 6-month PFS of 2% (47,48). Further studies are warranted to identify new therapeutic targets and novel agents that could treat patients who have relapsed following antiangiogenic therapy.

Because of the positive results with bevacizumab in recurrent GBM, recent research has focused on the therapeutic benefit of bevacizumab in conjunction with TMZ and radiation for newly diagnosed GBM. In a phase II trial of 70 newly diagnosed GBM patients, bevacizumab was administered with radiation treatment and TMZ (49). The median OS and PFS were 19.6 and 13.6 months, respectively. The authors concluded that the addition of bevacizumab improved PFS but not OS when compared to historical control. In another phase II trial of 125 patients, bevacizumab was given in addition to standard radiation therapy and TMZ followed by bevacizumab, TMZ, and irinotecan (50). The median OS was 21.2 months, and median PFS was 12.6 months, suggesting improved efficacy compared with historical controls (1,50,51). Two phase III studies have been performed so far evaluating bevacizumab in addition to radiation and TMZ in newly diagnosed GBMs (RTOG 0825 and AVAGlio). The RTOG 0825 trial is closed and results are pending. The AVAGlio trial is currently open (52). These studies will define the role of bevacizumab in frontline treatment for GBM.

Other VEGF-Targeted Therapy

In a phase I trial with Aflibercept, the VEGF and PlGF targeting agent, the drug was well tolerated. Maximal VEGF-bound aflibercept complex levels were reached at doses of 2 mg/kg or higher. Radiographic responses were observed at 3 mg/kg or higher (53). The recommended phase II dose was recommended as 4 mg/kg. A new formulation of subcutaneously administered aflibercept has also been evaluated (54). However, in a phase II study of recurrent malignant glioma trial by the North American Brain Tumor Consortium, aflibercept monotherapy showed minimal evidence of single-agent activity (55). The 6-month PFS was only 7.7% for the recurrent GBM cohort, and 25% for anaplastic glioma patients. In this study, molecular analysis of baseline tumor tissue identified tumor-associated markers of response and resistance. Genes associated with a longer time to progression included carbonic anhydrase 9 (CA9), HIF-1α, and SMAD2. Conversely, expression of CXCL16, CXCR4, ZAP70, CD27, CD84, and VEGF-B were associated with a short time to progression (55). However, these results require further validation studies. Future trials could be enriched with patients most likely to obtain the greatest benefit.

VEGFR-Targeted Therapy

Targeting VEGFR is another attractive strategy to suppress the VEGF-mediated angiogenesis process. Currently, there are two main classes of compounds that are under active development: (a) VEGFR TKIs, and (b) antibody or peptide-based agents (42).

Small molecule VEGFR TKIs are viewed as the most promising agents for GBMs. There are several VEGFR TKIs currently under evaluation in GBM (Table 2). Although these TKIs are considered to primarily target VEGFR, they also have varying potencies against other tyrosine kinases.

Cediranib is one of the most advanced TKIs in development (56). Cediranib showed promising results in several phase I clinical trials in patients with various solid tumors (57–62). It normalized tumor vasculature and alleviated edema in GBM patients (23). In a phase II trial of 31 patients with recurrent GBM, cediranib was administered as a 45 mg daily dose (63). The regimen was well tolerated with moderate toxicities. The 6-month PSF was 25.8%. Radiographic partial responses were observed by MRI in 17 (56.7%) of 30 evaluable patients using three-dimensional measurements

TABLE 2 Tyrosine kinase inhibitors and their targets

TKI	VEGFR-1	VEGFR-2	VEGFR-3	PDGFR	EGFR	KIT	Other
Vandetanib		+	+		+		RET
Cediranib	+	+	+	+		+	
Sorafenib	+	+	+	+		+	RAF, FLT3
Sunitinib	+	+	+	+		+	FLT3, RET
Axitinib	+	+	+				
Vatalanib	+	+	+	+		+	
Motesanib	+	+	+	+		+	RET
Pazopanib	+	+	+	+		+	
Nintedanib		+		+			FGFR
Brivanib	+	+	+				FGFR
Lenvatinib		+					FGFR, SCFR
Cabozantinib		+					cMET

Abbreviations: EGFR = epidermal growth factor receptor; FGFR = fibroblast growth factor receptor; PDGFR = platelet-derived growth factor; TKI = tyrosine kinase inhibitors; VEGFR = vascular endothelial growth factor receptor.

and in eight (27%) of 30 evaluable patients using two-dimensional measurements. It also resulted in a significant reduction of tumor-associated vasogenic edema, and for the 15 patients who entered the study taking corticosteroids, the dose was reduced (n = 10) or discontinued (n = 5) (63). Based on these results, a randomized phase III trial compared cediranib monotherapy, cediranib with lomustine, or lomustine alone in patients with recurrent GBM (64). Currently, there is also a phase II trial comparing TMZ and radiation therapy with or without cediranib in treating patients with newly diagnosed GBM (RTOG 0837, NCT01062425).

Sorafenib is approved by the FDA for the treatment of advanced renal cell carcinoma and hepatocellular carcinoma (65,66). It showed antitumor efficacy in glioma tumor models (67–69). A phase I study established the maximum tolerated dose (MTD) of sorafenib given orally BID on a continuous basis as 600 mg BID in patients with malignant glioma who were concurrently receiving enzyme-inducing antiseizure drugs and 800 mg BID in those who were not (70). A phase II study evaluated the efficacy of concurrent RT and TMZ followed by TMZ and sorafenib (400 mg BID) in the first-line treatment of patients with GBM (71). The median PFS for the entire group was 6 months. The median OS was 12 months. The addition of sorafenib did not appear to improve the efficacy of treatment when compared with the results expected with standard therapy, though 40% of patients did not receive any maintenance sorafenib, most often because of early disease progression (71). A phase II study combining TMZ with sorafenib in patients with recurrent GBM also failed to show significant efficacy (72). The 6-month PFS was only 9.4%.

Sunitinib has also been evaluated in glioma patients. A phase I study evaluated the MTD for sunitinib alone or in combination with irinotecan (73). The combination of sunitinib and irinotecan was associated with moderate toxicity and limited antitumor activity. A phase II trial of sunitinib monotherapy in 21 recurrent malignant glioma patients showed an OS and PFS of 3.8 m and 1.6 months, respectively. These results suggest that single-agent sunitinib has insufficient activity for recurrent high-grade glioma (74).

Pazopanib was evaluated as monotherapy in patients with recurrent gliomas. A phase II trial included 35 patients with recurrent GBM. Daily administration of 800 mg pazopanib was well tolerated. Radiographic responses were noted in only 6% of the patients, and the 6-month PFS was 3% (75). Thus, pazopanib appears to have limited activity as monotherapy for recurrent gliomas.

Vandetanib has been tested in a phase I setting with radiation and TMZ in patients with newly diagnosed GBM (76). It was found that vandetanib can be safely combined with RT and TMZ in GBM patients. A phase II study in which patients are randomized to vandetanib 100 mg daily with RT and TMZ or RT and TMZ alone is underway (NCT00128700). Vandetanib has also been evaluated with fractionated radiosurgery in patients with recurrent malignant gliomas (77). Fractionated radiosurgery is given at 36 Gy in three consecutive fractions. The MTD of vandetanib with SRS in recurrent malignant glioma is 100 mg daily. Further studies are needed to establish the efficacy of this combination.

A phase I study evaluating vatalanib with imatinib and hydroxyurea among patients with recurrent malignant glioma showed these agents can be safely combined at full-dose levels, and have modest antitumor activity (78). A phase I study of vatalanib in patients with newly diagnosed GBM treated with enzyme-inducing antiepileptic drugs and standard radiation and TMZ showed vatalanib was well tolerated and can be safely combined with standard radiation and TMZ in newly diagnosed GBM patients (79). In a phase I/II study by EORTC, once daily administration of up to 1000 mg of vatalanib in conjunction with concomitant TMZ and RT was feasible and safe. Prolonged administration of this oral agent is manageable. However, the planned randomized phase II trial was discontinued right at its onset due to industry decision not to further develop this agent (80).

There are several other VEGFR TKIs in clinical development, such as brivanib, lenvatinib (E7080), cabozantinib (XL-184), axitinib, motesanib, and nintedanib (BIBF1120). However, experience with these TKIs for high-grade glioma patients is very limited.

Currently, there are at least two antibody/peptide compounds against VEGF ligand binding that are being evaluated in GBM. Ramucirumab (IMC-1121B) is a monoclonal antibody that competitively binds the VEGFR ligand-binding site (81). It is being evaluated in a phase II trial for patients with recurrent GBM (NCT00895180). Angiocept (CT-322) is a novel, recombinant pegylated, 94-amino acid peptide that binds to and inhibits VEGFR-2 activation (82). It is being evaluated in a phase I trial for patients with newly diagnosed GBM in combination with radiation and TMZ (NCT00768911). It is also being evaluated in a phase I trial for patients with current GBM in combination with irinotecan (NCT00562419).

Other Antiangiogenic Strategies

Cilengitide

Cilengitide is a synthetic Arg-Gly-Asp (RGD) pentapeptide recognizing the RGD ligand-binding motif on the integrin receptors $\alpha V\beta 3$ and $\alpha V\beta 5$ (33,83). It inhibits integrin ligand binding. Preclinical studies showed it inhibits angiogenesis *in vivo* (84). It was also found to suppress tumor growth in an orthotopic brain tumor model (85). However, it has no effect on heterotopic tumor model, suggesting the brain environment is particularly susceptible to integrin inhibition (85). Cilengitide has been tested in two phase I studies (86,87). It is overall well tolerated, with no dose limiting toxicity up to 2400 mg/m^2. In a randomized phase II trial of 81 patients with recurrent GBM, cilengitide monotherapy (500 mg daily, and 2000 mg daily) was well tolerated. Objective responses were achieved in 5% or 13% of patients treated with 500 mg or 2000 mg, respectively. PFS after 6 months was 10% and 15%, whereas OS was 6.5 versus 9.9 months, respectively (88). Another phase II randomized trial (NABTC 03–02) also evaluated tumor delivery along with efficacy of cilengitide added to TMZand RT in recurrent GBM (89). The 6-month PFS rate was 12%. Cilengitide concentrations were several-fold higher in the tumor than the corresponding plasma concentrations, demonstrating both excellent penetration through the blood-tumor barrier and retention within the tumor. Cilengitide has also been evaluated in newly diagnosed GBM patients (90,91). In a multicenter pilot study on 52 patients, treatment was well tolerated with no identifiable added toxicity. The PFS at 6 months and 12 months were 69% and 33%, respectively, comparing favorably with historical controls (1,92). The median survival was 16.1 months, with a 2-year survival rate of 35%. Most interestingly, the PFS and OS were longer in patients with tumors with O^6-methylguanine-DNA methyltransferase (*MGMT*) promoter methylation. Such patients were previously identified to particularly benefit from TMZ chemotherapy (93). These findings are consistent with the working hypothesis that antiangiogenic therapy may enhance chemotherapy through normalization of tumor vasculature, decrease of hypoxia, improved drug delivery and enhanced cytotoxicity. On the basis of the results of this trial and supportive data from complementary trials and preclinical and clinical studies, a randomized phase III trial (CENTRIC, EORTC26071–22072, NCT00689221) was launched in 2008 for patients with a methylated MGMT. In parallel, a separate phase II trial has been designed for patients with MGMT unmethylated tumors (CORE study, NCT00813943). Here, an intensified high-dose daily cilengitide administration before RT is being explored.

Thalidomide and Analogs

Thalidomide was developed in the 1950s as a sedative medicine. It has recently been shown to inhibit angiogenesis, though the mechanism of action is poorly understood. It may be mediated through inhibition of TNF-α, VEGF, and bFGF expression by tumor cells, inhibition of cell surface receptors, and/or effects on the immune system (94,95). A phase II study of thalidomide alone in 39 recurrent high-grade glioma patients showed thalidomide is a generally well-tolerated drug that may have antitumor activity in a minority of patients (96). The median PFS and OS were 2.5 and 7.5 months, respectively. Similar findings were reported by another trial (97). Further trials were carried out to assess the efficacy of combining thalidomide with chemotherapy agents in recurrent GBM patients. A phase II study combining thalidomide with carmustine (BCNU) showed this regimen is well tolerated, and may be more active than either agent alone. The response rate was 24% and median PFS was 3.3 months (98). Thalidomide with concurrent TMZ was evaluated in the NABTC 99–04 trial for patients with recurrent GBM (99). This drug combination was reasonably safe, but with little indication of improvement compared to TMZ alone. The objective response rate was 7%. The estimated probability of being progression-free at 6 months with this therapy is 24%. A phase II study of combining thalidomide with irinotecan was also reported recently for recurrent anaplastic glioma patients (100). Unfortunately, the combination of thalidomide and irinotecan did not achieve sufficient efficacy to warrant further investigation. The use of thalidomide has also been evaluated in newly diagnosed GBM patients. A phase II trial of 67 patients, combining thalidomide with TMZ and radiation treatment resulted in a median survival of 73 weeks, which is favorable (101). In addition, a similar study of combining thalidomide with TMZ and radiation in children with newly diagnosed GBM and brainstem glioma showed benefit over historical control (102). The combination of thalidomide with radiation and 13-cis-retinoic acid was also studied in a phase II trial (103). The combined therapy was relatively well tolerated, but there was no survival advantage compared with historical studies without thalidomide. Similarly, a phase II study of combining thalidomide and celecoxib with TMZ after radiation treatment for newly diagnosed GBM failed to meet the primary endpoint of improvement of 4-month PFS (104). These results indicate that thalidomide plus cytotoxic agents seem to have limited antitumor activity when compared with thalidomide alone in patients with recurrent or newly diagnosed GBM

Lenalidomide is a potent structural and functional analog of thalidomide (105). It has been tested in phase I trials for brain tumors. A pilot study of lenalidomide with radiation in 23 patients with newly diagnosed GBM patients showed the MTD was 15 mg/m^2/d (106). In a phase I study of patients with recurrent central nervous system tumors, lenalidomide was well tolerated in doses up to 20 mg/m^2 (107). Preliminary data suggest that single-agent activity may be limited in patients with recurrent GBM. The median 6-month PFS was 12.5%. Further larger studies are needed to evaluate the antitumor activity of lenalidomide in patients with GBM.

PDGFR Inhibitors

PDGF also plays a role in angiogenesis. PDGF has been shown to be essential for the stability of normal blood vessel formation by recruiting pericytes and smooth muscle cells (108). The autocrine activation of PDGF is an important pathogenetic mechanism involved in different brain tumors (109–111). PDGFR inhibitors have been evaluated in clinical trials.

Imatinib is a multitargeted tyrosine kinase inhibitor that blocks PDGF receptor α, β, and c-Kit receptor (112). When imatinib was used alone in recurrent glioma patients, the dose range of 600 to 1,000 mg/d was well tolerated but had limited antitumor activity in patients with recurrent gliomas (113). The 6-month PFS was 16%. Imatinib in combination with hydroxyurea has also been evaluated in phase II trials. Imatinib in addition to hydroxyurea was well tolerated among patients with recurrent GBM but did not show clinically meaningful antitumor activity (114,115). A multicenter, randomized phase III trial including 240 recurrent GBM patients treated with hydroxyurea with or without imatinib also showed no clinical benefit of imatinib (116).

Dasatinib is an oral, multitargeted inhibitor of receptor tyrosine kinases, including BCR-ABL fusion protein, c-KIT, PDGFR, and Src family kinases (117). RTOG is conducting a phase II trial of dasatinib in patients with recurrent GBM (RTOG 0627).

Tandutinib

Tandutinib is a relatively selective inhibitor of type 3 tyrosine kinase receptor kinases with promising activity in some tumors (118). It is also in early clinical development in patients with recurrent glioma.

Cyclooxygenase 2 inhibitors

Cyclooxygenase 2 (COX2), an enzyme that is involved in prostaglandin synthesis, is frequently upregulated in nonsmall cell lung cancer, and may be a marker of worse prognosis (119). It also may promote angiogenesis, prevent apoptosis, and induce resistance to radiation therapy. Inhibitors of COX2 have been widely used for inflammatory conditions, and their anticancer activity has only recently begun to be explored. Preclinical studies showed celecoxib significantly enhanced GBM radiosensitivity, reduced clonogenic survival, and prolonged survival of GBM-implanted mice by inhibition of tumor angiogenesis with extensive tumor necrosis (120). In a phase II trial of 37 patients with recurrent GBM, it was found that irinotecan plus celecoxib could be safely administered concurrently at full-dose levels, and that this regimen had encouraging activity among heavily pretreated patients (121). The 6-month PFS was 25.1%.

Matrix Metalloproteinases Inhibitors

To form new blood vessels, endothelial cells of existing blood vessels must degrade the underlying basement membrane and invade into the stroma of the neighboring tissue. These processes of endothelial cell invasion and migration require the cooperative activity of plasminogen activators and matrix metalloproteinases (MMPs) (122). Marimastat was the first orally administrated synthetic MMP inhibitor (123). In a phase II trial of 44 patients with recurrent GBM, TMZ plus marimastat, the combination resulted in a 6-month PFS of 39%, which compared very favorably to historical control (124,125). However, in a randomized, double-blind, placebo-controlled trial of marimastat in GBM multiforme patients following surgery and irradiation, marimastat did not improve survival (126). Other matrix metalloproteinases inhibitors, such as prinomastat, CGS 27023A, BAY12–9566, Neovastat, and BMS-275291, are in early clinical development.

AMG 386

Angiopoietins and their receptors are key mediators of tumor angiogenesis (127). AMG 386 is an engineered peptibody composed of a truncated human IgG1 Fc domain covalently linked to two copies of a synthetic antiangiopoietin peptide. It suppresses angiogenesis through binding to and sequestering Ang-1 and Ang-2 (31,128). It is currently being tested in a phase II trial for patients with recurrent GBM. The first cohort will be single agent with AMG 386, and a second cohort will be AMG 386 in combination with bevacizumab (NCT01290263).

■ CHALLENGES AND FUTURE DIRECTIONS IN THE APPLICATION OF ANTIANGIOGENIC THERAPY

Resistance to Antiangiogenic Therapy

Despite the significant advance in the treatment of patients with recurrent GBM with the introduction of bevacizumab, most patients eventually become nonresponsive, and benefits in progression-free and OS are measured only in months (129). The underlying reasons for resistance to antiangiogenic therapy reside in the realization that tumor angiogenesis is a complex genetically heterogeneous process involving both tumor-mediated and host-mediated mechanisms (130). Preclinical and clinical studies indicate that during tumor angiogenesis as well as during VEGF-based antiangiogenic therapy, proangiogenic signaling pathways are upregulated in multiple cells, including endothelial cells, pericytes, bone marrow circulating cells, as well as cancer and other stromal cells. In particular, the process of tumor angiogenesis recruits several bone marrow–derived proangiogenic cells (BMDCs), including endothelial progenitor cells (EPCs), pericyte progenitor cells (131), which support tumor vessels, and $CD45^+$ "vascular modulatory" myeloid cells (132). BMDCs are recruited, in part through increases in HIF1α (133) which through induction of stromal-derived factor 1a (SDF1a), promotes tumor progression by recruiting vascular modulatory bone marrow–derived cells (BMDCs) to stimulate angiogenesis (134,135). Tumor microenvironmental stresses such as hypoxia and treatments with cytotoxic agents such as radiation therapy or chemotherapy contribute to recruitment of BMDCs into GBMs and their levels are increased in patients with malignant glioma (136).

Although VEGF is the prominent angiogenic factor, GBM frequently expresses other proangiogenic factors involved in different aspects of angiogenesis, such as PlGF, Ang-1 and Ang-2, PDGF, bFGF, SDF-1, IL-8, hepatocyte growth factor (HGF), and Delta-like 4 (Dll4) (137). In GBM patients treated with cediranib, bFGF, SDF-1, and viable circulating endothelial cells increase when tumors escape treatment (23). Thus, the existence of multiple vascularization mechanisms and angiogenic signaling pathways can compensate for the loss of VEGF activity under VEGF-based therapies such as bevacizumab treatment (130,137).

In addition to the above mechanisms of resistance, clinical studies indicate there is a population of patients who are intrinsically resistant, that is, do not respond at all to VEGF-targeted therapy, possibly indicating that their tumor cells may already express multiple proangiogenic pathways prior to antiangiogenic drug exposure because of the hypoxic microenvironment they are often found in.

Strategies for Overcoming Resistance to Antiangiogenic Therapy

Identification of Novel Targets for Antiangiogenic Therapy

Several exciting new investigations into the fundamental biology of tumor angiogenesis that may lead to novel targets include studies on the mechanisms that underlie formation of vascular tubes (138), identification of a dual endothelin-1/VEGF-signal peptide (DEspR) as playing a key role in vasculogenesis and angiogenesis (139) and the role of GPR124/TEM5, an orphan G protein-coupled receptor, in central nervous system angiogenesis (140).

Combination With Molecular Targeted Agents Inhibiting Other Relevant Targets

GBM formation is driven by many genetic and molecular alterations. Among the key pathways that are altered are the PI3K-AKT and EGFR-RAS-MEK-MAPK pathways with alterations in *EGFR, PI3K, PTEN, NF1,* and *RAS*; the p53 tumor suppressor pathway with alterations in *TP53, MDM2, MDM4, p14^ARF^*, RB, and cell cycle regulators with alterations in *RB1, CDK4, p16^INK4A^, CDKN2B*; and metabolic alterations in isocitrate dehydrogenase *(IDH1/IDH2)* (30). These pathways and their altered genes and products represent potential targeting areas for molecular targeted strategies. In addition, DNA repair mechanisms (Parp repair enzyme), tumor hypoxia (i.e., HIF-1α, carbonic anhydrase IX, glucose transporter 1), and the tumor microenvironment (i.e., tranforming growth factor-β, VEGF, and CXCR4) also provide targets for the development of molecular therapeutics for GBM. Combinations of antiangiogenic agents with molecular targeted agents may overcome the resistance that develops with single-agent therapy and could be incorporated either as part of initial therapy or later when disease resistance develops.

Combination of Antiangiogenic Therapy With Radiation and Chemotherapy

Currently there are a number of clinical trials which are combining antiangiogenic agents with chemotherapy or RT both in the frontline and recurrent settings (see section on clinical experience above). Bevacizumab, cediranib, vandetanib, aflibercept, XL184, and cilengitide are being evaluated in combination with standard therapy in newly diagnosed GBM patients. Other trials are evaluating combinations of antiangiogenic therapy with different cytotoxic agents or targeted agents in recurrent GBM patients in attempts to improve upon the efficacy gains already observed (141). Ultimately, optimal scheduling will depend upon a better understanding of mechanisms of interaction.

Multitargeting of More Than One Angiogenic Cytokine

There are many RTKIs currently in clinical trials that target more than one angiogenic cytokine. Examples are: sorafinib, sunitinib, cediranib, pazopanib, and vatalanib (see Table 2 and [30]).

Metronomic Angiogenic Chemotherapy

The concept, first reported in 2000, refers to the close regular administration of relatively low doses of conventional chemotherapy drugs with no prolonged breaks. Antitumor mechanisms of action include antiangiogenesis (e.g., by targeting dividing endothelial cells in the tumor neovasculature, as well as circulating host bone marrow–derived cells, and tumor cell HIF-1) (142). Metronomic chemotherapy is now undergoing randomized phase III clinical trial evaluation.

Interference With the Recruitment by Angiogenic Factors of Bone Marrow–Derived Cells (BMDCs) to Tumor Tissue for Revascularization

It has been shown preclinically that irradiation induces recruitment of proangiogenic BMDCs into intracranially implanted GBM xenografts, thereby restoring the radiation-damaged vasculature (134) and promoting tumor regrowth. This recruitment is in part stimulated through the interaction between the HIF-1-dependent stromal cell–derived factor-1 (SDF-1) and its receptor, CXCR4. AMD3100

(Plerixafor), a small molecule CXCR4 antagonist and an FDA-approved orphan drug, promotes the mobilization of BMDCs from the bone marrow niche to peripheral blood by inhibiting the interaction of SDF-1 with CXCR4 (134) and, therefore, has the potential to inhibit GBM revascularization following RT and improve tumor control.

Specific Targeting of Glioma Stem Cells in Combination With Antiangiogenic Drugs

GBM stem cells (GSCs) have been shown to overexpress VEGF and promote tumor angiogenesis and may therefore contribute to intrinsic resistance to antiangiogenic therapy (25). They have the potential to provide useful therapeutic targets in the treatment of recurrent or progressive GBMs. GSCs are regulated by molecular signaling pathways distinct from the bulk tumor (143). In particular, the Notch-mediated signaling pathway is very active in GSCs. It is dependent on the gamma secretase complex. Inhibition of Notch signaling by a gamma secretase inhibitor (GSI) impaired GSC tumorigenic potential in preclinical studies (144), thereby implicating GSIs as useful chemotherapeutic reagents to target GSCs in malignant gliomas. GSIs are in early clinical development for brain tumors (for a review of other signaling pathways in GSCs, see reference [143]).

Biomarkers of Response

A major challenge for improving the effectiveness of antiangiogenic therapy is how to best measure tumor response. This will depend on the identification and clinical validation of biomarkers to guide treatment for those individuals most likely to benefit from them. Currently no validated clinical biomarkers exist to stratify GBM patients to specific antiangiogenic drugs. However, a number of potential candidates are currently being studied in clinical trials. These candidates fall into different categories as follows: (a) *Imaging parameters:* Radiographic changes that occur after treatment with anti-VEGF agents; these changes are difficult to interpret because of the effect of these agents on vascular permeability, which results in diminished contrast enhancement on computed tomography or MRI scans. Current MRI techniques cannot clearly distinguish infiltrative tumor versus vasogenic edema (5). (b) *Candidate circulating biomarkers:* These include VEGF, which is elevated after anti-VEGF therapy; PlGF, a VEGF family member, also elevated after anti-VEGF therapy; circulating EPCs (136), which are also elevated following therapy; and soluble VEGFR-2, which decreases after therapy (145). The clinical significance and mechanisms regulating these changes are not well understood. (c) *Tissue biomarkers*: Tumor markers of hypoxia (Hif-1α, Hif-2α, carbonic anhydrase, Glut-1) (146,147). (d) *Systemic biomarkers:* Hypertension as a marker of VEGF pathway inhibition occurs in about 25% of cancer patients (147). (See review by Duda et al. for a more detailed discussion of putative biomarkers [147].)

Activation and Enhancement of Invasion and Metastasis by Antiangiogenic Therapy

Preclinical studies have shown that anti-VEGF treatment might enhance the migration of cancer cells from the primary tumor along adjacent preexisting blood vessels by mechanisms including cooption of normal blood vessels (vascular cooption) (148). In particular, in both clinical and preclinical studies, bevacizumab has been shown to induce an invasive tumor phenotype expressing insulin-like growth factor binding protein-2 and matrix metalloprotease-2 in GBM (149). Hypoxia induced by vessel regression after VEGF blockade can also switch on a more invasive and metastatic program. It has therefore been proposed that antiangiogenic agents may select for more invasive phenotypes and require the addition of alternative agents to overcome this invasive resistance.

■ CONCLUSIONS

A great deal of progress has been made in the biological understanding of tumor angiogenesis, the identification of angiogenic targets, and the development of antiangiogenic agents for these targets. Antiangiogenic therapy with bevacizumab has been validated for patients with recurrent GBM. However, despite these advances, the survival benefits of antiangiogenic treatments are relatively modest (usually measured in months) Among major challenges in the application of antiangiogenic therapy for GBM are (a) identifying better targets; it is now known that a variety of cell types in the tumor stroma and bone marrow participate in tumor angiogenesis and promotion and potentially provide new and better targets for antiangiogenesis development; (b) overcoming resistance to existing antiangiogenic agents; the upregulation of multiple proangiogenic pathways requires the development of alternative antiangiogenic strategies; (c) determining optimal scheduling, timing, and dosing of these agents with cytotoxic therapies; and (d) identifying clinically useful biomarkers that can predict the efficacy of these agents and guide treatment for those individuals most likely to benefit from them.

Antiangiogenic agents still hold great promise for alleviating GBM disease. Overcoming the existing challenges will require finetuning our understanding of GBM angiogenesis and the mechanisms of treatment resistance. Further preclinical and clinical studies should lead to more effective use of these agents to prolong the lives of GBM patients.

■ REFERENCES

1. Stupp R, Hegi ME, Mason WP, et al.; European Organisation for Research and Treatment of Cancer Brain Tumour and Radiation Oncology Groups; National Cancer Institute of Canada Clinical Trials Group. Effects of radiotherapy with concomitant and adjuvant temozolomide versus radiotherapy alone on survival in glioblastoma in a randomised phase III study: 5-year analysis of the EORTC-NCIC trial. *Lancet Oncol.* 2009;10(5):459–466.
2. Stupp R, Hegi ME, Gilbert MR, Chakravarti A. Chemoradiotherapy in malignant glioma: standard of care and future directions. *J Clin Oncol.* 2007;25(26):4127–4136.
3. Beal K, Abrey LE, Gutin PH. Antiangiogenic agents in the treatment of recurrent or newly diagnosed glioblastoma: analysis of single-agent and combined modality approaches. *Radiat Oncol.* 2011;6:2.
4. Dvorak HF, Nagy JA, Feng D, Brown LF, Dvorak AM. Vascular permeability factor/vascular endothelial growth factor and the significance of microvascular hyperpermeability in angiogenesis. *Curr Top Microbiol Immunol.* 1999;237:97–132.
5. Gerstner ER, Duda DG, di Tomaso E, et al. VEGF inhibitors in the treatment of cerebral edema in patients with brain cancer. *Nat Rev Clin Oncol.* 2009;6(4):229–236.
6. Sarkaria JN, Kitange GJ, James CD, et al. Mechanisms of chemoresistance to alkylating agents in malignant glioma. *Clin Cancer Res.* 2008;14(10):2900–2908.
7. Huang Q, Zhang QB, Dong J, et al. Glioma stem cells are more aggressive in recurrent tumors with malignant progression than in the primary tumor, and both can be maintained long-term *in vitro*. *BMC Cancer.* 2008;8:304.
8. Folkman J. Tumor angiogenesis: therapeutic implications. *N Engl J Med.* 1971;285(21):1182–1186.
9. Folkman J. The vascularization of tumors. *Sci Am.* 1976;234(5):58–64, 70.
10. Kaur B, Tan C, Brat DJ, Post DE, Van Meir EG. Genetic and hypoxic regulation of angiogenesis in gliomas. *J Neurooncol.* 2004;70(2):229–243.
11. Ferrara N. Role of vascular endothelial growth factor in physiologic and pathologic angiogenesis: therapeutic implications. *Semin Oncol.* 2002;29(6 Suppl 16):10–14.
12. Takano S, Yoshii Y, Kondo S, et al. Concentration of vascular endothelial growth factor in the serum and tumor tissue of brain tumor patients. *Cancer Res.* 1996;56(9):2185–2190.
13. Goussia AC, Bruner JM, Kyritsis AP, Agnantis NJ, Fuller GN. Cytogenetic and molecular genetic abnormalities in primitive neuroectodermal tumors of the central nervous system. *Anticancer Res.* 2000;20(1A):65–73.
14. Brat DJ, Van Meir EG. Glomeruloid microvascular proliferation orchestrated by VPF/VEGF: a new world of angiogenesis research. *Am J Pathol.* 2001;158(3):789–796.
15. Zundel W, Schindler C, Haas-Kogan D, et al. Loss of PTEN facilitates HIF-1-mediated gene expression. *Genes Dev.* 2000;14(4):391–396.
16. Duda DG, Jain RK, Willett CG. Antiangiogenics: the potential role of integrating this novel treatment modality with chemoradiation for solid cancers. *J Clin Oncol.* 2007;25(26):4033–4042.
17. Wachsberger P, Burd R, Dicker AP. Tumor response to ionizing radiation combined with antiangiogenesis or vascular targeting agents: exploring mechanisms of interaction. *Clin Cancer Res.* 2003;9(6):1957–1971.
18. Kerbel R, Folkman J. Clinical translation of angiogenesis inhibitors. *Nat Rev Cancer.* 2002;2(10):727–739.
19. Moeller BJ, Cao Y, Li CY, Dewhirst MW. Radiation activates HIF-1 to regulate vascular radiosensitivity in tumors: role of reoxygenation, free radicals, and stress granules. *Cancer Cell.* 2004;5(5):429–441.
20. Moeller BJ, Dreher MR, Rabbani ZN, et al. Pleiotropic effects of HIF-1 blockade on tumor radiosensitivity. *Cancer Cell.* 2005;8(2):99–110.
21. Jain RK. Normalization of tumor vasculature: an emerging concept in antiangiogenic therapy. *Science* 2005;307(5706):58–62.
22. Winkler F, Kozin SV, Tong RT, et al. Kinetics of vascular normalization by VEGFR2 blockade governs brain tumor response to radiation: role of oxygenation, angiopoietin-1, and matrix metalloproteinases. *Cancer Cell* 2004;6(6):553–563.
23. Batchelor TT, Sorensen AG, di Tomaso E, et al AZD2171, a pan-VEGF receptor tyrosine kinase inhibitor, normalizes tumor vasculature and alleviates edema in glioblastoma patients. *Cancer Cell.* 2007;11(1):83–95.
24. Garcia-Barros M, Paris F, Cordon-Cardo C, et al. Tumor response to radiotherapy regulated by endothelial cell apoptosis. *Science.* 2003;300(5622):1155–1159.
25. Bao S, Wu Q, Sathornsumetee S, et al. Stem cell-like glioma cells promote tumor angiogenesis through vascular endothelial growth factor. *Cancer Res.* 2006;66(16):7843–7848.

26. Folkins C, Shaked Y, Man S, et al. Glioma tumor stem-like cells promote tumor angiogenesis and vasculogenesis via vascular endothelial growth factor and stromal-derived factor 1. *Cancer Res.* 2009;69(18):7243–7251.

27. Hasumi Y, Mizukami H, Urabe M, et al. Soluble FLT-1 expression suppresses carcinomatous ascites in nude mice bearing ovarian cancer. *Cancer Res.* 2002;62(7):2019–2023.

28. Holash J, Davis S, Papadopoulos N, et al. VEGF-Trap: a VEGF blocker with potent antitumor effects. *Proc Natl Acad Sci USA.* 2002;99(17):11393–11398.

29. Wachsberger PR, Burd R, Cardi C, et al. VEGF trap in combination with radiotherapy improves tumor control in u87 glioblastoma. *Int J Radiat Oncol Biol Phys.* 2007;67(5):1526–1537.

30. Bai RY, Staedtke V, Riggins GJ. Molecular targeting of glioblastoma: Drug discovery and therapies. *Trends Mol Med.* 2011;17(6):301–312.

31. Oliner J, Min H, Leal J, et al. Suppression of angiogenesis and tumor growth by selective inhibition of angiopoietin-2. *Cancer Cell.* 2004;6(5):507–516.

32. D'Abaco GM, Kaye AH. Integrins: molecular determinants of glioma invasion. *J Clin Neurosci.* 2007;14(11):1041–1048.

33. Xiong JP, Stehle T, Zhang R, et al. Crystal structure of the extracellular segment of integrin alpha Vbeta3 in complex with an Arg-Gly-Asp ligand. *Science.* 2002;296(5565):151–155.

34. Van Meter ME, Kim ES. Bevacizumab: current updates in treatment. *Curr Opin Oncol.* 2010;22(6):586–591.

35. Vredenburgh JJ, Desjardins A, Herndon JE 2nd, et al. Bevacizumab plus irinotecan in recurrent glioblastoma multiforme. *J Clin Oncol.* 2007;25(30):4722–4729.

36. Vredenburgh JJ, Desjardins A, Herndon JE 2nd, et al. Phase II trial of bevacizumab and irinotecan in recurrent malignant glioma. *Clin Cancer Res.* 2007;13(4):1253–1259.

37. Hurwitz H, Fehrenbacher L, Novotny W, et al. Bevacizumab plus irinotecan, fluorouracil, and leucovorin for metastatic colorectal cancer. *N Engl J Med.* 2004;350(23):2335–2342.

38. Desjardins A, Vredenburgh JJ, Reardon DA, et al. Long-term survival from the initial trial of bevacizumab and irinotecan. *J Clin Oncol.* 2010;28:191S.

39. Kreisl TN, Kim L, Moore K, et al. Phase II trial of single-agent bevacizumab followed by bevacizumab plus irinotecan at tumor progression in recurrent glioblastoma. *J Clin Oncol.* 2009;27(5):740–745.

40. Friedman HS, Prados MD, Wen PY, et al. Bevacizumab alone and in combination with irinotecan in recurrent glioblastoma. *J Clin Oncol.* 2009;27(28):4733–4740.

41. Wick W, Weller M, van den Bent M, Stupp R. Bevacizumab and recurrent malignant gliomas: a European perspective. *J Clin Oncol.* 2010;28(12):e188–9; author reply e190.

42. Reardon DA, Turner S, Peters KB, et al. A review of VEGF/VEGFR-targeted therapeutics for recurrent glioblastoma. *J Natl Compr Canc Netw.* 2011;9(4):414–427.

43. Raizer JJ, Grimm S, Chamberlain MC, et al. A phase 2 trial of single-agent bevacizumab given in an every-3-week schedule for patients with recurrent high-grade gliomas. *Cancer.* 2010;116(22):5297–5305.

44. Fogh SE, Andrews DW, Glass J, et al. Hypofractionated stereotactic radiation therapy: an effective therapy for recurrent high-grade gliomas. *J Clin Oncol.* 2010;28(18):3048–3053.

45. Gutin PH, Iwamoto FM, Beal K, et al. Safety and efficacy of bevacizumab with hypofractionated stereotactic irradiation for recurrent malignant gliomas. *Int J Radiat Oncol Biol Phys.* 2009;75(1):156–163.

46. Cuneo KC, Vredenburgh JJ, Sampson JH, et al. Safety and efficacy of stereotactic radiosurgery and adjuvant bevacizumab in patients with recurrent malignant gliomas. *Int J Radiat Oncol Biol Phys.* 2012;82(5):2018–2024.

47. Ananthnarayan S, Bahng J, Roring J, et al. Time course of imaging changes of GBM during extended bevacizumab treatment. *J Neurooncol.* 2008;88(3):339–347.

48. Quant EC, Norden AD, Drappatz J, et al. Role of a second chemotherapy in recurrent malignant glioma patients who progress on bevacizumab. *Neuro-oncology.* 2009;11(5):550–555.

49. Lai A, Tran A, Nghiemphu PL, et al. Phase II study of bevacizumab plus temozolomide during and after radiation therapy for patients with newly diagnosed glioblastoma multiforme. *J Clin Oncol.* 2011;29(2):142–148.

50. Vredenburgh JJ, Desjardins A, Reardon DA, et al. The addition of bevacizumab to standard radiation therapy and temozolomide followed by bevacizumab, temozolomide, and irinotecan for newly diagnosed glioblastoma. *Clin Cancer Res.* 2011;17(12):4119–4124.

51. Vredenburgh JJ, Desjardins A, Kirkpatrick JP, et al. Addition of bevacizumab to standard radiation therapy and daily temozolomide is associated with minimal toxicity in newly diagnosed glioblastoma multiforme. *Int J Radiat Oncol Biol Phys.* 2012;82(1):58–66.

52. Chinot OL, de La Motte Rouge T, Moore N, et al. AVAglio: Phase 3 trial of bevacizumab plus temozolomide and radiotherapy in newly diagnosed glioblastoma multiforme. *Adv Ther.* 2011;28(4):334–340.

53. Lockhart AC, Rothenberg ML, Dupont J, et al. Phase I study of intravenous vascular endothelial growth factor trap, aflibercept, in patients with advanced solid tumors. *J Clin Oncol.* 2010;28(2):207–214.

54. Wang-Gillam A, Tew WP, Rothenberg ML, et al. A phase I study of subcutaneously administered aflibercept (VEGF trap) in a new formulation in patients with advanced solid tumors. *Invest New Drugs.* 2011;doi: 10.1007/s10637-011-9753-y.

55. de Groot JF, Lamborn KR, Chang SM, et al. Phase II study of aflibercept in recurrent malignant glioma: a North American Brain Tumor Consortium study. *J Clin Oncol.* 2011;29(19):2689–2695.

56. Dietrich J, Wang D, Batchelor TT. Cediranib: profile of a novel anti-angiogenic agent in patients with glioblastoma. *Expert Opin Investig Drugs.* 2009;18(10):1549–1557.

57. Drevs J, Siegert P, Medinger M, et al. Phase I clinical study of AZD2171, an oral vascular endothelial growth factor signaling inhibitor, in patients with advanced solid tumors. *J Clin Oncol.* 2007;25(21):3045–3054.

58. Ryan CJ, Stadler WM, Roth B, et al. Phase I dose escalation and pharmacokinetic study of AZD2171, an inhibitor of the vascular endothelial growth factor receptor tyrosine kinase, in patients with hormone refractory prostate cancer (HRPC). *Invest New Drugs.* 2007;25(5):445–451.

59. Fox E, Aplenc R, Bagatell R, et al. A phase 1 trial and pharmacokinetic study of cediranib, an orally bioavailable pan-vascular endothelial growth factor receptor inhibitor, in children and adolescents with refractory solid tumors. *J Clin Oncol.* 2010;28(35):5174–5181.

60. Lorusso P, Shields AF, Gadgeel S, et al. Cediranib in combination with various anticancer regimens: results of a phase I multi-cohort study. *Invest New Drugs.* 2011;29(6):1395–1405.

61. Yamamoto N, Tamura T, Yamamoto N, et al. Phase I, dose escalation and pharmacokinetic study of cediranib (RECENTIN), a highly potent and selective VEGFR signaling inhibitor, in Japanese patients with advanced solid tumors. *Cancer Chemother Pharmacol.* 2009;64(6):1165–1172.

62. Laurie SA, Gauthier I, Arnold A, et al. Phase I and pharmacokinetic study of daily oral AZD2171, an inhibitor of vascular endothelial growth factor tyrosine kinases, in combination with carboplatin and paclitaxel in patients with advanced non-small-cell lung cancer: the National Cancer Institute of Canada clinical trials group. *J Clin Oncol.* 2008;26(11):1871–1878.

63. Batchelor TT, Duda DG, di Tomaso E, et al. Phase II study of cediranib, an oral pan-vascular endothelial growth factor receptor tyrosine kinase inhibitor, in patients with recurrent glioblastoma. *J Clin Oncol.* 2010;28(17):2817–2823.

64. Batchelor T, Mulholland P, Neyns B, et al. A phase III randomized study comparing the efficacy of cediranib as monotherapy, and in combination with lomustine, with lomustine alone in recurrent glioblastoma patients. *Ann Oncol.* 2010;21(suppl 8):2817–2823.

65. Tomuleasa C, Cristea V, Irimie A. Sorafenib for advanced-stage hepatocellular carcinoma. *Eur J Gastroenterol Hepatol.* 2012;24(3):346–347.

66. Strumberg D. Sorafenib for the treatment of renal cancer. *Expert Opin Pharmacother.* 2012;13(3):407–419.

67. Jane EP, Premkumar DR, Pollack IF. Coadministration of sorafenib with rottlerin potently inhibits cell proliferation and migration in human malignant glioma cells. *J Pharmacol Exp Ther.* 2006;319(3):1070–1080.

68. Yang F, Brown C, Buettner R, et al. Sorafenib induces growth arrest and apoptosis of human glioblastoma cells through the dephosphorylation of signal transducers and activators of transcription 3. *Mol Cancer Ther.* 2010;9(4):953–962.

69. Siegelin MD, Raskett CM, Gilbert CA, Ross AH, Altieri DC. Sorafenib exerts anti-glioma activity *in vitro* and in vivo. *Neurosci Lett.* 2010;478(3):165–170.

70. Nabors LB, Supko JG, Rosenfeld M, et al.; New Approaches to Brain Tumor Therapy (NABTT) CNS Consortium. Phase I trial of sorafenib in patients with recurrent or progressive malignant glioma. *Neuro-oncology.* 2011;13(12):1324–1330.

71. Hainsworth JD, Ervin T, Friedman E, et al. Concurrent radiotherapy and temozolomide followed by temozolomide and sorafenib in the first-line treatment of patients with glioblastoma multiforme. *Cancer.* 2010;116(15):3663–3669.

72. Reardon DA, Vredenburgh JJ, Desjardins A, et al. Effect of CYP3A-inducing anti-epileptics on sorafenib exposure: results of a phase II study of sorafenib plus daily temozolomide in adults with recurrent glioblastoma. *J Neurooncol.* 2011;101(1):57–66.

73. Reardon DA, Vredenburgh JJ, Coan A, et al. Phase I study of sunitinib and irinotecan for patients with recurrent malignant glioma. *J Neurooncol.* 2011;105(3):621–627.

74. Neyns B, Sadones J, Chaskis C, et al. Phase II study of sunitinib malate in patients with recurrent high-grade glioma. *J Neurooncol.* 2011;103(3):491–501.

75. Iwamoto FM, Lamborn KR, Robins HI, et al. Phase II trial of pazopanib (GW786034), an oral multi-targeted angiogenesis inhibitor, for adults with recurrent glioblastoma (North American Brain Tumor Consortium Study 06–02). *Neuro-oncology.* 2010;12(8):855–861.

76. Drappatz J, Norden AD, Wong ET, et al. Phase I study of vandetanib with radiotherapy and temozolomide for newly diagnosed glioblastoma. *Int J Radiat Oncol Biol Phys.* 2010;78(1):85–90.

77. Fields EC, Damek D, Gaspar LE, et al. Phase I dose escalation trial of vandetanib with fractionated radiosurgery in patients with recurrent malignant gliomas. *Int J Radiat Oncol Biol Phys.* 2012;82(1):51–57.

78. Reardon DA, Egorin MJ, Desjardins A, et al. Phase I pharmacokinetic study of the vascular endothelial growth factor receptor tyrosine kinase inhibitor vatalanib (PTK787) plus imatinib and hydroxyurea for malignant glioma. *Cancer.* 2009;115(10):2188–2198.

79. Gerstner ER, Eichler AF, Plotkin SR, et al. Phase I trial with biomarker studies of vatalanib (PTK787) in patients with newly diagnosed glioblastoma treated with enzyme inducing anti-epileptic drugs and standard radiation and temozolomide. *J Neurooncol.* 2011;103(2):325–332.

80. Brandes AA, Stupp R, Hau P, et al. EORTC study 26041–22041: phase I/II study on concomitant and adjuvant temozolomide (TMZ) and radiotherapy (RT) with PTK787/ZK222584 (PTK/ZK) in newly diagnosed glioblastoma. *Eur J Cancer.* 2010;46(2):348–354.

81. Spratlin J. Ramucirumab (IMC-1121B): Monoclonal antibody inhibition of vascular endothelial growth factor receptor-2. *Curr Oncol Rep.* 2011;13(2):97–102.

82. Mamluk R, Carvajal IM, Morse BA, et al. Anti-tumor effect of CT-322 as an adnectin inhibitor of vascular endothelial growth factor receptor-2. *MAbs.* 2010;2(2):199–208.

83. Smith JW. Cilengitide Merck. *Curr Opin Investig Drugs.* 2003;4(6):741–745.

84. Nisato RE, Tille JC, Jonczyk A, Goodman SL, Pepper MS. Alphav beta 3 and alphav beta 5 integrin antagonists inhibit angiogenesis *in vitro*. *Angiogenesis*. 2003;6(2):105–119.

85. MacDonald TJ, Taga T, Shimada H, et al. Preferential susceptibility of brain tumors to the antiangiogenic effects of an alpha(v) integrin antagonist. *Neurosurgery*. 2001;48(1):151–157.

86. Nabors LB, Mikkelsen T, Rosenfeld SS, et al. Phase I and correlative biology study of cilengitide in patients with recurrent malignant glioma. *J Clin Oncol*. 2007;25(13):1651–1657.

87. MacDonald TJ, Stewart CF, Kocak M, et al. Phase I clinical trial of cilengitide in children with refractory brain tumors: Pediatric Brain Tumor Consortium Study PBTC-012. *J Clin Oncol*. 2008;26(6):919–924.

88. Reardon DA, Fink KL, Mikkelsen T, et al. Randomized phase II study of cilengitide, an integrin-targeting arginine-glycine-aspartic acid peptide, in recurrent glioblastoma multiforme. *J Clin Oncol*. 2008;26(34):5610–5617.

89. Gilbert MR, Kuhn J, Lamborn KR, et al. Cilengitide in patients with recurrent glioblastoma: the results of NABTC 03–02, a phase II trial with measures of treatment delivery. *J Neurooncol*. 2012;106(1):147–153.

90. Stupp R, Hegi ME, Neyns B, et al. Phase I/IIa study of cilengitide and temozolomide with concomitant radiotherapy followed by cilengitide and temozolomide maintenance therapy in patients with newly diagnosed glioblastoma. *J Clin Oncol*. 2010;28(16):2712–2718.

91. Nabors LB, Mikkelsen T, Batchelor T, et al. A randomized phase II trial of EMD 121974 in conjunction with concomitant and adjuvant temozolomide with radiation therapy in patients with newly diagnosed glioblastoma multiforme (GBM). *J Clin Oncol*. 2006;27:15s, suppl:abstract 2001.

92. Stupp R, Mason WP, van den Bent MJ, et al.; European Organisation for Research and Treatment of Cancer Brain Tumor and Radiotherapy Groups; National Cancer Institute of Canada Clinical Trials Group. Radiotherapy plus concomitant and adjuvant temozolomide for glioblastoma. *N Engl J Med*. 2005;352(10):987–996.

93. Hegi ME, Diserens AC, Gorlia T, et al. MGMT gene silencing and benefit from temozolomide in glioblastoma. *N Engl J Med*. 2005;352(10):997–1003.

94. Paravar T, Lee DJ. Thalidomide: mechanisms of action. *Int Rev Immunol*. 2008;27(3):111–135.

95. D'Amato RJ, Loughnan MS, Flynn E, Folkman J. Thalidomide is an inhibitor of angiogenesis. *Proc Natl Acad Sci USA*. 1994;91(9):4082–4085.

96. Fine HA, Figg WD, Jaeckle K, et al. Phase II trial of the antiangiogenic agent thalidomide in patients with recurrent high-grade gliomas. *J Clin Oncol*. 2000;18(4):708–715.

97. Marx GM, Pavlakis N, McCowatt S, et al. Phase II study of thalidomide in the treatment of recurrent glioblastoma multiforme. *J Neurooncol*. 2001;54(1):31–38.

98. Fine HA, Wen PY, Maher EA, et al. Phase II trial of thalidomide and carmustine for patients with recurrent high-grade gliomas. *J Clin Oncol*. 2003;21(12):2299–2304.

99. Groves MD, Puduvalli VK, Chang SM, et al. A North American brain tumor consortium (NABTC 99–04) phase II trial of temozolomide plus thalidomide for recurrent glioblastoma multiforme. *J Neurooncol*. 2007;81(3):271–277.

100. Giglio P, Dhamne M, Hess KR, et al. Phase 2 trial of irinotecan and thalidomide in adults with recurrent anaplastic glioma. *Cancer*. 2011;doi: 10.1002/cncr.26663.

101. Chang SM, Lamborn KR, Malec M, et al. Phase II study of temozolomide and thalidomide with radiation therapy for newly diagnosed glioblastoma multiforme. *Int J Radiat Oncol Biol Phys*. 2004;60(2):353–357.

102. Turner CD, Chi S, Marcus KJ, et al. Phase II study of thalidomide and radiation in children with newly diagnosed brain stem gliomas and glioblastoma multiforme. *J Neurooncol*. 2007;82(1):95–101.

103. Butowski N, Prados MD, Lamborn KR, et al. A phase II study of concurrent temozolomide and cis-retinoic acid with radiation for adult patients with newly diagnosed supratentorial glioblastoma. *Int J Radiat Oncol Biol Phys*. 2005;61(5):1454–1459.

104. Kesari S, Schiff D, Henson JW, et al. Phase II study of temozolomide, thalidomide, and celecoxib for newly diagnosed glioblastoma in adults. *Neuro-oncology*. 2008;10(3):300–308.

105. Tageja N. Lenalidomide—current understanding of mechanistic properties. *Anticancer Agents Med Chem*. 2011;11(3):315–326.

106. Drappatz J, Wong ET, Schiff D, et al. A pilot safety study of lenalidomide and radiotherapy for patients with newly diagnosed glioblastoma multiforme. *Int J Radiat Oncol Biol Phys*. 2009;73(1):222–227.

107. Fine HA, Kim L, Albert PS, et al. A phase I trial of lenalidomide in patients with recurrent primary central nervous system tumors. *Clin Cancer Res*. 2007;13(23):7101–7106.

108. Lindahl P, Johansson BR, Levéen P, Betsholtz C. Pericyte loss and microaneurysm formation in PDGF-B-deficient mice. *Science*. 1997;277(5323):242–245.

109. Adams EF, Todo T, Schrell UM, Thierauf P, White MC, Fahlbusch R. Autocrine control of human meningioma proliferation: secretion of platelet-derived growth-factor-like molecules. *Int J Cancer*. 1991;49(3):398–402.

110. Hermanson M, Funa K, Hartman M, et al. Platelet-derived growth factor and its receptors in human glioma tissue: expression of messenger RNA and protein suggests the presence of autocrine and paracrine loops. *Cancer Res*. 1992;52(11):3213–3219.

111. Nistér M, Libermann TA, Betsholtz C, et al. Expression of messenger RNAs for platelet-derived growth factor and transforming growth factor-alpha and their receptors in human malignant glioma cell lines. *Cancer Res*. 1988;48(14):3910–3918.

112. Savage DG, Antman KH. Imatinib mesylate–a new oral targeted therapy. *N Engl J Med*. 2002;346(9):683–693.

113. Raymond E, Brandes AA, Dittrich C, et al.; European Organisation for Research and Treatment of Cancer Brain Tumor Group Study. Phase II study of imatinib in patients with recurrent gliomas of various histologies: a European Organisation for Research and Treatment of Cancer Brain Tumor Group Study. *J Clin Oncol.* 2008;26(28):4659–4665.

114. Reardon DA, Dresemann G, Taillibert S, et al. Multicentre phase II studies evaluating imatinib plus hydroxyurea in patients with progressive glioblastoma. *Br J Cancer.* 2009;101(12):1995–2004.

115. Reardon DA, Egorin MJ, Quinn JA, et al. Phase II study of imatinib mesylate plus hydroxyurea in adults with recurrent glioblastoma multiforme. *J Clin Oncol.* 2005;23(36):9359–9368.

116. Dresemann G, Weller M, Rosenthal MA, et al. Imatinib in combination with hydroxyurea versus hydroxyurea alone as oral therapy in patients with progressive pre-treated glioblastoma resistant to standard dose temozolomide. *J Neurooncol.* 2010;96(3):393–402.

117. Olivieri A, Manzione L. Dasatinib: a new step in molecular target therapy. *Ann Oncol.* 2007;18(Suppl 6):vi42–46.

118. Cheng Y, Paz K. Tandutinib, an oral, small-molecule inhibitor of FLT3 for the treatment of AML and other cancer indications. *IDrugs.* 2008;11(1):46–56.

119. Altorki NK, Keresztes RS, Port JL, et al. Celecoxib, a selective cyclo-oxygenase-2 inhibitor, enhances the response to preoperative paclitaxel and carboplatin in early-stage non-small-cell lung cancer. *J Clin Oncol.* 2003;21(14):2645–2650.

120. Kang KB, Wang TT, Woon CT, et al. Enhancement of glioblastoma radioresponse by a selective COX-2 inhibitor celecoxib: inhibition of tumor angiogenesis with extensive tumor necrosis. *Int J Radiat Oncol Biol Phys.* 2007;67(3):888–896.

121. Reardon DA, Quinn JA, Vredenburgh J, et al. Phase II trial of irinotecan plus celecoxib in adults with recurrent malignant glioma. *Cancer.* 2005;103(2):329–338.

122. Roy R, Yang J, Moses MA. Matrix metalloproteinases as novel biomarkers and potential therapeutic targets in human cancer. *J Clin Oncol.* 2009;27(31):5287–5297.

123. (No authors listed) Marimastat: BB 2516, TA 2516. *Drugs R D.* 2003;4:198–203.

124. Groves MD, Puduvalli VK, Hess KR, et al. Phase II trial of temozolomide plus the matrix metalloproteinase inhibitor, marimastat, in recurrent and progressive glioblastoma multiforme. *J Clin Oncol.* 2002;20(5):1383–1388.

125. Groves MD, Puduvalli VK, Conrad CA, et al. Phase II trial of temozolomide plus marimastat for recurrent anaplastic gliomas: a relationship among efficacy, joint toxicity and anticonvulsant status. *J Neurooncol.* 2006;80(1):83–90.

126. Levin VA, Phuphanich S, Yung WK, et al. Randomized, double-blind, placebo-controlled trial of marimastat in glioblastoma multiforme patients following surgery and irradiation. *J Neurooncol.* 2006;78(3):295–302.

127. Huang H, Bhat A, Woodnutt G, Lappe R. Targeting the ANGPT-TIE2 pathway in malignancy. *Nat Rev Cancer.* 2010;10(8):575–585.

128. Neal J, Wakelee H. AMG-386, a selective angiopoietin-1/-2-neutralizing peptibody for the potential treatment of cancer. *Curr Opin Mol Ther.* 2010;12(4):487–495.

129. Iwamoto FM, Abrey LE, Beal K, et al. Patterns of relapse and prognosis after bevacizumab failure in recurrent glioblastoma. *Neurology.* 2009;73(15):1200–1206.

130. Ebos JM, Lee CR, Kerbel RS. Tumor and host-mediated pathways of resistance and disease progression in response to antiangiogenic therapy. *Clin Cancer Res.* 2009;15(16):5020–5025.

131. Lamagna C, Bergers G. The bone marrow constitutes a reservoir of pericyte progenitors. *J Leukoc Biol.* 2006;80(4):677–681.

132. Yang L, DeBusk LM, Fukuda K, et al. Expansion of myeloid immune suppressor Gr+CD11b+ cells in tumor-bearing host directly promotes tumor angiogenesis. *Cancer Cell.* 2004;6(4):409–421.

133. Du R, Lu KV, Petritsch C, et al. HIF1alpha induces the recruitment of bone marrow-derived vascular modulatory cells to regulate tumor angiogenesis and invasion. *Cancer Cell.* 2008;13(3):206–220.

134. Kioi M, Vogel H, Schultz G, Hoffman RM, Harsh GR, Brown JM. Inhibition of vasculogenesis, but not angiogenesis, prevents the recurrence of glioblastoma after irradiation in mice. *J Clin Invest.* 2010;120(3):694–705.

135. Kozin SV, Kamoun WS, Huang Y, Dawson MR, Jain RK, Duda DG. Recruitment of myeloid but not endothelial precursor cells facilitates tumor regrowth after local irradiation. *Cancer Res.* 2010;70(14):5679–5685.

136. Rafat N, Beck GCh, Schulte J, Tuettenberg J, Vajkoczy P. Circulating endothelial progenitor cells in malignant gliomas. *J Neurosurg.* 2010;112(1):43–49.

137. Bergers G, Hanahan D. Modes of resistance to anti-angiogenic therapy. *Nat Rev Cancer.* 2008;8(8):592–603.

138. Xu K, Cleaver O. Tubulogenesis during blood vessel formation. *Semin Cell Dev Biol.* 2011;22(9):993–1004.

139. Herrera VL, Ponce LR, Bagamasbad PD, VanPelt BD, Didishvili T, Ruiz-Opazo N. Embryonic lethality in Dear gene-deficient mice: new player in angiogenesis. *Physiol Genomics.* 2005;23(3):257–268.

140. Kuhnert F, Mancuso MR, Shamloo A, et al. Essential regulation of CNS angiogenesis by the orphan G protein-coupled receptor GPR124. *Science.* 2010;330(6006):985–989.

141. Chi A, Norden AD, Wen PY. Inhibition of angiogenesis and invasion in malignant gliomas. *Expert Rev Anticancer Ther.* 2007;7(11):1537–1560.

142. Kerbel RS, Kamen BA. The anti-angiogenic basis of metronomic chemotherapy. *Nat Rev Cancer.* 2004;4(6):423–436.

143. Huang Z, Cheng L, Guryanova OA, Wu Q, Bao S. Cancer stem cells in glioblastoma–molecular signaling and therapeutic targeting. *Protein Cell.* 2010;1(7):638–655.

144. Fan X, Khaki L, Zhu TS, et al. NOTCH pathway blockade depletes CD133-positive glioblastoma cells and inhibits growth of tumor neurospheres and xenografts. *Stem Cells.* 2010;28(1):5–16.

145. Jubb AM, Oates AJ, Holden S, Koeppen H. Predicting benefit from anti-angiogenic agents in malignancy. *Nat Rev Cancer.* 2006;6(8):626–635.

146. Sathornsumetee S, Cao Y, Marcello JE, et al. Tumor angiogenic and hypoxic profiles predict radiographic response and survival in malignant astrocytoma patients treated with bevacizumab and irinotecan. *J Clin Oncol.* 2008;26(2):271–278.

147. Duda DG, Ancukiewicz M, Jain RK. Biomarkers of antiangiogenic therapy: how do we move from candidate biomarkers to valid biomarkers? *J Clin Oncol.* 2010;28(2):183–185.

148. Rubenstein JL, Kim J, Ozawa T, et al. Anti-VEGF antibody treatment of glioblastoma prolongs survival but results in increased vascular cooption. *Neoplasia.* 2000;2(4):306–314.

149. de Groot JF, Fuller G, Kumar AJ, et al. Tumor invasion after treatment of glioblastoma with bevacizumab: radiographic and pathologic correlation in humans and mice. *Neuro-oncology.* 2010;12(3):233–242.

150. Reardon DA, Desjardins A, Vredenburgh JJ, et al. Metronomic chemotherapy with daily, oral etoposide plus bevacizumab for recurrent malignant glioma: a phase II study. *Br J Cancer.* 2009;101(12):1986–1994.

151. Hasselbalch B, Lassen U, Hansen S, et al. Cetuximab, bevacizumab, and irinotecan for patients with primary glioblastoma and progression after radiation therapy and temozolomide: a phase II trial. *Neuro-oncology.* 2010;12(5):508–516.

152. Sathornsumetee S, Desjardins A, Vredenburgh JJ, et al. Phase II trial of bevacizumab and erlotinib in patients with recurrent malignant glioma. *Neuro-oncology.* 2010;12(12):1300–1310.

153. Reardon DA, Desjardins A, Peters KB, et al. Phase II study of carboplatin, irinotecan, and bevacizumab for bevacizumab naive, recurrent glioblastoma. *J Neurooncol.* 2011.

154. Desjardins A, Reardon DA, Coan A, et al. Bevacizumab and daily temozolomide for recurrent glioblastoma. *Cancer.* 2012;118(5):1302–1312.

demos MEDICAL

RADIATION MEDICINE ROUNDS

Kinase Inhibitors in the Treatment of Malignant Gliomas: Current Indications and New Directions

Adam Maier[1] and Arnab Chakravarti[2]

[1]*Clinical Resident, Department of Radiation Oncology, Arthur G. James Comprehensive Cancer Center and Richard L. Solove Research Institute, The Wexner Medical Center at The Ohio State University, Columbus, OH*

[2]*Chair and Professor, Department of Radiation Oncology, Arthur G. James Comprehensive Cancer Center and Richard L. Solove Research Institute, The Wexner Medical Center at The Ohio State University, Columbus, OH*

ABSTRACT

Receptor tyrosine kinases (RTKs) are cell-signaling proteins that regulate growth, metabolism, differentiation, survival, and cell-cycle control. RTK activity has been shown to be dysregulated in malignant gliomas. This chapter provides an overview of major known abnormal signaling pathways in malignant glioma. We discuss clinical data from a representative group of tyrosine kinase inhibitors being studied in malignant gliomas. Blocking RTK activity has shown promise in preclinical trials, but success has yet to be realized in randomized phase III trials. We also review the theory of vascular normalization and methods of measuring tumor response utilizing imaging and biomarker studies.

Keywords: tyrosine kinase inhibitors, malignant glioma, GBM, vascular normalization

Receptor tyrosine kinases (RTKs) are a diverse group of signaling proteins that serve as a bridge between the external and internal cellular environments. RTKs regulate instrumental activities including growth, metabolism, differentiation, cell survival, and cell-cycle control. There are over 50 known RTKs that can be further characterized into 20 subfamilies. There are also many non-RTKs that play a role in cancer development and proliferation. RTKs typically consist of an extracellular domain, an α-helix component located within the cell membrane, and an intracellular protein kinase domain (1,2).

The activation of a RTK typically involves a ligand binding to the extracellular domain, thereby inducing receptor dimerization. This conformational change results in autophosphorylation of the cytoplasmic domain of the RTK, ultimately leading to the activation of intracellular signaling pathways. Interestingly, exceptions to the strict dimerization-to-activation hypothesis have been shown to include receptor oligomerization and receptor cross-communication. For example, insulin-like growth factor-1 (IGF-1) may transduce epithelial growth factor (EGF) pathway signaling in glioblastoma multiforme (GBM) (3–5).

The discovery of RTKs, many of which are oncogenes, paved the way for a renaissance in our

*Corresponding author, Department of Radiation Oncology, Arthur G. James Comprehensive Cancer Center and Richard L. Solove Research Institute, The Ohio State University, Columbus, OH

E-mail address: adam.maier@osumc.edu

Radiation Medicine Rounds 3:2 (2012) 261–274.

DOI: 10.5003/2151–4208.3.2.261

understanding of cancer (2). Agents that successfully target aberrant RTK activity have jumped into the spotlight as effective treatments for a variety of cancers. Imatinib is a tyrosine kinase inhibitor (TKI) used in gastrointestinal stromal tumor (GIST) and Philadelphia chromosome-positive chronic myelogenous leukemia (Ph^+ CML) (6–8). Erlotinib is TKI with activity against human epidermal growth factor receptor 1 (HER1/EGFR) that improves outcomes in non-small cell lung cancer (NSCLC) patients with mutant EGFR (9). Crizotinib, a TKI that targets anaplastic lymphoma kinase (ALK), improves survival in NSCLC patients with chromosomal rearrangements of ALK (10,11).

Targeted therapies are efficacious because the aberrant processes they disrupt are specific to and necessary for the proliferation of the diseases they treat. The apparent lack of dependence of GBM on any one individual pathway for survival makes finding a single-agent "cure" unlikely. Glioblastoma has many well-described genetic alterations. Mutations in the RTK/RAS/PI3K, retinoblastoma (RB), and p53 signaling pathways are present in 88%, 78%, and 87% of GBM, respectively (12). Blocking these pathways individually has shown promise in preclinical trials, but success has yet to be realized in randomized phase III trials.

Although targeted therapies for GBM hold the promise of improving therapeutic outcomes, radiation combined with a "nontargeted" cytotoxic agent, temozolomide (TMZ), is the current standard of care. TMZ is effective through a global alkylating mechanism of action. Concurrent chemoradiation followed with six months of maintenance TMZ remains the current standard of care in the treatment of newly diagnosed GBM. The addition of concurrent and maintenance TMZ to radiation therapy in newly diagnosed GBM increases median survival from 12.1 to 14.6 months and boosts survival at 5 years from roughly 2% to 10% (13,14).

Outcomes of patients with GBM in the recurrent setting are correspondingly dismal. Even with the addition of the targeted vascular endothelial growth factor (VEGF) antibody bevacizumab, 6-month progression-free survival (PFS) in recurrent GBM (rGBM) is roughly 40% to 50%. The median overall survival (OS) is approximately 9 months (15,16). RTOG 0825, a phase III randomized study, is underway examining bevacizumab in conjunction with TMZ and radiation in the upfront setting for newly diagnosed GBM patients.

Early data for TKI use in treating GBM has been encouraging. Improvements in outcomes have failed, however, to materialize into survival gains in randomized clinical trials. Despite the obvious theoretical advantage of targeted therapies, impairing DNA replication through alkylation remains the most efficacious systemic therapy in GBM. Although they are often referred to as targeted therapy, many TKIs actually show activity against multiple tyrosine kinases.

This chapter will provide an overview of relevant signaling pathways being targeted by TKIs in malignant gliomas. We review the evolving theory of vascular normalization as well as methods to measure response to therapy via advanced imaging techniques and biomarker studies. We finally discuss clinical data from a representative group of TKIs across various signaling pathways.

■ KEY PATHWAY: VEGF

In 1983, Ferrara and colleagues discovered a compound secreted by tumor cells they termed the vascular permeability factor (VPF) (17). VPF was highly conserved, found in several species, and induced a "rapid and completely reversible increase in micro vascular permeability" (18). Leung and colleagues reported the VEGF later that same decade. VEGF was "specific for vascular endothelial cells" and was "able to induce angiogenesis in vivo" (19) VEGF and VPF were eventually found to be the same protein (20). VEGF binds with high affinity to the RTK KDR/Flk-1, also known as the VEGF receptor 2 (VEGFR-2), and is mediator of endothelial cell related angiogenesis (21,22).

The expression of VEGF in glioblastoma is an independent prognostic marker and is associated with poor survival (23,24). Levels of VEGF have been shown to correlate with microvessel density and tumor grade in GBM (25,26). The binding of VEGF to VEGFR-2 results in endothelial cell contraction, weakening of the vascular endothelial to cadherin linkage, and promotion of the migration of endothelial cells (27). Thus, in the presence of VEGF the integrity of the already weakened foundation of tumor vessels becomes even less stable. These vessel infrastructure changes make tumor vessels highly permeable and raise interstitial fluid pressures in gliomas (28). Paradoxically, the basement membrane (BM) thickness in GBM is increased relative to other malignancies. The BM in GBM has been observed to decrease in thickness during treatment with anti-VEGF therapy (29).

VEGF production and VEGFR expression are regulated by various factors including response to hypoxia, damage to vascular endothelium, cytokine signaling, growth factors, and aberrant gene expression (30). Even in the absence of hypoxia, VEGF expression in GBM can be upregulated by other pathways, such as EGF signaling (31). The hypoxia inducible factor-1 (HIF-1) system serves as a cellular oxygen sensor. Low intracellular oxygen levels impair the breakdown of HIF-1α. This excess HIF-1α is available to bind HIF-1β. The HIF-1α/HIF-1β dimer translocates to the nucleus and promotes increased transcription of VEGF. Angiogenesis in GBM is regulated through both VEGF-independent mechanisms. The HIF-1 pathway increases expression of many proangiogenic growth factors including transforming growth factors α and β (TGF-α/β), inducible nitric oxide synthase, matrix metalloproteinases, and angiopoietin. HIF-1 activity also upregulates the Tie receptor pathway (32).

■ KEY PATHWAY: PI3K/Akt/mTOR

The PI3K/Akt/mTOR pathway regulates a myriad of cellular functions. These include adhesion-independent cell survival, migration, cell-cycle progression, protein synthesis, and growth (33). Over 80% of GBM have dysregulation of the PI3K/Akt/mTOR axis (12). Phosphatidylinositol-3 kinases are a group of membrane-associated lipid kinases. We are most familiar with class IA PI3Ks (hereafter referred to as PI3K) that are activated by cell membrane-bound RTKs. Other classes of phosphatidylinositol 3 kinases can be activated by G protein-linked receptors (i.e., Ras) and cytoplasmic protein kinases (i.e., Src) (2,34). The PI3K complex is comprised of a catalytically active protein, p110α, and the p85α regulatory protein. The p110α and p85α subunits are encoded by PI3KCA and PIK3R1 genes, respectively (35,36). Mutation in either gene can result in aberrant PI3K/Akt regulation (37). Activating missense mutations in PIK3CA are by far the most common, occurring in approximately 15% of GBM (35).

PI3K is activated by translocation to the cell membrane where SH2 domains on p85 interact with activated RTKs. PI3K then converts phosphatidylinositol 4, 5 bisphosphonate (PIP2) into the active phosphatidylinositol 3, 4, 5-triphosphate (PIP3). The now active PIP3 is able to activate multiple downstream signaling pathways. To counter PIP3 activity, phosphatase and tensin homologue deleted on chromosome ten (PTEN) halts PI3K signaling by dephosphorylating PIP3 into PIP2. Thus, the loss of PTEN results in dysregulation of the PI3K pathway (38). PTEN is mutated or deleted in 36% of GBM (12).

One of the better-known downstream effectors of PIP3 is Akt (sometimes referred to as protein kinase B), a plekstrin-homology domain protein with serine-threonine kinase activity. Akt lies at the intersection of multiple pathways. Increased Akt activity can serve to amplify signaling which may lead to resistance to apoptosis, uncontrolled growth, and aggressive invasive behavior (33,39). Amplified Akt pathway activity is commonly seen in GBM. In fact, nearly 90% of the endothelial cells of GBM show increased expression of phosphorylated Akt (40). Akt also plays a role in angiogenesis and stem-like cell formation in GBM (41).

Akt continues signal transduction through a variety of downstream intermediaries including the highly conserved protein kinase mammalian target of rapamycin (mTOR). mTOR is known to form two complexes, mTORC1 and mTORC2, that play a role in essential cellular functions. Protein translation, cell growth, and proliferation are promoted by activated mTORC1 in response to upstream signaling (42). mTORC2 is known to phosphorylate Akt, thereby influencing proliferation and survival (43).

■ KEY PATHWAY: Met

Early in embryogenesis, select cells undergo a transformation from an epithelial phenotype into a mesenchymal one. This epithelial-mesenchymal transition (EMT) is a crucial step that precedes cell migration and morphogenesis. A similar process occurs in normal wound repair in adults. Without these processes, normal growth, development, and tissue repair cannot occur (44,45).

Met plays a crucial role in the cellular migration process by modulating cell dissociation from its tissue of origin, degrading the extracellular matrix, and promoting survival (46). Both Met and its ligand, hepatocyte growth factor (HGF) (sometimes referred to as scatter factor [SF]), regulate the expression of matrix metalloproteinases, cadherins, and integrins (47). HGF activity has been implicated in angiogenesis in GBM (25). It is not surprising that, deregulation of Met is associated with metastatic propensity, an invasive phenotype, decreased survival, and poor response to treatment in glioblastoma (48). PTEN has been shown to oppose gene expression induced by the SF/HGF/Met signaling pathway in human glioblastoma cells (49).

■ KEY PATHWAY: EGFR

EGFR activity has been shown to be increased in approximately half of all GBM patients. This can result from gene amplification or mutation (12,50). An in-frame deletion of exons 2–7 in the EGFR gene alters the expressed receptor's extracellular domain. The result is EGFRvIII, a constitutively activated mutant EGFR receptor. In addition to increasing proliferative ability, EGFRvIII activity makes glioblastoma cells resistant to apoptosis (51). EGFR signaling is able to increase the expression of VEGF, even in the absence of hypoxia (31). Activity in the EGFR pathway plays a role in both forming and sustaining glioma stem cells (41,52).

It is well known that GBM are resistant to chemotherapy and radiation, and research has shown that EGFR activity can promote resistance to therapy. In glioblastoma cell lines, EGFR activates both the PI3K/Akt and MAPK pathways. The upregulation of the PI3K/Akt and MAPK pathways by chemotherapy and radiation is associated with impaired apoptosis. Chakravarti and colleagues showed that inhibition of EGFR was able to improve glioblastoma cell response to sequential chemotherapy and radiation (53). Bredel and colleagues demonstrated that the loss of a key inhibitory factor in the EGFR pathway, NFκBIα (nuclear factor of κ-light peptide enhancer in B-cells inhibitor-α), was associated with poor prognosis in patients with structurally normal EGFR (54).

■ VASCULAR NORMALIZATION, PERFUSION, EDEMA, AND SURVIVAL IN GBM

The term "vascular normalization" was coined by Jain and colleagues to refer to a phenomenon observed in tumor blood vessels following therapy with anti-VEGF antibodies. There is a temporary period, or "window" when perictye coverage and BM thickness normalizes thereby promoting more physiologic, functional tumor vasculature. This normalization window is associated with an increased response to radiation and chemotherapy postulated to arise from improved oxygenation and drug delivery to tumor tissue (29,55).

Recent developments further support that vascular normalization, increased tumor perfusion, and response to therapy are intimately linked. Tumor blood perfusion seen on proton magnetic resonance spectroscopy (^{1}H-MRS) was increased in a small series of patients treated with cediranib, a pan-VEGF TKI inhibitor. This increase in perfusion was durable for at least 1 month and was associated with improved median survival: 348 days in patients that had an increase in tumor perfusion compared to 213 days in those without increased perfusion (56).

In an orthotopic GBM mouse model, treatment with cediranib resulted in less permeable tumor blood vessels (57). Although unable to control tumor growth, cediranib succeeded in decreasing cerebral edema and improving survival. This data suggested that cediranib's effect on survival arises, at least in part, from alleviation of cerebral edema (57).

Batchelor and colleagues showed in patients with rGBM, treatment with cediranib promoted the normalization of tumor blood vessels, decreased edema, and resulted in reduced corticosteroid requirements. Increasing levels of SDF1α, bFGF, and circulating endothelial cells coincided with tumor progression during cediranib treatment. Following the interruption of cediranib, an increase in the level of circulating progenitor cells (CPCs) corresponded with tumor progression (58).

■ MECHANISM OF FAILURE FOLLOWING ANTI-VEGF THERAPY

It has been previously noted that anti-VEGF therapy in malignant gliomas produces a more aggressive and infiltrative phenotype (59,60). Following treatment with bevacizumab, some patients develop tumors that do not contrast enhance on MRI. This nonenhancing phenotype is purportedly associated with poor survival (59). It has also been shown that under hypoxic conditions, and in the presence of VEGF blockade, alternative angiogenic pathways are recruited in GBM (61,62). Recent findings in rGBM patients suggest that alternate mechanisms may underlie treatment failure following treatment with the anti-VEGF TKI cediranib.

Tumor blood vessel structure was studied in a small series of rGBM patients. Patients underwent surgical resection of their tumors at the time of recurrence. The resected tumor specimens from each patient were later compared to tumor specimens obtained at autopsy. Patients receiving cediranib therapy were compared to patients naïve to anti-VEGF therapy. In the group exposed to cediranib, autopsy tumor vasculature was essentially normal—both structurally and by molecular expression profiling. Furthermore, tumor cellularity was decreased in cediranib-treated patients. The greatest decrease in cellularity occurred at the infiltrating edge of the tumor as opposed to the perivascular region. These findings suggest that the mechanism of failure following VEGF therapy may be more complex than previously thought (63).

■ MEASURING RESPONSE TO THERAPY ON IMAGING

Traditionally, response of GBM to therapy was measured using the McDonald criteria that included examining contrast enhancing tumor on cross-sectional imaging, measuring corticosteroid requirements, and monitoring a patient's clinical performance status (64). These criteria have evolved to include more comprehensive reporting of clinical data, biomarkers, and the volumetric and mechanistic analysis of imaging studies (65,66). Antiangiogenic therapy (AAT) can make it difficult, however, to characterize changes on contrast-enhanced T1 MRI as either disease response to treatment or vascular stabilization. Advances in proton magnetic resonance spectroscopy have allowed to "see past" contrast enhancement by utilizing functional imaging (67).

Active disease is often missed by standard contrast-enhanced T1 MRI when compared to ^{1}H-MRS (68). An increase in the ratio of N-acetylaspartate (NAA), a marker of neuronal integrity, to choline, a cell membrane component increased in rapidly dividing tumors, signifies a response to treatment that can be visualized on ^{1}H-MRS. This relationship between choline and NAA can be utilized to more accurately identify areas of active disease for purposes of radiation treatment planning (67–69).

^{1}H-MRS was able to predict outcomes in recurrent glioblastoma patients treated with cediranib. The ratio of NAA to choline was compared prior to, shortly after beginning, and following the cessation of cediranib. The ratio was stable during the first 28 days of treatment, increased on days 28 through 56, and then decreased as treatment continued signifying an eventual decrease in efficacy leading to treatment failure. The NAA to choline ratio was able to predict 6-month survival in patients treated with cediranib. Noninvasive measurement of these metabolites proved to be a feasible method of monitoring patient response to therapy and suggested that cediranib can directly influence tumor metabolism (70).

Batchelor and colleagues showed a combination of two parameters measurable by MRI and one blood biomarker were predictive of both overall and PFS in rGBM patients. The imaging parameters included the volume transfer coefficient or K^{trans} (which measures the ratio of vascular permeability to blood flow) and microvessel volume. The level of circulating collagen IV, a component of the vascular BM, was a biomarker measurable in patient blood (71).

Cediranib

As previously noted, cediranib is a pan-VEGF receptor TKI being studied in malignant gliomas. Phase I studies evaluating cediranib demonstrated decreases in soluble VEGF-2 receptors that were both time- and dose-dependent (72). Cediranib is being evaluated in a phase II study, RTOG 0837, in combination with the current standard of care concurrent RT and TMZ in newly diagnosed GBM [NCT01062425]. Cediranib is also being combined with Cilengitide, a $\alpha v\beta 3$ and $\alpha v\beta 5$ integrin inhibitor, in progressive or rGBM as well as in combination with bevacizumab and gefitinib.

Erlotinib

Erlotinib is an EGFR/HER1 TKI that has shown activity in pancreatic cancer and NSCLC that have failed first- or second-line chemotherapy (74). Initial phase I trials of erlotinib with TMZ, without the use of concurrent radiation therapy, showed acceptable toxicity profile and efficacy (75). In a phase II study of 27 newly diagnosed GBM patients, erlotinib was combined with standard concurrent radiation and TMZ followed by maintenance TMZ with an extension of maintenance TMZ from 6 to 12 months. Eighteen left for progression of disease and four went off study for adverse events that included anemia, thrombocytopenia, lymphopenia, febrile neutropenia, and fatigue. Unfortunately, the median OS was 8.6 months, much lower than in recent trials. There were three treatment-related deaths and the trial was terminated before completing accrual (76).

Gefitinib (Iressa)

Gefitinib is an EGFR TKI that used in the treatment of NSCLC outside of the United States. Phase I and II studies combining gefitinib with radiotherapy in GBM showed OS and PFS in line with historical controls but did not show improvement from the addition of gefitinib (77,78). These trials completed accrual before the results of the Stupp trial were available. Uhm did note an improved survival in a subset of patients with side effects attributed to gefitinib, specifically diarrhea or rash (77). A similar phenomenon has been seen in cetuximab and anti-EGFR monoclonal antibody used in the treatment of head and neck cancers (79). In a small phase I trial, gefitinib was shown to be safe in rGBM and anaplastic astrocytomas when used in conjunction with stereotactic radiotherapy (80). There is an ongoing phase II trial of cediranib with and without gefitinib in rGBM [NCT01310855].

Intedanib (VARGATEF) (BIBF 1120)

Intedanib (VARGATEF) (BIBF 1120, Boehringer Ingelheim) is a new TKI with activity against VEGFR, platelet derived growth factor receptor (PDGFR), and fibroblast growth factor receptor. It inhibits the MAPK and Akt pathways and induces apoptosis. Intedanib has effects on both endothelial cells and perivascular cells (vascular smooth muscle and pericytes) (81). The drug is currently being evaluated with cediranib in rGBM [NCT01251484] as well as in the treatment of idiopathic pulmonary fibrosis (82) and multiple other cancers including colon, ovarian, and non-small cell lung carcinoma (83–86).

Imatinib (Gleevec) STI571

Imatinib is a TKI with activity against c-Kit, PDGFR and the Bcr-Abl tyrosine kinase. Imatinib is approved for the treatment of Ph$^+$ CML and c-Kit positive GIST (6–8). It has been studied in both newly diagnosed and rGBM. A phase II trial of neoadjuvant imatinib prior to surgical resection in GBM showed minimal effectiveness but did confirm that the drug was present in biopsy specimens on mass spectroscopy. A median survival of 6.2 months was reported. Staining for Ki67 showed no evidence of decreased cellular proliferation with administration of imatinib. In a subset of patients, the drug appeared to decrease the activity of Akt and MAPK (87).

The North American Brain Tumor Consortium Study 99–08, a phase I/II study in recurrent malignant gliomas, proved disappointing (88). Phase II data on imatinib in combination with hydroxyurea in the recurrent disease setting showed PFS at 6 months and median PFS of 27% and 14.4 weeks, respectively (89). The most common side effects of imatinib are neutropenia, elevated liver transaminases, rash, edema, and thrombocytopenia (88,89).

Dasatinib (Sprycel) BMS-354825

Dasatinib is an ATP competitive small TKI currently used to treat Ph$^+$ CML in patients who cannot tolerate imatinib (90). Dasatinib exhibits activity against PDGFRβ, Src, Bcr-Abl, and c-Kit (91). Src is a nonreceptor cytoplasmic kinase that is being evaluated as a therapeutic target in both GBMs and brain metastases (92). Dasatinib is readily absorbed orally with side effects of fatigue, lethargy, nausea, diarrhea, anorexia, proteinuria (93). The drug may cause QT prolongation in patients taking CYP3A4 (cytochrome P450 3A4) inhibitors (94).

Dasatinib induces autophagy, but not apoptosis or cell cycle arrest, in glioma cells. Treatment with nanomolar concentrations of dasatinib led to decreased concentrations of phosphorylated-Src, phosphorylated-Akt, and phosphorylated ribosomal protein S. These changes in molecular intermediates occurred both before and after stimulation with EGF. A synergistic therapeutic effect is seen with a combination of TMZ and dasatinib. Glioma cells with intact PTEN had increased sensitivity to the effects of dasatinib relative to PTEN-deficient cells (95). Retrospective data on combining dasatinib with bevacizumab in rGBM patients who had failed multiple prior treatment regimens showed no significant activity (91).

Pazopanib (GW786034)

Pazopanib (GW786034) is a TKI with activity against VEGFR-1, VEGFR-2, VEGFR-3, PDGRF α and β, and c-Kit. Phase II data from North American Brain tumor consortium study 06–02 examined the drug's effect in patients with recurrent glioblastoma naïve to anti-VEGF/R therapies. No improvement in 6-month PFS (the study's primary endpoint) was found. Median PFS and median OS were 12 and 35 weeks, respectively. Investigators did find radiographic evidence of activity manifest as decreased edema and a decrease in contrast enhancement. Pazopanib was well tolerated with toxicities that are seen with similar anti-VEGF therapies (96).

Sorafenib (Nexavar) BAY 43–9006

Sorafenib inhibits the b-Raf (wild type and V600E mutant) and c-Raf kinases, VEGFR-2, VEGFR-3, PDGFR-β, and c-Kit. The drug also inhibits the phosphorylation of MEK and ERK (97).

Preclinical studies of sorafenib showed a reduction in the phosphorylation of Akt and signal transducers and activators of transcription 3 (STAT3). There was additional inhibition of STAT3 via inhibition of JAK1 and JAK2. Levels of cyclin D and cyclin E as well as Mcl-1 were decreased upon treatment with Sorafenib. These effects were achieved at concentrations at or below 10 μmol/L (98). The main side effects of sorafenib are dermatological and gastrointestinal in nature (99). The drug's half-life has been reported as ranging between 24 and 38 hours (99,100). Concurrent TMZ, sorafenib, and radiation followed by maintenance TMZ with sorafenib were studied in newly diagnosed patients with GBM. PFS and median OS of 6 and 12 months, respectively, did not show improvement relative to the standard of care (101).

Sunitinib

Sunitinib is a small-molecule TKI that targets VEGFR-2, PDRFR-α, Ret, FLT1, FLT3, FLK1/KDR, and c-Kit. It has shown efficacy in many solid tumors, including renal cell carcinoma and GIST refractory to imatinib (102). Sunitinib has not, however, shown efficacy in malignant glioma. A phase II trial of single-agent sunitinib in 21 patients with high-grade gliomas that had recurred following radiation and chemotherapy did not show sufficient activity to warrant further study. Unfortunately, combination therapy with sunitinib did not fare better. A phase I study of combination sunitinib and irinotecan reported moderate toxicity and unremarkable antitumor activity in recurrent malignant glioma (103).

Valatanib (PTK787) (ZK222584)

Valatanib is an orally available VEGFR TKI with activity against RTKs, including PDGFR-β, c-Kit, and c-Fms. There has been no demonstrated activity in other RTK families. Valatanib does not appear to have cytotoxic or antiproliferative effects on cells lacking the VEGFR. Wound-healing problems have not been associated with this drug (104). Preclinical data in C6 rat glioma cells showed impressive reductions in vessel density, necrosis, proliferation index, and tumor size on MRI volumetry (105).

A phase I trial evaluated valatanib in 13 patients with newly diagnosed GBM. Patients received the standard of care per the Stupp regimen with the addition of EIAEDs and valatanib. Partial response and stable disease were observed in two and nine patients, respectively. Levels of soluble VEGFR-1 increased while on treatment. A decrease was seen in levels of soluble VEGFR-2 and Tie2. Dose-limiting toxicities were thrombocytopenia and transaminitis (106). Phase I data has shown valatanib combined with imatinib and hydroxyurea is well tolerated with GI, hematological, hepatic, and renal dose-limiting toxicities (107). Conrad and colleagues showed phase I/II results showing patients treated with valatanib and TMZ in rGBM showed partial response and stable disease in 4% and 56% of those treated (108).

Vandetinib ZD6474

Vandetanib is an orally available inhibitor of EGFR, VEGFR-2, and Ret that has been shown to counteract angiogenesis and tumor growth in glioblastoma cells. The drug is believed to augment the efficacy of radiotherapy and has shown promising preclinical results (109–112). Drappatz and colleagues examined dose escalation of vandetanib in 13 newly diagnosed GBM patients. The drug was combined with standard of care radiation and TMZ. No dose-limiting toxicities were observed during the trial, although there was a high incidence of pulmonary embolism observed. A follow-up phase II trial of vandetinib is ongoing (113). Vandetinib is also being evaluated in conjunction with fractionated radiotherapy in adults and pontine glioma in children (114,115).

NVP-BEZ235

NVP-BEZ235 is a dual PI3K and mTOR inhibitor. Treatment with NVP-BEZ235 induces differentiation and decreased tumorigenicity in A172 cancer stem-like cells (CSLCs) (116). By attaching to the ATP binding region cleft of mTOR and PI3K, NVP-BEZ235 is able to interrupt aberrant signaling of the PI3K/Akt/mTOR cascade. At nanomolar concentrations, this compound was able to inhibit the activity of the pathway members Akt, S6, S6K 1, and 4EBP1 in human glioma cells. NVP-BEZ235 induces G_1 cell cycle arrest, autophagy, and decreased expression of VEGF with a subsequent reduction in angiogenesis (117,118).

LY294002

Another PI3K inhibitor, LY294002, is being studied in human glioma cell lines. The combination of

TMZ and LY294002 resulted in decreased proliferation, increased apoptosis, and decreased invasiveness compared to TMZ monotherapy. Researchers noted decreases levels of phosphorylated Akt and Bcl-2 when LY294002 and TMZ were used in combination. This suggested that LY294002, by inhibiting the PI3K/Akt pathway, may be able to decrease glioma cell resistance to TMZ (119). Another experiment examined the effect of pairing LY294002 with 17-allyl-aminogeldanamycin (17-AAG), an inhibitor of heat shock protein 90, in human glioma cells. The combination decreased the activity of Akt, MAPK, EGFR, and Raf-1 while showing increases in several apoptotic markers. Together, LY294002 and 17-AAG induced cell death and irreversibly inhibited glioma proliferation (120). When used on glioblastoma stem-like cells in conjunction with rapamycin, LY294002 increased βIII tubulin expression, suggesting it promotes neuronal differentiation (116).

XL765 and XL147

There is phase I dose-escalation study with the PI3K inhibitor XL765 (SAR245409) in GBM patients with stable disease who are on maintenance TMZ (NCT00704080). XL765 is also being evaluated as monotherapy in patients with recurrent disease who are candidates for surgical resection. This trial will examine the in vivo effects of XL765 on the PI3K/mTOR pathway in resected tumor specimens. A parallel trial using a similar drug XL147 is also being conducted (NCT01240460).

Cabozantinib BMS-907351 (XL-184)

Cabozantinib BMS-907351 (XL-184) is a TKI that primarily targets Met, Ret, and VEGFR-2. The compound is reported to additionally inhibit TEK, FLT3, and c-Kit. Cabozantinib is orally available and able to cross the blood–brain barrier. In mice, cabozantinib promoted apoptosis and decreased the proliferation of both tumor and endothelial cells in a dose-dependent manner (121,122). An ongoing phase II trial is assessing cabozantinib in recurrent GBM. Interim analyses showed over half of patients requiring corticosteroids at the start of the study required fewer steroids following initiation of cabozantinib. In patients naïve to AAT, preliminary results show overall response rates of 21% to 30%. The 6-month PFS ranged between 10% and 25%. The median PFS was 16 weeks. Results are less impressive in patients who had received AAT previously (123). A phase I trial is examining the addition of cabozantinib to standard of care concurrent radiation with TMZ followed by adjuvant TMZ (NCT00960492).

Crizotinib (PF02341066)

Crizotinib (PF02341066) is a recently FDA-approved therapy marketed as an ALK inhibitor in ALK-rearranged NSCLC. Interestingly, the drug was originally designed to target the Met tyrosine kinase, and was only secondarily found to have activity against ALK (124–126). Crizotinib has shown activity in U87MG glioblastoma xenografts. Data suggests that a high portion of inhibition of Met phosphorylation is required to inhibit tumor growth in GBM: The dose at which the EC_{90} for Met phosphorylation was reached resulted in the EC_{50} for tumor growth (127).

■ RATIONAL DESIGN AND IMPLEMENTATION OF TARGETED THERAPIES

The effectiveness of current kinase inhibitors lies in their ability to target various signaling pathways. Each TKI impacts these signaling pathways in subtly different ways. This is evidenced by distinctive temporal, qualitative, and quantitative changes in cellular intermediaries. Researchers prospectively monitor biomarkers they believe appropriate, but these often vary widely between studies. How can we identify new relationships within signaling pathways to assist with drug design and research?

Contemporary clinical trials must collect, analyze, and archive tissue from all trial participants. Examining tissue facilitates the prospective and retrospective analysis of patient outcomes data in the context of genomic, transcriptomic, and proteomic tumor profiles. The confirmation of the prognostic significance of MGMT promoter methylation in GBM is a salient example of how retrospective analysis is facilitated when patient tissue is available for study (128). We can never anticipate every important variable prospectively. It is vital, therefore, to consistently have the resources to retrospectively investigate them.

We suggest, in addition to any particular biomarker of interest, that researchers collect and report on a standard comprehensive panel of biomarkers in all TKI trials. This evolving list would allow for an "apples to apples" comparison between various candidate therapies across different labs. The aggregation of data could lead to the identification novel relationships that would otherwise go unnoticed in small phase I and II trials. In this way, researchers could avoid discarding compounds that, by themselves show no activity, but may prove effective when combined with other agents. Once large amounts of data are collected, a molecular response map can be compiled for each TKI.

Much like pharmacodynamics and pharmacokinetics facilitate our understanding of pharmacology, it may be helpful to evaluate tumor response to a targeted therapy in terms of biomarker dynamics and biomarker kinetics. Understanding biomarker kinetics and biomarker dynamics would allow for the pairing of complementary therapies. Take, for example, a hypothetical TKI, ABC-inib, that exhibits good initial anti-VEGF activity but eventually fails, perhaps through an upregulation of EGFR and Met. On the other hand, a second hypothetical TKI, XYZ-inib, primarily inhibits EGFR and Met but also has secondary antiangiogenic activity through a VEGF-independent mechanism (i.e., by blocking the angiopoietin pathway). It would be rational to pair ABC-inib with XYZ-inib.

Just as in antibiotic therapy, there will be synergistic and antagonistic combinations of agents. As was astutely suggested by Huang, significant improvements in GBM therapy will likely require combination therapy, just as was the case with HIV. Initially, single agents resulted in short periods of clinical efficacy with the disease escaping control with near certainty. Combination therapy in HIV, however, significantly prolongs survival in what had previously been a near-universally fatal disease (129).

GBM is an aggressive malignancy characterized by numerous genetic mutations. These mutations result in aberrant cellular signaling via multiple redundant pathways (12). This has made finding effective targeted therapies a challenge. The targeted anti-VEGF antibody bevacizumab has shown promise in GBM but patient outcomes are still dismal (15,16,130). Once delineated, the redundant secondary and tertiary pathways GBM utilizes to sustain proliferation could be preemptively blocked. These alternate pathways may be less hardy and more easily interrupted. Effective therapy for GBM might even include temporary inhibition of canonical pathways, with the expectation that normal cells can withstand a greater degree of physiologic insult. Tumor cells, just as any other, are ultimately limited by cellular physiology.

Biomarker analysis will permit the real-time selection, monitoring and adjustment of therapy in tumor. The initial biomarker pattern of a patient's tumor will be obtained from preoperative serum measurements. Resected tumors will be interrogated in xenograft systems to guide the selection of initial therapy or establish eligibility for clinical trial. Following the initiation of treatment, markers of response will be monitored in the patient's serum. Spectral MRI and molecular imaging will allow for further timely adjustment of therapy. Advancements in imaging and molecular diagnostics will help predict outcomes before clinical treatment failure is manifest allowing us to refine systemic and local therapies.

Real-time selection and adjustment of targeted therapies in patients undergoing treatment for GBM is not currently feasible on a large scale. As any technology advances, the initial gains will be incremental and the resources required extensive. Keep in mind, however, that it recently became possible to commercially sequence an individual human genome in one day for one-thousand U.S. dollars. This happened nearly after 60 years following Watson and Crick's characterization of DNA in April 1953, but less than 10 years following the "completion" of sequencing of the Human Genome Project in April 2003. Personalized medicine is, rightly so, the future of medicine. With coordinated efforts and the rational application of therapies, in our lifetimes we hope to see significant improvements in outcomes of patients fighting GBM.

REFERENCES

1. Ullrich A, Schlessinger J. Signal transduction by receptors with tyrosine kinase activity. *Cell*. 1990;61(2):203–212.
2. Blume-Jensen P, Hunter T. Oncogenic kinase signalling. *Nature*. 2001;411(6835):355–365.
3. Clayton AH, Walker F, Orchard SG, et al. Ligand-induced dimer-tetramer transition during the activation of the cell surface epidermal growth factor receptor-A multidimensional microscopy analysis. *J Biol Chem*. 2005;280(34):30392–30399.
4. Gadella TW Jr, Jovin TM. Oligomerization of epidermal growth factor receptors on A431 cells studied by time-resolved fluorescence imaging microscopy. A stereochemical model for tyrosine kinase receptor activation. *J Cell Biol*. 1995;129(6):1543–1558.
5. Chakravarti A, Loeffler JS, Dyson NJ. Insulin-like growth factor receptor I mediates resistance to anti-epidermal growth factor receptor therapy in primary human glioblastoma cells through continued activation of phosphoinositide 3-kinase signaling. *Cancer Res*. 2002;62(1):200–207.

6. Thiesing JT, Ohno-Jones S, Kolibaba KS, Druker BJ. Efficacy of STI571, an abl tyrosine kinase inhibitor, in conjunction with other antileukemic agents against bcr-abl-positive cells. *Blood.* 2000;96(9):3195–3199.

7. Druker BJ, Sawyers CL, Kantarjian H, et al. Activity of a specific inhibitor of the BCR-ABL tyrosine kinase in the blast crisis of chronic myeloid leukemia and acute lymphoblastic leukemia with the Philadelphia chromosome. *N Engl J Med.* 2001;344(14):1038–1042.

8. Verweij J, Casali PG, Zalcberg J, et al. Progression-free survival in gastrointestinal stromal tumours with high-dose imatinib: randomised trial. *Lancet.* 2004;364(9440):1127–1134.

9. Zhou C, Wu YL, Chen G, et al. Erlotinib versus chemotherapy as first-line treatment for patients with advanced EGFR mutation-positive non-small-cell lung cancer (OPTIMAL, CTONG-0802): a multicentre, open-label, randomised, phase 3 study. *Lancet Oncol.* 2011;12(8):735–742.

10. Shaw AT, Yeap BY, Solomon BJ, et al. Effect of crizotinib on overall survival in patients with advanced non-small-cell lung cancer harbouring ALK gene rearrangement: a retrospective analysis. *Lancet Oncol.* 2011;12(11):1004–1012.

11. Kwak EL, Bang YJ, Camidge DR, et al. Anaplastic lymphoma kinase inhibition in non-small-cell lung cancer. *N Engl J Med.* 2010;363(18):1693–1703.

12. The Cancer Genome Atlas Network. Comprehensive genomic characterization defines human glioblastoma genes and core pathways. *Nature.* 2008;455(7216):1061–1068.

13. Stupp R, Hegi ME, Mason WP, et al.; European Organisation for Research and Treatment of Cancer Brain Tumour and Radiation Oncology Groups; National Cancer Institute of Canada Clinical Trials Group. Effects of radiotherapy with concomitant and adjuvant temozolomide versus radiotherapy alone on survival in glioblastoma in a randomised phase III study: 5-year analysis of the EORTC-NCIC trial. *Lancet Oncol.* 2009;10(5):459–466.

14. Stupp R, Mason WP, van den Bent MJ, et al.; European Organisation for Research and Treatment of Cancer Brain Tumor and Radiotherapy Groups; National Cancer Institute of Canada Clinical Trials Group. Radiotherapy plus concomitant and adjuvant temozolomide for glioblastoma. *N Engl J Med.* 2005;352(10):987–996.

15. Vredenburgh JJ, Desjardins A, Herndon JE 2nd, et al. Bevacizumab plus irinotecan in recurrent glioblastoma multiforme. *J Clin Oncol.* 2007;25(30):4722–4729.

16. Friedman HS, Prados MD, Wen PY, et al. Bevacizumab alone and in combination with irinotecan in recurrent glioblastoma. *J Clin Oncol.* 2009;27(28):4733–4740.

17. Senger DR, Galli SJ, Dvorak AM, Perruzzi CA, Harvey VS, Dvorak HF. Tumor cells secrete a vascular permeability factor that promotes accumulation of ascites fluid. *Science.* 1983;219(4587):983–985.

18. Senger DR, Perruzzi CA, Feder J, Dvorak HF. A highly conserved vascular permeability factor secreted by a variety of human and rodent tumor cell lines. *Cancer Res.* 1986;46(11):5629–5632.

19. Leung DW, Cachianes G, Kuang WJ, Goeddel DV, Ferrara N. Vascular endothelial growth factor is a secreted angiogenic mitogen. *Science.* 1989;246(4935):1306–1309.

20. Keck PJ, Hauser SD, Krivi G, et al. Vascular permeability factor, an endothelial cell mitogen related to PDGF. *Science.* 1989;246(4935):1309–1312.

21. Millauer B, Wizigmann-Voos S, Schnürch H, et al. High affinity VEGF binding and developmental expression suggest Flk-1 as a major regulator of vasculogenesis and angiogenesis. *Cell.* 1993;72(6):835–846.

22. Terman BI, Dougher-Vermazen M, Carrion ME, et al. Identification of the KDR tyrosine kinase as a receptor for vascular endothelial cell growth factor. *Biochem Biophys Res Commun.* 1992;187(3):1579–1586.

23. Zhou YH, Tan F, Hess KR, Yung WK. The expression of PAX6, PTEN, vascular endothelial growth factor, and epidermal growth factor receptor in gliomas: relationship to tumor grade and survival. *Clin Cancer Res.* 2003;9(9):3369–3375.

24. Flynn JR, Wang L, Gillespie DL, et al. Hypoxia-regulated protein expression, patient characteristics, and preoperative imaging as predictors of survival in adults with glioblastoma multiforme. *Cancer.* 2008;113(5):1032–1042.

25. Schmidt NO, Westphal M, Hagel C, et al. Levels of vascular endothelial growth factor, hepatocyte growth factor/scatter factor and basic fibroblast growth factor in human gliomas and their relation to angiogenesis. *Int J Cancer.* 1999;84(1):10–18.

26. Samoto K, Ikezaki K, Ono M, et al. Expression of vascular endothelial growth factor and its possible relation with neovascularization in human brain tumors. *Cancer Res.* 1995;55(5):1189–1193.

27. Dejana E, Tournier-Lasserve E, Weinstein BM. The control of vascular integrity by endothelial cell junctions: molecular basis and pathological implications. *Dev Cell.* 2009;16(2):209–221.

28. Boucher Y, Salehi H, Witwer B, Harsh GR 4th, Jain RK. Interstitial fluid pressure in intracranial tumours in patients and in rodents. *Br J Cancer.* 1997;75(6):829–836.

29. Winkler F, Kozin SV, Tong RT, et al. Kinetics of vascular normalization by VEGFR2 blockade governs brain tumor response to radiation: role of oxygenation, angiopoietin-1, and matrix metalloproteinases. *Cancer Cell.* 2004;6(6):553–563.

30. Vogelstein B, Kinzler KW. Cancer genes and the pathways they control. *Nat Med.* 2004;10(8):789–799.

31. Maity A, Pore N, Lee J, Solomon D, O'Rourke DM. Epidermal growth factor receptor transcriptionally up-regulates vascular endothelial growth factor expression in human glioblastoma cells via a pathway involving phosphatidylinositol 3'-kinase and distinct from that induced by hypoxia. *Cancer Res.* 2000;60(20):5879–5886.

32. Kaur B, Khwaja FW, Severson EA, Matheny SL, Brat DJ, Van Meir EG. Hypoxia and the hypoxia-inducible-factor

pathway in glioma growth and angiogenesis. *Neuro-oncology.* 2005;7(2):134–153.

33. Vivanco I, Sawyers CL. The phosphatidylinositol 3-Kinase AKT pathway in human cancer. *Nat Rev Cancer.* 2002;2(7):489–501.

34. Wymann MP, Zvelebil M, Laffargue M. Phosphoinositide 3-kinase signalling–which way to target? *Trends Pharmacol Sci.* 2003;24(7):366–376.

35. Gallia GL, Rand V, Siu IM, et al. PIK3CA gene mutations in pediatric and adult glioblastoma multiforme. *Mol Cancer Res.* 2006;4(10):709–714.

36. Samuels Y, Wang Z, Bardelli A, et al. High frequency of mutations of the PIK3CA gene in human cancers. *Science.* 2004;304(5670):554.

37. Mizoguchi M, Nutt CL, Mohapatra G, Louis DN. Genetic alterations of phosphoinositide 3-kinase subunit genes in human glioblastomas. *Brain Pathol.* 2004;14(4):372–377.

38. Maehama T, Dixon JE. The tumor suppressor, PTEN/MMAC1, dephosphorylates the lipid second messenger, phosphatidylinositol 3,4,5-trisphosphate. *J Biol Chem.* 1998;273(22):13375–13378.

39. McDowell KA, Riggins GJ, Gallia GL. Targeting the AKT pathway in glioblastoma. *Curr Pharm Des.* 2011;17(23):2411–2420.

40. Sihto H, Tynninen O, Bützow R, Saarialho-Kere U, Joensuu H. Endothelial cell KIT expression in human tumours. *J Pathol.* 2007;211(4):481–488.

41. Jin X, Yin J, Kim SH, et al. EGFR-AKT-Smad signaling promotes formation of glioma stem-like cells and tumor angiogenesis by ID3-driven cytokine induction. *Cancer Res.* 2011;71(22):7125–7134.

42. Fingar DC, Blenis J. Target of rapamycin (TOR): an integrator of nutrient and growth factor signals and coordinator of cell growth and cell cycle progression. *Oncogene.* 2004;23(18):3151–3171.

43. Sarbassov DD, Guertin DA, Ali SM, Sabatini DM. Phosphorylation and regulation of Akt/PKB by the rictor-mTOR complex. *Science.* 2005;307(5712):1098–1101.

44. Keller R. Cell migration during gastrulation. *Curr Opin Cell Biol.* 2005;17(5):533–541.

45. Shook D, Keller R. Mechanisms, mechanics and function of epithelial-mesenchymal transitions in early development. *Mech Dev.* 2003;120(11):1351–1383.

46. Birchmeier C, Birchmeier W, Gherardi E, Vande Woude GF. Met, metastasis, motility and more. *Nat Rev Mol Cell Biol.* 2003;4(12):915–925.

47. Trusolino L, Comoglio PM. Scatter-factor and semaphorin receptors: cell signalling for invasive growth. *Nat Rev Cancer.* 2002;2(4):289–300.

48. Kong DS, Song SY, Kim DH, et al. Prognostic significance of c-Met expression in glioblastomas. *Cancer.* 2009;115(1):140–148.

49. Abounader R, Reznik T, Colantuoni C, Martinez-Murillo F, Rosen EM, Laterra J. Regulation of c-Met-dependent gene expression by PTEN. *Oncogene.* 2004;23(57):9173–9182.

50. Libermann TA, Nusbaum HR, Razon N, et al. Amplification, enhanced expression and possible rearrangement of EGF receptor gene in primary human brain tumours of glial origin. *Nature.* 1985;313(5998):144–147.

51. Nagane M, Coufal F, Lin H, Bögler O, Cavenee WK, Huang HJ. A common mutant epidermal growth factor receptor confers enhanced tumorigenicity on human glioblastoma cells by increasing proliferation and reducing apoptosis. *Cancer Res.* 1996;56(21):5079–5086.

52. Lee J, Kotliarova S, Kotliarov Y, et al. Tumor stem cells derived from glioblastomas cultured in bFGF and EGF more closely mirror the phenotype and genotype of primary tumors than do serum-cultured cell lines. *Cancer Cell.* 2006;9(5):391–403.

53. Chakravarti A, Chakladar A, Delaney MA, Latham DE, Loeffler JS. The epidermal growth factor receptor pathway mediates resistance to sequential administration of radiation and chemotherapy in primary human glioblastoma cells in a RAS-dependent manner. *Cancer Res.* 2002;62(15):4307–4315.

54. Bredel M, Scholtens DM, Yadav AK, et al. NFKBIA deletion in glioblastomas. *N Engl J Med.* 2011;364(7):627–637.

55. Jain RK. Normalizing tumor vasculature with anti-angiogenic therapy: a new paradigm for combination therapy. *Nat Med.* 2001;7(9):987–989.

56. Sorensen AG, Emblem KE, Polaskova P, et al. Increased survival of glioblastoma patients who respond to antiangiogenic therapy with elevated blood perfusion. *Cancer Res.* 2012;72(2):402–407.

57. Kamoun WS, Ley CD, Farrar CT, et al. Edema control by cediranib, a vascular endothelial growth factor receptor-targeted kinase inhibitor, prolongs survival despite persistent brain tumor growth in mice. *J Clin Oncol.* 2009;27(15):2542–2552.

58. Batchelor TT, Sorensen AG, di Tomaso E, et al. AZD2171, a pan-VEGF receptor tyrosine kinase inhibitor, normalizes tumor vasculature and alleviates edema in glioblastoma patients. *Cancer Cell.* 2007;11(1):83–95.

59. Iwamoto FM, Abrey LE, Beal K, et al. Patterns of relapse and prognosis after bevacizumab failure in recurrent glioblastoma. *Neurology.* 2009;73(15):1200–1206.

60. Pàez-Ribes M, Allen E, Hudock J, et al. Antiangiogenic therapy elicits malignant progression of tumors to increased local invasion and distant metastasis. *Cancer Cell.* 2009;15(3):220–231.

61. Rubenstein JL, Kim J, Ozawa T, et al. Anti-VEGF antibody treatment of glioblastoma prolongs survival but results in increased vascular cooption. *Neoplasia.* 2000;2(4):306–314.

62. Kunkel P, Ulbricht U, Bohlen P, et al. Inhibition of glioma angiogenesis and growth *in vivo* by systemic treatment with a monoclonal antibody against vascular endothelial growth factor receptor-2. *Cancer Res.* 2001;61(18):6624–6628.

63. di Tomaso E, Snuderl M, Kamoun WS, et al. Glioblastoma recurrence after cediranib therapy in patients: lack of "rebound" revascularization as mode of escape. *Cancer Res.* 2011;71(1):19–28.
64. Macdonald DR, Cascino TL, Schold SC Jr, Cairncross JG. Response criteria for phase II studies of supratentorial malignant glioma. *J Clin Oncol.* 1990;8(7):1277–1280.
65. Sorensen AG, Batchelor TT, Wen PY, Zhang WT, Jain RK. Response criteria for glioma. *Nat Clin Pract Oncol.* 2008;5(11):634–644.
66. Wen PY, Macdonald DR, Reardon DA, et al. Updated response assessment criteria for high-grade gliomas: response assessment in neuro-oncology working group. *J Clin Oncol.* 2010;28(11):1963–1972.
67. Howe FA, Opstad KS. 1H MR spectroscopy of brain tumours and masses. *NMR Biomed.* 2003;16(3):123–131.
68. Oh J, Henry RG, Pirzkall A, et al. Survival analysis in patients with glioblastoma multiforme: predictive value of choline-to-N-acetylaspartate index, apparent diffusion coefficient, and relative cerebral blood volume. *J Magn Reson Imaging.* 2004;19(5):546–554.
69. Glunde K, Ackerstaff E, Mori N, Jacobs MA, Bhujwalla ZM. Choline phospholipid metabolism in cancer: consequences for molecular pharmaceutical interventions. *Mol Pharm.* 2006;3(5):496–506.
70. Kim H, Catana C, Ratai EM, et al. Serial magnetic resonance spectroscopy reveals a direct metabolic effect of cediranib in glioblastoma. *Cancer Res.* 2011;71(11):3745–3752.
71. Sorensen AG, Batchelor TT, Zhang WT, et al. A "vascular normalization index" as potential mechanistic biomarker to predict survival after a single dose of cediranib in recurrent glioblastoma patients. *Cancer Res.* 2009;69(13):5296–5300.
72. Drevs J, Siegert P, Medinger M, et al. Phase I clinical study of AZD2171, an oral vascular endothelial growth factor signaling inhibitor, in patients with advanced solid tumors. *J Clin Oncol.* 2007;25(21):3045–3054.
73. Gilbert MR, Kuhn J, Lamborn KR, et al. Cilengitide in patients with recurrent glioblastoma: the results of NABTC 03–02, a phase II trial with measures of treatment delivery. *J Neurooncol.* 2012;106(1):147–153.
74. Shepherd FA, Rodrigues Pereira J, Ciuleanu T, et al.; National Cancer Institute of Canada Clinical Trials Group. Erlotinib in previously treated non-small-cell lung cancer. *N Engl J Med.* 2005;353(2):123–132.
75. Prados MD, Lamborn KR, Chang S, et al. Phase 1 study of erlotinib HCl alone and combined with temozolomide in patients with stable or recurrent malignant glioma. *Neuro-oncology.* 2006;8(1):67–78.
76. Peereboom DM, Shepard DR, Ahluwalia MS, et al. Phase II trial of erlotinib with temozolomide and radiation in patients with newly diagnosed glioblastoma multiforme. *J Neurooncol.* 2010;98(1):93–99.
77. Uhm JH, Ballman KV, Wu W, et al. Phase II evaluation of gefitinib in patients with newly diagnosed Grade 4 astrocytoma: Mayo/North Central Cancer Treatment Group Study N0074. *Int J Radiat Oncol Biol Phys.* 2011;80(2):347–353.
78. Chakravarti A, Berkey B, Robins HI, Guha A et al. An update of phase II results from RTOG 0211: A phase I/II study of gefitinib with radiotherapy in newly diagnosed glioblastoma [Abstract]. *J Clin Oncol.* 2006;24(18S):1527. *ASCO Annual Meeting Proceedings*, Part I, 2006.
79. Bonner JA, Harari PM, Giralt J, et al. Radiotherapy plus cetuximab for locoregionally advanced head and neck cancer: 5-year survival data from a phase 3 randomised trial, and relation between cetuximab-induced rash and survival. *Lancet Oncol.* 2010;11(1):21–28.
80. Schwer AL, Damek DM, Kavanagh BD, et al. A phase I dose-escalation study of fractionated stereotactic radiosurgery in combination with gefitinib in patients with recurrent malignant gliomas. *Int J Radiat Oncol Biol Phys.* 2008;70(4):993–1001.
81. Hilberg F, Roth GJ, Krssak M, et al. BIBF 1120: triple angiokinase inhibitor with sustained receptor blockade and good antitumor efficacy. *Cancer Res.* 2008;68(12):4774–4782.
82. Richeldi L, Costabel U, Selman M, et al. Efficacy of a tyrosine kinase inhibitor in idiopathic pulmonary fibrosis. *N Engl J Med.* 2011;365(12):1079–1087.
83. Bouche O, Maindrault-Goebel F, Ducreux M, et al. Phase II trial of weekly alternating sequential BIBF 1120 and afatinib for advanced colorectal cancer. *Anticancer Res.* 2011;31(6):2271–2281.
84. Ellis PM, Kaiser R, Zhao Y, Stopfer P, Gyorffy S, Hanna N. Phase I open-label study of continuous treatment with BIBF 1120, a triple angiokinase inhibitor, and pemetrexed in pretreated non-small cell lung cancer patients. *Clin Cancer Res.* 2010;16(10):2881–2889.
85. Ledermann JA, Hackshaw A, Kaye S, et al. Randomized phase II placebo-controlled trial of maintenance therapy using the oral triple angiokinase inhibitor BIBF 1120 after chemotherapy for relapsed ovarian cancer. *J Clin Oncol.* 2011;29(28):3798–3804.
86. Reck M, Kaiser R, Eschbach C, et al. A phase II double-blind study to investigate efficacy and safety of two doses of the triple angiokinase inhibitor BIBF 1120 in patients with relapsed advanced non-small-cell lung cancer. *Ann Oncol.* 2011;22(6):1374–1381.
87. Razis E, Selviaridis P, Labropoulos S, et al. Phase II study of neoadjuvant imatinib in glioblastoma: evaluation of clinical and molecular effects of the treatment. *Clin Cancer Res.* 2009;15(19):6258–6266.
88. Wen PY, Yung WK, Lamborn KR, et al. Phase I/II study of imatinib mesylate for recurrent malignant gliomas: North American Brain Tumor Consortium Study 99–08. *Clin Cancer Res.* 2006;12(16):4899–4907.
89. Reardon DA, Egorin MJ, Quinn JA, et al. Phase II study of imatinib mesylate plus hydroxyurea in adults with recurrent glioblastoma multiforme. *J Clin Oncol.* 2005;23(36):9359–9368.

90. Brave M, Goodman V, Kaminskas E, et al. Sprycel for chronic myeloid leukemia and Philadelphia chromosome-positive acute lymphoblastic leukemia resistant to or intolerant of imatinib mesylate. *Clin Cancer Res.* 2008;14(2):352–359.

91. Lu-Emerson C, Norden AD, Drappatz J, et al. Retrospective study of dasatinib for recurrent glioblastoma after bevacizumab failure. *J Neurooncol.* 2011;104(1):287–291.

92. Ahluwalia MS, de Groot J, Liu WM, Gladson CL. Targeting SRC in glioblastoma tumors and brain metastases: rationale and preclinical studies. *Cancer Lett.* 2010;298(2):139–149.

93. Demetri GD, Lo Russo P, MacPherson IR, et al. Phase I dose-escalation and pharmacokinetic study of dasatinib in patients with advanced solid tumors. *Clin Cancer Res.* 2009;15(19):6232–6240.

94. Johnson FM, Agrawal S, Burris H, et al. Phase 1 pharmacokinetic and drug-interaction study of dasatinib in patients with advanced solid tumors. *Cancer.* 2010;116(6):1582–1591.

95. Milano V, Piao Y, LaFortune T, de Groot J. Dasatinib-induced autophagy is enhanced in combination with temozolomide in glioma. *Mol Cancer Ther.* 2009;8(2):394–406.

96. Iwamoto FM, Lamborn KR, Robins HI, et al. Phase II trial of pazopanib (GW786034), an oral multi-targeted angiogenesis inhibitor, for adults with recurrent glioblastoma (North American Brain Tumor Consortium Study 06–02). *Neuro-oncology.* 2010;12(8):855–861.

97. Adnane L, Trail PA, Taylor I, Wilhelm SM. Sorafenib (BAY 43–9006, Nexavar), a dual-action inhibitor that targets RAF/MEK/ERK pathway in tumor cells and tyrosine kinases VEGFR/PDGFR in tumor vasculature. *Meth Enzymol.* 2006;407:597–612.

98. Yang F, Brown C, Buettner R, et al. Sorafenib induces growth arrest and apoptosis of human glioblastoma cells through the dephosphorylation of signal transducers and activators of transcription 3. *Mol Cancer Ther.* 2010;9(4):953–962.

99. Nabors LB, Supko JG, Rosenfeld M, et al.; New Approaches to Brain Tumor Therapy (NABTT) CNS Consortium. Phase I trial of sorafenib in patients with recurrent or progressive malignant glioma. *Neuro-oncology.* 2011;13(12):1324–1330.

100. Strumberg D, Richly H, Hilger RA, et al. Phase I clinical and pharmacokinetic study of the Novel Raf kinase and vascular endothelial growth factor receptor inhibitor BAY 43–9006 in patients with advanced refractory solid tumors. *J Clin Oncol.* 2005;23(5):965–972.

101. Hainsworth JD, Ervin T, Friedman E, et al. Concurrent radiotherapy and temozolomide followed by temozolomide and sorafenib in the first-line treatment of patients with glioblastoma multiforme. *Cancer.* 2010;116(15):3663–3669.

102. Chow LQ, Eckhardt SG. Sunitinib: from rational design to clinical efficacy. *J Clin Oncol.* 2007;25(7):884–896.

103. Reardon DA, Vredenburgh JJ, Coan A, et al. Phase I study of sunitinib and irinotecan for patients with recurrent malignant glioma. *J Neurooncol.* 2011;105(3):621–627.

104. Wood JM, Bold G, Buchdunger E, et al. PTK787/ZK 222584, a novel and potent inhibitor of vascular endothelial growth factor receptor tyrosine kinases, impairs vascular endothelial growth factor-induced responses and tumor growth after oral administration. *Cancer Res.* 2000;60(8):2178–2189.

105. Goldbrunner RH, Bendszus M, Wood J, Kiderlen M, Sasaki M, Tonn JC. PTK787/ZK222584, an inhibitor of vascular endothelial growth factor receptor tyrosine kinases, decreases glioma growth and vascularization. *Neurosurgery.* 2004;55(2):426–32; discussion 432.

106. Gerstner ER, Eichler AF, Plotkin SR, et al. Phase I trial with biomarker studies of vatalanib (PTK787) in patients with newly diagnosed glioblastoma treated with enzyme inducing anti-epileptic drugs and standard radiation and temozolomide. *J Neurooncol.* 2011;103(2):325–332.

107. Reardon DA, Egorin MJ, Desjardins A, et al. Phase I pharmacokinetic study of the vascular endothelial growth factor receptor tyrosine kinase inhibitor vatalanib (PTK787) plus imatinib and hydroxyurea for malignant glioma. *Cancer.* 2009;115(10):2188–2198.

108. Conrad C, Friedman H, Reardon D, et al. A phase I/II trial of single-agent PTK 787/ZK 222584 (PTK/ZK), a novel, oral angiogenesis inhibitor, in patients with recurrent glioblastoma multiforme (GBM) [Abstract]. *J Clin Oncol.* 2004;22(14S (July 15, suppl):1512. *ASCO Annual Meeting Proceedings* (postmeeting edition).

109. Sandström M, Johansson M, Andersson U, Bergh A, Bergenheim AT, Henriksson R. The tyrosine kinase inhibitor ZD6474 inhibits tumour growth in an intracerebral rat glioma model. *Br J Cancer.* 2004;91(6):1174–1180.

110. Rich JN, Sathornsumetee S, Keir ST, et al. ZD6474, a novel tyrosine kinase inhibitor of vascular endothelial growth factor receptor and epidermal growth factor receptor, inhibits tumor growth of multiple nervous system tumors. *Clin Cancer Res.* 2005;11(22):8145–8157.

111. Wedge SR, Ogilvie DJ, Dukes M, et al. ZD6474 inhibits vascular endothelial growth factor signaling, angiogenesis, and tumor growth following oral administration. *Cancer Res.* 2002;62(16):4645–4655.

112. Carlomagno F, Vitagliano D, Guida T, et al. ZD6474, an orally available inhibitor of KDR tyrosine kinase activity, efficiently blocks oncogenic RET kinases. *Cancer Res.* 2002;62(24):7284–7290.

113. Drappatz J, Norden AD, Wong ET, et al. Phase I study of vandetanib with radiotherapy and temozolomide for newly diagnosed glioblastoma. *Int J Radiat Oncol Biol Phys.* 2010;78(1):85–90.

114. Fields EC, Damek D, Gaspar LE, et al. Phase I dose escalation trial of vandetanib with fractionated radiosurgery in patients with recurrent malignant gliomas. *Int J Radiat Oncol Biol Phys.* 2012;82(1):51–57.

115. Broniscer A, Baker JN, Tagen M, et al. Phase I study of vandetanib during and after radiotherapy in children

with diffuse intrinsic pontine glioma. *J Clin Oncol.* 2010;28(31):4762–4768.

116. Sunayama J, Sato A, Matsuda K, et al. Dual blocking of mTor and PI3K elicits a prodifferentiation effect on glioblastoma stem-like cells. *Neuro-oncology.* 2010;12(12):1205–1219.

117. Liu TJ, Koul D, LaFortune T, et al. NVP-BEZ235, a novel dual phosphatidylinositol 3-kinase/mammalian target of rapamycin inhibitor, elicits multifaceted antitumor activities in human gliomas. *Mol Cancer Ther.* 2009;8(8):2204–2210.

118. Maira SM, Stauffer F, Brueggen J, et al. Identification and characterization of NVP-BEZ235, a new orally available dual phosphatidylinositol 3-kinase/mammalian target of rapamycin inhibitor with potent *in vivo* antitumor activity. *Mol Cancer Ther.* 2008;7(7):1851–1863.

119. Chen L, Han L, Shi Z, et al. LY294002 enhances cytotoxicity of temozolomide in glioma by down-regulation of the PI3K/Akt pathway. *Mol Med Report.* 2012;5(2):575–579.

120. Premkumar DR, Arnold B, Jane EP, Pollack IF. Synergistic interaction between 17-AAG and phosphatidylinositol 3-kinase inhibition in human malignant glioma cells. *Mol Carcinog.* 2006;45(1):47–59.

121. Yakes FM, Chen J, Tan J, et al. Cabozantinib (XL184), a novel MET and VEGFR2 inhibitor, simultaneously suppresses metastasis, angiogenesis, and tumor growth. *Mol Cancer Ther.* 2011;10(12):2298–2308.

122. Zhang Y, Guessous F, Kofman A, Schiff D, Abounader R. XL-184, a MET, VEGFR-2 and RET kinase inhibitor for the treatment of thyroid cancer, glioblastoma multiforme and NSCLC. *IDrugs.* 2010;13(2):112–121.

123. Wen PY, Prados M, Schiff D, et al. Phase II study of XL184 (BMS 907351), an inhibitor of MET, VEGFR2, and RET, in patients (pts) with progressive glioblastoma (GB) [abstract]. *J Clin Oncol.* 2010;28(15 suppl):181s.

124. Cui JJ, Tran-Dubé M, Shen H, et al. Structure based drug design of crizotinib (PF-02341066), a potent and selective dual inhibitor of mesenchymal-epithelial transition factor (c-MET) kinase and anaplastic lymphoma kinase (ALK). *J Med Chem.* 2011;54(18):6342–6363.

125. Shaw AT, Yasothan U, Kirkpatrick P. Crizotinib. *Nat Rev Drug Discov.* 2011;10(12):897–898.

126. Zou HY, Li Q, Lee JH, et al. An orally available small-molecule inhibitor of c-Met, PF-2341066, exhibits cytoreductive antitumor efficacy through antiproliferative and antiangiogenic mechanisms. *Cancer Res.* 2007;67(9):4408–4417.

127. Yamazaki S, Skaptason J, Romero D, et al. Pharmacokinetic-pharmacodynamic modeling of biomarker response and tumor growth inhibition to an orally available cMet kinase inhibitor in human tumor xenograft mouse models. *Drug Metab Dispos.* 2008;36(7):1267–1274.

128. Hegi ME, Diserens AC, Gorlia T, et al. MGMT gene silencing and benefit from temozolomide in glioblastoma. *N Engl J Med.* 2005;352(10):997–1003.

129. Huang TT, Sarkaria SM, Cloughesy TF, Mischel PS. Targeted therapy for malignant glioma patients: lessons learned and the road ahead. *Neurotherapeutics.* 2009;6(3):500–512.

130. Vredenburgh JJ, Desjardins A, Herndon JE 2nd, et al. Phase II trial of bevacizumab and irinotecan in recurrent malignant glioma. *Clin Cancer Res.* 2007;13(4):1253–1259.

demos MEDICAL

RADIATION MEDICINE ROUNDS

Gene Therapy for Malignant Gliomas

Ahmed Mohyeldin and E. Antonio Chiocca*

Department of Neurological Surgery, Dardinger Laboratory for Neurooncology and Neurosciences, The James Comprehensive Cancer Center and Wexner Medical Center at The Ohio State University, Columbus, OH

ABSTRACT

Over the last two decades, research has been improving the efficiency and safety of using genes as anticancer and antiglioma therapy. In gene therapy, replication-incompetent viral vectors are utilized to deliver anticancer genes. In virotherapy, genetically engineered or mutated strains of viruses are generated to replicate and lyse tumor cells. In this chapter, we will review some of the approaches employed in both of these strategies, at the preclinical and the clinical level. We will also discuss the challenges of effective gene or virus biodistribution in tumors, including effects that the glioma microenvironment, the immune system, and the vascular system may have on injected viruses and vectors. The use of drug adjuvants to improve the efficiency of therapy will also be reviewed.

Keywords: oncolytic viral therapy, gene therapy, glioma, astrocytoma, immune system, clinical trial, HSV-1, adenovirus

INTRODUCTION

Primary malignant brain tumors remain a daunting challenge in medicine, with glioblastoma multiforme (GBM) being the most common and aggressive of these cancers (1). GBM epitomizes a class of brain tumors called gliomas that represent a broad diagnostic category with diffuse malignant cells known for their ability to infiltrate surrounding brain parenchyma. Their notorious invasive capacity makes complete surgical resection impossible (2). So devastating is the prognosis of this disease that, despite aggressive surgical resection followed with optimized radiation and chemotherapy treatment, the median survival for a GBM patient today continues to be 14.6 months (3). To put the dismal prognosis of this cancer more into perspective, a majority of patients succumb to their disease within 2 years and nearly all that survive die by 5 years, making GBM an inevitably fatal cancer (4). Despite the volume of literature on the extent of resection and GBMs, the aggressive biology of this neoplasm, as evidenced by clinical survival metrics and basic science data, has led some experts to insightfully point out that "significant

*Corresponding author, Dardinger Laboratory for Neurooncology and Neurosciences, Department of Neurological Surgery, James Comprehensive Cancer Center and The Ohio State University Medical Center, 410 W. 10th Avenue, N-1017 Doan Hall, Columbus, OH 43210.

E-mail address: EA.Chiocca@osumc.edu

Radiation Medicine Rounds 3:2 (2012) 275–288.

DOI: 10.5003/2151–4208.3.2.275

improvements in survival will not result from extensive surgery" (5). Although advances in imaging (6), surgical technique (7), drug delivery (8), and molecular stratification of these cancers (9,10) have demonstrated modest improvements in our management of GBM patients in the past three decades, significant breakthroughs in treatment are still lacking and will come from better insight into the disease process and more rational molecular targeting.

Progress in improving the prognosis of patients with GBM has been modest and has predominantly relied on informative imaging, optimization of medical and surgical treatment, and approval of new drugs with modest benefits on overall and/or progression-free survival. This has frustrated clinicians and demoralized patients but has underscored the importance of pursuing novel treatment strategies in hopes of mounting a decisive assault on this disease. Although initially not intuitive, the use of a pathogen to treat cancer has become a radical and sophisticated strategy to combat the aggressive phenotype of this disease. In fact, the engineering of viruses to fight cancer is a field that has now reached scientific maturity and has rapidly progressed from preclinical stages to clinical testing with considerable safety but disappointing efficacy. In this chapter, we review the milestones of this therapy focusing on landmark clinical trials, shed light on the limitations of this approach, and describe the recent and future strategies aimed at bringing promising efficacy to this mode of therapy.

■ CANCER AND VIROLOGY: A BRIEF HISTORY

Experimental use of viruses to combat cancer is a fairly old concept that has found contemporary scientific interest. The earliest documented studies fundamentally linking viruses to cancer treatment date back to the early 1900s. These early case reports described transient regression of blood cancers during a time when patients harbored natural viral infections (11,12). At the turn of the 20th century, although many scientists were describing the use of viruses to combat cancer, their association with cancer genesis fascinated others. In fact these two bodies of research would develop in parallel over the next 100 years and ironically, the Nobel Prize would be awarded five times to discoveries that elucidated the mechanisms of viral oncogenesis (13). Like most novel therapies, viral therapy showed early promise with reports of tumor regression but unfortunately disease progression often prevailed. As a consequence, enthusiasm among clinicians and scientists would waver leading many to abandon this mode of therapy for a period of time (12). Remarkably, advances in virology, molecular biology and profound insight gained from research on viral oncogenesis subsequently reinvigorated interest in this approach, and has now led to a blossoming and exciting area of cancer research.

The use of viral therapy in the treatment of cancer has emerged as one of many novel experimental approaches for cancer and in particular, extremely aggressive cancers like gliomas (14). This hypothesis of using viruses to combat cancer would be interrogated in the future with the development of more sophisticated viral engineering, controlled animal studies, and clinical testing that ultimately would converge on a major milestone in viral therapy and the introduction of the first genetically modified oncolytic virus (adenovirus H101) approved for cancer therapy in November of 2005 (15) in China.

Like many cancers that are refractory to treatment, the evaluation of the susceptibility of GBM to viral therapy has been an area that has received great scientific interest. It has rapidly progressed from preclinical evaluation to clinical testing in patients with a remarkably well-accepted safety profile. Viral therapeutics in the treatment of GBM has predominantly relied on utilizing two distinct strategies: (a) Replication-incompetent viruses that can be used as vectors for therapeutic gene delivery. Their therapeutic effect is harnessed through the delivery of transgenes that exert their cytotoxicity through multiple mechanisms. (b) Replication-competent viruses, also known as oncolytic viruses (OVs), are engineered to preferentially target tumor cells over normal cells of the brain and were initially designed to exert their cytotoxicity via replication lysis, and subsequent spread from host cell to neighboring cells. The vast majority of studies that have reached clinical testing for these two approaches have been phase I/II safety trials. In this chapter, we will attempt to review published clinical trials, discuss their rationale and outcomes. We also will discuss possible physiologic responses, including tumor microenvironment and immune system surveillance that may affect successful delivery of viral particles. In the context of these challenges, we will highlight emerging strategies to circumvent these obstacles and the rationale behind the engineering of future viruses to combat this relentless disease.

■ GENE THERAPY AND REPLICATION-INCOMPETENT VIRUSES

Retroviruses and adenoviruses (AdVs) were among the earliest viruses used for the delivery of genes in gliomas. These viruses were rendered replication-incompetent through the deletion of early regions of the viral genome and the strategic insertion of therapeutic transgenes (16). Initially, they were engineered to express the prodrug-converting enzyme herpes simplex virus thymidine kinase (HSV-TK). This was an ingenious proposal that achieved widespread preclinical appeal and efficacy because it was the first time tumor cells were rendered biochemically unique through the insertion of a single gene that would be later exploited through the administration of a cytotherapeutic drug (17). The prodrug used was ganciclovir (GCV), which served as a substrate for phosphorylation by HSV-TK, converting GCV to GCV-monophosphate. The subsequent conversion to GCV-triphosphate via other cellular kinases would deliver the lethal blow to cancer cells because this product incorporates into DNA and inhibits DNA polymerase ultimately halting proliferation and also inhibiting DNA repair (18,19).The transduction of the HSV-TK system and the subsequent treatment with GCV in glioma cells and other cancers proved to be an exciting breakthrough in cancer biology as data from animal models demonstrated regression and even complete eradication of malignant gliomas (19–22). These early seminal observations laid down the foundation for clinical testing.

In 1997, investigators at the National Institutes of Health (NIH) used replication-incompetent retroviruses engineered to harbor the HSV-TK transgene as the first gene therapy vectors to be tested in clinical trials for GBM patients (23). The study involved 15 patients, 12 with malignant gliomas, who received intratumoral stereotactic injections of vector producing cells (VPCs) that released retroviruses engineered with the HSV-TK gene. With a median survival of 8.1 months, modest antitumor activity was observed in four patients and documented responses were observed only in small tumors, with one GBM patient free of recurrence for 50 months following initial treatment (23). It was initially hypothesized that not all tumor cells needed to be transduced as neighboring cells that lack that HSV-TK genes were found to be apoptotic. Mechanistically, this was explained by *the bystander effect*, where toxic accumulation of the GCV metabolite permeated via cell-to-cell passage, killing neighboring cells (24). The authors of the NIH study cautiously concluded that improved transduction efficiency was required for this technology to reach therapeutic efficacy. This conclusion would set up the rationale for the design of the next generation of vectors used for clinical trials. In the subsequent years, investigators began to work with vectors that generated 100-fold higher titers than those used previously and viruses that were able to transduce tumor cells with a higher efficiency (25). In addition, experimentation with different delivery systems and scheduling (26,27) as well as the use of an Ommaya reservoir (28). to permit multiple treatments were employed with the intent to deliver a higher viral load to tumors. However, it was not until a series of elegant studies and careful neuropathological examination using gene-marking strategies to evaluate transduction efficiency that it became clear the retroviral VPC strategy was not a suitable mode of therapy (29,30).

The results of the initial NIH study documented an increase in seizure activity as the main adverse side effect. However, over the next several years other clinical trials with phase I/II/III status and safer engineered vectors would underscore the remarkable safety and low toxicity of this mode of therapy (for an excellent review on these trials, using other viruses, see Pulkkanen and Yla-Herrtuala, 2005) (31). With 248 patients with previously untreated newly diagnosed GBM, Rainov and his colleagues brought the first phase III randomized control trial evaluating the efficacy of the HSV-TK and GCV system as an adjuvant to surgical resection and radiation (32). The trial was a milestone in gene therapy but evidence of efficacy was not forthcoming, as no statistically significant measure was found between the gene therapy arms and standard therapy in progression-free survival or median survival (32). However, the study, for the first time, convincingly demonstrated the safety of this therapeutic modality as no difference in safety was appreciated between the two arms.

Although the retrovirus VPC approach has for the most part been abandoned as a vehicle to deliver genes to tumors, newly engineered AdVs and HSVs have emerged to maintain this line of work. Work with AdVs in primary or recurrent glioma patients reinvigorated hope in this therapeutic approach when a phase IIb clinical trial (n = 36) with engineered AdV expressing HSV-TK showed a statistically significant difference in median survival from 37.7 to 62.4 weeks (33). However, although the results of the phase III trial have not been published, the lack of European regulatory approval suggests that efficacy may not have been as evident: http://investors.arktherapeutics.com/servlet/HsPublic?context=ir.access&ir_option=RNS_NEWS&item=315695128659129&ir_client_id=4553.

Although many of these viruses continue to be engineered with HSV-TK, new technologies and transgenes are being explored. The next generation of gene therapy vectors to reach clinical trials may include (a) other gene-directed enzyme/prodrug systems such as cytosine deaminase (34); (b) wild-type 53 and other frequently mutated or deleted tumor suppressor genes in GBM (35); (c) antiangiogenic gene products that act as decoy vascular endothelial growth factor (VEGF) receptors (36); (d) immune modifying genes, that enhance our natural antitumor defense mechanisms (37); (e) resistance-modifying genes that protect hematopoietic cells and allow for intensified dosing of chemotherapeutic agents (38); and (f) antisense oligonucleotides for inhibition of key protein regulators cell growth (39).

■ ONCOLYTIC VIRAL THERAPY AND REPLICATION—COMPETENT VIRUSES

The tempered enthusiasm from the limited efficacy experienced from clinical trials using replication-incompetent viruses prompted investigators to consider other paradigms (40). OVs became an attractive tool to circumvent those shortcomings with hopes to improve transduction efficiency and local spread to other tumor cells via viral progeny after lysis. OV therapy uses replication-competent viruses that are engineered to preferential target and destroy cancer cells. This form of therapy relies on the viruses' ability to infect, reproduce, propagate, and subsequently spread to adjacent tumor cells to achieve oncolysis (16–41). Although new viruses are frequently being engineered and tested in a variety of cancers and in vitro systems, four OVs have reached clinical stage testing in gliomas: (a) HSV, (b) Newcastle disease virus (NDV), (c) AdV, and (d) reovirus (41). There are additional clinical trials in progress, using different types of AdVs, measles virus, and replicating retroviruses, but because data has not been published, we will not discuss them here.

For OVs to be safe, they had to be attenuated to be relatively avirulent in normal cells and avoid the associated neurotoxicity, at the same time be toxic to cancer cells. This remarkable achievement in virology continues to be an exciting and rapidly growing field but one that is made possible by exploiting the aberrant molecular/genetic pathways in tumors thus limiting viral replication and lytic destruction in cancer cells only (42). Most of the molecular strategies used to achieve this rely on three major mechanisms: (a) deletion of components of the viral genome necessary for viral replication that appear not to be expressed in normal cells but aberrantly expressed in cancer cells (16); (b) the insertion of promoter sequences into the viral genome that drive the expression-replication genes under the control of unique transcription factors found to be overexpressed in cancer (43); and (c) engineering viral capsid proteins to selectively transduce targeted cancer cells via unique molecular targeting (44).

HSV-1 Clinical Trials

Two replication-competent HSV-1 viruses have been engineered and clinical testing in human patients with GBMs related to this use has been published. These are G207 and 1716. Deletions of ICP6/RR, a ribonucleotide reductase essential for viral replication, rendered HSV-1 (G207) neuroattenuated (i.e., replication-incompetent in nondividing cells such as neurons). This allowed for intratumoral injection testing with hopes of specific replication within tumor cells followed by pan-tumoral dissemination to attack other cancer cells. Two phase I studies have tested the safety of this virus in patients (45,46). Using 21 patients, Markert et al. demonstrated that administration of HSV-1 (G207) at doses as high as 3×10^9 pfu was safe but never reached a maximum tolerated dose (MTD). Of the 21 patients, 6 patients showed improvement in neurological status and 3 showed volume decrease on MRI (45). In a more recent phase Ib study in 2009 that included six patients aimed to look at replication competency, this group of investigators demonstrated that HSV replication within the tumor occurred in some patients and a multiple dose injection paradigm was indeed safe (46).

Continued work with the HSV led to the engineering of HSV-1 (1716), another attenuated virus selective for rapidly dividing cells and unable to replicate in terminally differentiated cells (47). Preclinical testing in animals exhibited remarkable selectivity with minimal cytotoxicity in surrounding brain parenchyma (48,49). In 2002, nine patients underwent the first dose escalation study using HSV-1 (1716). Of the nine patients there were three responders, one showed progression-free survival for 3 years and two others were alive at 4 years posttreatment (50). No toxicity or serious adverse side effects were associated with the treatment and MTD was never reached (50). In a proof of principle study, Papanstassiou et al. administered intratumoral injections of HSV-1 (1716) in 12 glioma patients and assayed replication capacity from resected tumor 4 to 9 days after inoculation. Their study detected HSV DNA via polymerase chain reaction at tumor sites distal to the inoculation site in 4/12 patients and were able to detect the virus at the inoculation site in 10/12 patients. Furthermore, they were able to measure immune responses to HSV-1 (1716) with IgG and IgM antibody titers (51). A third trial in 2004 using the same viral injection dose (1×10^5 pfu) in newly diagnosed or recurrent high-grade glioma patients ($n = 12$) showed that three patients exhibited long-term survival (15–22 months) and underscored the safety of this virus as minimal toxicities were observed (52).

AdV Clinical Trials

AdVs offer unique advantages over other viruses in that they can be produced to high titers, replicate without direct integration into the genome of the host cell and have an ability to infect dividing and nondividing cells maximizing transduction efficiency (16). ONYX-015 is a conditionally replicating AdV with a deletion in its E1B gene, which allows to replicate in cells defective in viral RNA export (53,54), This unique feature led to testing of the virus with 24 recurrent GBM patients (55). Although no efficacy was appreciated (median time to progression was 46 days), MTDs were never reached and two patients who underwent a second resection 3 months after inoculation showed lymphocytic and plasmacytoid cellular infiltrates in perivascular spaces (55).

Reovirus Clinical Trials

Reoviruses are double-stranded RNA viruses with efficient capacities to infect mammalian cells. Furthermore, strong antiviral defense mechanisms keep viral replication in check thus minimizing associated cytotoxicity to normal cells (42). Remarkably, the commonly activated Ras signaling pathway in glioma cells overcomes antiviral defenses and permits for the replication of the virus in neoplastic cells (56). A phase I trial using reovirus was performed in 2008. Single intratumoral injections in 12 recurrent malignant glioma patients with escalating doses from 1×10^7 to 1×10^{10} pfu were administered. One of the twelve patients demonstrated disease-free survival for more than 6 years. The treatment was well tolerated with minimal side effects and the MTD was never reached (57).

NDV Clinical Trials

NDV is a virus known for its toxicity in most avian species with minimal toxicity exhibited by humans. It is a single-stranded RNA virus that first reached notoriety as an OV when it was found to selectively target and kill human and rat neuroblastoma cells without effect on normal fibroblasts in vitro (58). Since then two NDV strains have been used in clinical trials, MTH-68/H and NDV-HUJ. Only NDV-HUJ has reached clinical trial testing with a recent phase I/II clinical trial where 14 MRI-confirmed recurrent high-grade glioma patients received 8 cycles of NDV-HUJ via intravenous dosing (59). Toxicity was minimal among the patients treated, and 3 of the 14 were considered "long-term" survivors, and 1 patient had a complete tumor response. Although there have been no formal clinical trials with MTH-68/H strain there have been three published case reports incorporating six patients total that have also demonstrated early promise (60–62).

For a complete overview of all clinical trials to date using oncolytic viral therapy in gliomas, see Table 1.

■ VIRAL THERAPY AND THE TUMOR MICROENVIRONMENT

Spatial Barriers and Extracellular Matrix

One of the physical challenges that limits spread of the virus after intratumoral injection is the positive interstitial pressure within the tumor that thwarts viral particles from permeating to more distant sites within the tumor bulk (29). This problem could be possibly circumvented with convection-enhanced delivery resulting in a wider area of viral distribution. It works by giving a slow continuous infusion with a microinfusion pump connected to a microcatheter inserted in the tumor, with a slightly positive pressure gradient. This technology has been tested in humans and shown to be well tolerated and feasible (63). Inefficient dispersal of OV particles is further exacerbated by tumor extracellular matrix (ECM). Appreciation for structural ECM components such as collagens and proteoglycans hindering distribution of large therapeutic molecules has prompted investigators to consider novel ECM-modulating

TABLE 1. Clinical trials for high-grade gliomas using replication-competent oncolytic viruses

Study Type	Virus (Strain)	Patient (n)	Delivery Site	Dosing and Schedule	Efficacy	Toxicities	Reference
Phase I	HSV-l (G207)	21	Intratumoral	(SI) 1×10^6 to 3×10^9 pfu	6/21 improved neurological status, 8/21 decreased in tumor volume (MRI)	No toxicities appreciated	(44)
Phase I	HSV-l (G207)	9	Intratumoral	(MI) 1.5×10^8 to 1×10^9 pfu	No significant difference found	Seizures	(45)
Phase I	HSV-l (1716)	9	Intratumoral	(SI) 1×10^3 to 3×10^5 pfu	3/9 responded, 5/9 stable (MRI), 1/9 smaller, 2/9 stable (SPECT)	No toxicities appreciated	(49)
Phase I	HSV-l (1716)	12	Intratumoral	(SI) 1×10^5 pfu	No significant difference found	No toxicities appreciated	(48)
Phase I	HSV-l (1716)	12	Intratumoral	(SI) 1×10^5 pfu	3/12 disease-free for 15–22 months	No toxicities appreciated	(50)
Phase I	AdV (ONYX -015)	24	Resection cavity	(SI) 1×10^7 to 1×10^{10} pfu	No significant difference found	No toxicities appreciated	(54)
Phase I	Reovirus	12	Intratumoral	(SI) 1×10^7 to 1×10^{10} pfu	1/12 disease-free for > 6 years	No grade III/IV adverse effects	(56)
Case report	NDV (MTH-68/H)	1	Intravenous	(Dy) 2×10^7 to 2.5×10^8 pfu	First MRI, 95% tumor size decrease, second MRI stable disease	No toxicities appreciated	(59)
Case report	NDV (MTH-68/H)	4	Intravenous	(Dy) 2×10^7 to 2.5×10^8 pfu	4/4 Long-term survivors	No toxicities appreciated	(60)
Case report	NDV (MTH-68/H)	1	Inhalational	(DM) 4×10^8 pfu	Regression of thalamic tumor	No toxicities appreciated	(61)
Phase I/II	NDV (NDV-HUJ)	14	Intravenous	(MI) 0.1×10^9 to 11×10^9 IU	1/14 complete response, 3/14 long-term survival	Fevers 5/14	(58)

Abbreviations: DM = daily for months; Dy = daily for years; MI = multiple injections; SI = single injection.

enzymes to clear the path for viral particles. A recently engineered herpes simplex-1 virus designed to express Chondroitinase ABC, a bacterial enzyme that can cleave and remove elements of glioma ECM, showed enhanced OV spread and antitumor efficacy in orthotopic and in vivo animal models (64).

Preclinical testing in immunocompromised animal models has shed light on another barrier, the immune system. One of the reasons why preclinical studies have been so successful is that immune system is lacking in these animal models, underscoring the importance the immune system plays in eradicating therapeutic viruses from the body, effectively reducing viral load. Strategies aimed at bypassing this include direct intratumoral injection, careful selection of innate viruses that are known to have low antigenicity towards human immune systems, and more recently the identification of key cell populations implicated in the reduction of OVs viral titers within brain tumors that may be amenable to pharmacological inhibition (65). In fact, cyclophosphamide, an alkylating and immunosuppressive agent, has been shown to enhance glioma virotherapy by inhibiting innate immune responses leading to more efficient oncolytic viral transduction and cell killing (66).

Tumor Hypoxia and Angiogenesis

Hypoxia-induced necrosis and vascular proliferation are pathological hallmarks that distinguish GBM from other low-grade gliomas and is primarily a consequence of a rapidly proliferating tumor burden with slowly adapting and faulty vasculature (67). Hypoxia in GBM is associated with increased patient mortality, chemoresistance and radiation resistance, enhanced invasive phenotype, increased angiogenesis, and has more recently been identified to modulate cancer stem cell biology (67–71). Low-oxygen tension is known to affect viral replication and spatial distribution within the tumor bed because some viruses such as the AdVs are accustomed to higher oxygen tensions such as those found in the respiratory epithelium (72). To circumvent this, a family of viruses with tropism to brain paranchema and mucosa where oxygen tensions are substantially lower, appear to offer better strategies in tumor microenvironments where oxygen tensions can reach as low as 2 to 18 mmHg. In fact, in vitro studies have already established precedence for this as HSV-1, VV, and VSV have been shown to replicate efficiently in hypoxic malignant glioma cells (41).

Transcriptional biological responses, orchestrated as a consequence of decreasing oxygen tensions within cell systems, are mediated predominantly by the transcriptional regulator hypoxia inducible factor (HIF). Alternatively, a recent novel strategy in viral engineering differentially exploits hypoxic cancer cell signaling from surrounding normoxic tissue by inserting transcriptional driving domains that bind HIF in order to drive the viral replication apparatus (43,73,74). This allows viral replication to uniquely target hypoxic cancer cells and arrest much of the aggressive biology associated with GBM. In another approach, disrupting the functional network of vasculature that supplies rapidly dividing tumor cells, renders angiogenesis a highly attractive therapeutic target. In fact, it was demonstrated that in addition to impacting cancer cell growth, oncolytic AdVs reduce VEGF expression and disturb the orchestrated development of tumor-associated angiogenesis (75). Other viruses, such as oncolytic HSV-1, target proliferating tumor endothelial cells and have been shown to decrease microvessel density in treated tumors (76,77). More recently, novel strategies aimed at thwarting the angiogenic response used the combination of cleaved receptor molecules and OVs synergistically. Hardcastle and colleagues combined Vasculostatin (Vstat120), a cleaved and secreted fragment of angiogenic receptors in conjunction with OV therapy and demonstrated significant suppression of intracranial glioma growth in mice (78). Collectively, this body of work has underscored that combination therapy with oncolytic viral therapy and antiangiogenesis strategies reduce tumor vasculature density, promote viral spread and propagation leading to increased antitumor efficacy in several tumor models.

For an overview of viral engineering strategies and novel delivery systems, see Figure 1.

■ HARNESSING THE IMMUNE SYSTEM

The complex dynamic that exists between antiviral immunity and antitumor immunity has compelled several investigators to rethink the role the immune system plays in viral oncolysis (79). Upon injection of oncolytic viral particles, the innate immune system mounts its first assault limiting the therapeutic efficacy that OVs are designed to achieve. In contrast, the adaptive component of the immune system would result in antibody synthesis and T-cell responses that were antitumorigenic. A significant portion of the

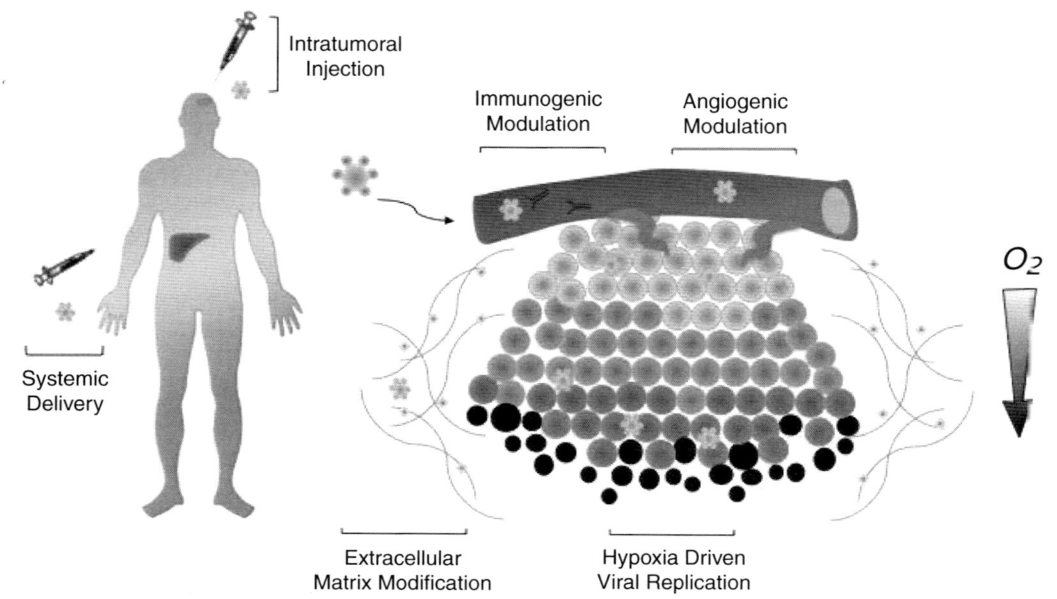

FIGURE 1 Tumor microenvironment, systemic barriers, and novel viral strategies. (a) Systemic delivery—strategies to deliver viruses systemically via blood and evade the immune system as well as liver clearance recently became available with the introduction of JX-594, a poxvirus that has naturally evolved for blood-borne systemic spread in mammals (43). (b) Intratumoral injection—intratumoral injection using positive pressure infusion pumps and the use of replication-competent viruses have helped enhance local spread within tumors (62). (c) Extracellular matrix modification—the introduction of viruses engineered to express matrix-modifying enzymes such as chondroitinase ABC has mediated enhancement of oncolytic virus spread and antitumor activity (63). (d) Immunogenic modulation—several strategies have emerged to modify and more particularly harness host immune responses to promote antitumor defense mechanisms (see section on Harnessing the Immune System). (e) Hypoxia-driven viral replication—engineering of viruses whose replication apparatus is driven by unique transcriptional promoter domains has led to exploitation of the commonly upregulated hypoxia pathway seen in GBMs (71). (f) Angiogenic modulation—viruses engineered to express cleaved extracellular fragments that inhibit angiogenesis have shown promise in preclinical testing (72).

efficacy exhibited by OVs is thought to be attributable to secondary immune defense mechanisms by the host and, as a result, investigators have begun to harness the synergy that exists between the immune system and virotherapy as a novel strategy to test in preclinical trials.

A recent study aimed to do this, utilized a vesicular stomatitis virus (VSV) vector carrying a cDNA library that expressed normal human prostate antigens that induced rejection of mouse prostate tumors via an immune-generated response. This approach worked but tumors often escaped immune selection and recurred at which point they were treated with a second-line therapy in which the VSV vector expressed a set of antigens derived from the recurrent tumor itself mounting another immune response to a different repertoire of antigens effectively curing animals of cancer (80). This specific strategy holds promise in the treatment of GBM, which displays high rates of recurrence and may help guide the future design of vaccines without the need for previous knowledge of tumor-associated antigens (79).

Other strategies aimed at engaging the immune system include viruses that have been engineered to express genes encoding for various immune-modulating cytokines such as Interleukins (IL)-2, 4, 12, and GM-CSF (81–84). Local tumor hypoxia has also been shown to stunt T-cell antitumor immune responses by inhibiting their proliferation and attenuating cytokine production. One recent strategy has been achieved where T cells were engineered to upregulate IL-2 production under a modified hypoxia response element thus promoting cytotoxic T-cell survival and proliferation in hypoxic tumors cells (85). This strategy showed promise in an in vivo lymphoma model where engineered T cells showed faster and more complete tumor regression (85). Of particular interest, is the study by Post et al. where inclusion of IL-4 gene therapy in hypoxia-driven oncolytic AdVs led to regression of human glioma xenografts in rodent models (82). Furthermore, some of these newly designed immune-modulating viruses have reached human clinical testing and have been shown to be safe for use as one study showed the therapeutic potential of a newly designed viral vector (pLIL-2-TK), which combined the expression of the suicide gene TK with the immunomodulatory gene IL-2 (37).

More recently, a phase Ib dose escalation trial using an AdV-TK in malignant gliomas aimed at capitalizing on the synergy between immunotherapy and radiation, in an early treatment paradigm, showed to be more effective in the upfront adjuvant setting in delaying recurrence, as survival at 2 years was 33% and at 3 years was 25% (86).

■ SYNERGY AMONG OVS, RADIOTHERAPY, AND CHEMOTHERAPY

There are currently several cancer therapeutics that have demonstrated promising potential in combination with oncolytic viral therapy. The Stupp Protocol has currently thrust radiation therapy with concomitant temozolomide treatment at the core of malignant glioma oncological management. As a result, several labs have started to test in preclinical and clinical stages combined efficacy of these approaches with oncolytic viral therapy, a strategy that offers quick translational promise. Radiation therapy has long been known to be staple in glioma therapy and investigators were optimistic when in vivo animal glioma models showed enhanced antitumor efficacy with HSV-1 treatment and coupled with radiation treatment (87). These findings have been demonstrated with other viruses (88,89) and clinical trials from other cancers have documented similar results, which have been elegantly reviewed previously (90). The proposed mechanism behind such synergy is thought to result from the increased replication potential of viruses within tumor cells leading to increased viral distribution with the tumor (91).

Chemotherapeutic drugs with potent immunosuppression achieved early notoriety in the field when Ikeda et al. demonstrated that oncolytic viral therapy, when delivered intravascularly, is significantly limited by antiviral activity predominantly through antibody and complement mediated mechanisms. Pretreatment with the immunosuppressive drug cyclophosphamide in animals and humans attenuated these defense mechanisms. In animals, in particular, it led to increased viral survival and propagation and ultimately tumor regression (92). Since those initial studies, several chemotherapeutic drugs have been tested including temozolomide, rapamycin, and valproic acid. Temozolomide treatment in combination with HSV-1 (G207) demonstrated increased efficacy when MGMT-positive cells were targeted in vivo (93). Similarly, rapamycin and valproic acid, two drugs that are commonly used clinically in malignant glioma patients, showed strong synergistic effects with oncolytic viral therapy (94,95).

The recent popularity of the antiangiogenic drug bevacizumab, a humanized anti-VEGF monoclonal antibody currently used in the management of recurrent glioma patients, has garnered some attention when combined with viral therapy. It has long been known that rapidly dividing tumors harbor a disturbed, tortuous, and leaky vasculature that leads to high interstitial pressures, poor circulation, and ultimately poor delivery of viral therapeutics. Recent studies have shown that bevacizumab results in normalization of tumor vasculature and enhanced drug delivery, leading investigators to speculate that combination therapy might aid in local viral distribution (96). This hypothesis was tested in a model of thyroid cancer where combined therapy significantly reduced tumor growth when compared with single treatment (97). The combined use of bevacizumab and oncolytic viral therapy has only recently been tested in gliomas by Martuza's group, who demonstrated strong synergy in controlling glioma invasion in mice (98). We suspect that combination treatment of bevacizumab and oncolytic viral therapy has a promising translational potential and speculate that it will rapidly move to human clinical testing as both agents have demonstrated a strong safety data, independently.

■ CONCLUSION: A CONVERGENCE OF STRATEGIES AND NOVEL DELIVERY MECHANISMS

A significant volume of human clinical trials has unequivocally underscored the safety associated with gene delivery and oncolytic viral therapy. Phase III studies demonstrating reproducible efficacy in curbing GBM median survival metrics have been disappointing but recent strategies focusing on ways to enhance viral spread, bypass the tumor microenvironment, and modulate and harness host immune defense mechanisms continue to keep this novel strategy highly attractive for clinical translation. These novel strategies have been achieved in part because of a convergence of ideas, as newly designed viruses offer multiple modalities of cell killing and OVs are now being engineered to deliver specific genes that allow for different modes of attack or immune modulation in addition to their cell lytic properties. Furthermore, recently engineered viruses that have genomes transcriptionally driven by unique promoter sequences will only improve the targeted specificity and killing of cancer cells. As genomic interrogation of GBM continues to define signaling hallmarks of this cancer, new promoter sequences will inevitably be explored and tested in the next generation of viral vectors.

Nearly all clinical trials in glioma patients have relied on intratumoral injection of OVs in part because of the significant reduction of viral load if injected via the blood stream and also because of the difficulties in getting past the blood–brain barrier. These inherent challenges to brain tumor therapy have compelled investigators to seek novel therapeutic delivery platforms for delivery. Remarkably, several groups have demonstrated neural and mesenchymal stem cell tropism towards gliomas (99–101). These cells can carry immune-modulating genes but more interestingly have recently been shown to deliver oncolytic AdV in mice bearing U87 glioma xenografts (100). A recently exciting discovery has introduced JX-594, a poxvirus that has naturally evolved for blood-borne systemic spread in mammals and was engineered for cancer-selective replication, transgene expression, and amplification in cancer cells harboring activation of the epidermal growth factor receptor (EGFR)/Ras pathway, a pathway that is aberrantly expressed in ~40% to 50% of primary GBMs (44). The virus can be used as a vehicle for intravenous delivery and expression of transgenes in tumors was recently demonstrated in clinical trials against several human cancers (44). Although not tested against gliomas it will be interesting to see if it has the capacity to breach the blood–brain barrier and reach brain tumor parenchyma.

Viral therapy is an exciting and blossoming field in cancer research. The rapid progress and safety that has been established as a consequence of preclinical and clinical testing has affirmed the scientific maturity of this therapeutic approach with hopes of providing the decisive assault that we so eagerly anticipate for this disease.

REFERENCES

1. CBTRUS Statistical Report: primary brain and central nervous system tumors diagnosed in the United States in 2004–2007 (February 2011).
2. Silbergeld DL, Chicoine MR. Isolation and characterization of human malignant glioma cells from histologically normal brain. *J Neurosurg.* 1997;86(3):525–531.
3. Stupp R, Mason WP, van den Bent MJ, et al.; European Organisation for Research and Treatment of Cancer Brain Tumor and Radiotherapy Groups; National Cancer Institute of Canada Clinical Trials Group. Radiotherapy plus concomitant and adjuvant temozolomide for glioblastoma. *N Engl J Med.* 2005;352(10):987–996.
4. Davis FG, Freels S, Grutsch J, Barlas S, Brem S. Survival rates in patients with primary malignant brain tumors stratified by patient age and tumor histological type: an analysis based on Surveillance, Epidemiology, and End Results (SEER) data, 1973–1991. *J Neurosurg.* 1998;88(1):1–10.
5. Piepmeier J. Comment on: extent of resection and survival in glioblastoma multiforme: identification of and adjustment for bias. *Neurosurgery.* 2008;62(3):564–76; discussion 64–76.
6. Dhermain FG, Hau P, Lanfermann H, Jacobs AH, van den Bent MJ. Advanced MRI and PET imaging for assessment of treatment response in patients with gliomas. *Lancet Neurol.* 2010;9(9):906–920.
7. Stummer W, Pichlmeier U, Meinel T, Wiestler OD, Zanella F, Reulen HJ; ALA-Glioma Study Group. Fluorescence-guided surgery with 5-aminolevulinic acid for resection of malignant glioma: a randomised controlled multicentre phase III trial. *Lancet Oncol.* 2006;7(5):392–401.
8. Westphal M, Hilt DC, Bortey E, et al. A phase 3 trial of local chemotherapy with biodegradable carmustine (BCNU) wafers (Gliadel wafers) in patients with primary malignant glioma. *Neuro-oncology.* 2003;5(2):79–88.
9. Hegi ME, Diserens AC, Gorlia T, et al. MGMT gene silencing and benefit from temozolomide in glioblastoma. *N Engl J Med.* 2005;352(10):997–1003.
10. Phillips HS, Kharbanda S, Chen R, et al. Molecular subclasses of high-grade glioma predict prognosis, delineate a pattern of disease progression, and resemble stages in neurogenesis. *Cancer Cell.* 2006;9(3):157–173.
11. Dock G. The influence of complicating diseases upon leukemia. *Amer J Med Sci.* 1904;127(4):563–592.
12. Kelly E, Russell SJ. History of oncolytic viruses: genesis to genetic engineering. *Mol Ther.* 2007;15(4):651–659.
13. Moore PS, Chang Y. Why do viruses cause cancer? Highlights of the first century of human tumour virology. *Nat Rev Cancer.* 2010;10(12):878–889.
14. Kaur B, Chiocca EA. Oncolytic viruses: extreme treatment for an extreme disease. *Future Microbiol.* 2006;1(4):351–353.
15. Garber K. China approves world's first oncolytic virus therapy for cancer treatment. *J Natl Cancer Inst.* 2006;98(5):298–300.

16. Cutter JL, Kurozumi K, Chiocca EA, Kaur B. Gene therapeutics: the future of brain tumor therapy? *Expert Rev Anticancer Ther.* 2006;6(7):1053–1064.

17. Moolten FL. Tumor chemosensitivity conferred by inserted herpes thymidine kinase genes: paradigm for a prospective cancer control strategy. *Cancer Res.* 1986;46(10):5276–5281.

18. Moolten FL, Wells JM. Curability of tumors bearing herpes thymidine kinase genes transferred by retroviral vectors. *J Natl Cancer Inst.* 1990;82(4):297–300.

19. Ezzeddine ZD, Martuza RL, Platika D, et al. Selective killing of glioma cells in culture and *in vivo* by retrovirus transfer of the herpes simplex virus thymidine kinase gene. *New Biol.* 1991;3(6):608–614.

20. Culver KW, Ram Z, Wallbridge S, Ishii H, Oldfield EH, Blaese RM. *In vivo* gene transfer with retroviral vector-producer cells for treatment of experimental brain tumors. *Science.* 1992;256(5063):1550–1552.

21. Izquierdo M, Cortés M, de Felipe P, et al. Long-term rat survival after malignant brain tumor regression by retroviral gene therapy. *Gene Ther.* 1995;2(1):66–69.

22. Ram Z, Culver KW, Walbridge S, Blaese RM, Oldfield EH. In situ retroviral-mediated gene transfer for the treatment of brain tumors in rats. *Cancer Res.* 1993;53(1):83–88.

23. Ram Z, Culver KW, Oshiro EM, et al. Therapy of malignant brain tumors by intratumoral implantation of retroviral vector-producing cells. *Nat Med.* 1997;3(12):1354–1361.

24. Freeman SM, Abboud CN, Whartenby KA, et al. The "bystander effect": tumor regression when a fraction of the tumor mass is genetically modified. *Cancer Res.* 1993;53(21):5274–5283.

25. Lyons RM, Forry-Schaudies S, Otto E, et al. An improved retroviral vector encoding the herpes simplex virus thymidine kinase gene increases antitumor efficacy in vivo. *Cancer Gene Ther.* 1995;2(4):273–280.

26. Shand N, Weber F, Mariani L, et al. A phase 1–2 clinical trial of gene therapy for recurrent glioblastoma multiforme by tumor transduction with the herpes simplex thymidine kinase gene followed by ganciclovir. GLI328 European-Canadian Study Group. *Hum Gene Ther.* 1999;10(14):2325–2335.

27. Packer RJ, Raffel C, Villablanca JG, et al. Treatment of progressive or recurrent pediatric malignant supratentorial brain tumors with herpes simplex virus thymidine kinase gene vector-producer cells followed by intravenous ganciclovir administration. *J Neurosurg.* 2000;92(2):249–254.

28. Prados MD, McDermott M, Chang SM, et al. Treatment of progressive or recurrent glioblastoma multiforme in adults with herpes simplex virus thymidine kinase gene vector-producer cells followed by intravenous ganciclovir administration: a phase I/II multi-institutional trial. *J Neurooncol.* 2003;65(3):269–278.

29. Puumalainen AM, Vapalahti M, Agrawal RS, et al. Beta-galactosidase gene transfer to human malignant glioma *in vivo* using replication-deficient retroviruses and adenoviruses. *Hum Gene Ther.* 1998;9(12):1769–1774.

30. Harsh GR, Deisboeck TS, Louis DN, et al. Thymidine kinase activation of ganciclovir in recurrent malignant gliomas: a gene-marking and neuropathological study. *J Neurosurg.* 2000;92(5):804–811.

31. Pulkkanen KJ, Yla-Herttuala S. Gene therapy for malignant glioma: current clinical status. *Mol Ther.* 2005;12(4):585–598.

32. Rainov NG. A phase III clinical evaluation of herpes simplex virus type 1 thymidine kinase and ganciclovir gene therapy as an adjuvant to surgical resection and radiation in adults with previously untreated glioblastoma multiforme. *Hum Gene Ther.* 2000;11(17):2389–2401.

33. Immonen A, Vapalahti M, Tyynelä K, et al. AdvHSV-tk gene therapy with intravenous ganciclovir improves survival in human malignant glioma: a randomised, controlled study. *Mol Ther.* 2004;10(5):967–972.

34. Miller CR, Williams CR, Buchsbaum DJ, Gillespie GY. Intratumoral 5-fluorouracil produced by cytosine deaminase/5-fluorocytosine gene therapy is effective for experimental human glioblastomas. *Cancer Res.* 2002;62(3):773–780.

35. Lang FF, Bruner JM, Fuller GN, et al. Phase I trial of adenovirus-mediated p53 gene therapy for recurrent glioma: biological and clinical results. *J Clin Oncol.* 2003;21(13):2508–2518.

36. Kaur B, Cork SM, Sandberg EM, et al. Vasculostatin inhibits intracranial glioma growth and negatively regulates *in vivo* angiogenesis through a CD36-dependent mechanism. *Cancer Res.* 2009;69(3):1212–1220.

37. Palù G, Cavaggioni A, Calvi P, et al. Gene therapy of glioblastoma multiforme via combined expression of suicide and cytokine genes: a pilot study in humans. *Gene Ther.* 1999;6(3):330–337.

38. Raffel C, Culver K, Kohn D, et al. Gene therapy for the treatment of recurrent pediatric malignant astrocytomas with *in vivo* tumor transduction with the herpes simplex thymidine kinase gene/ganciclovir system. *Hum Gene Ther.* 1994;5(7):863–890.

39. Hau P, Jachimczak P, Schlingensiepen R, et al. Inhibition of TGF-beta2 with AP 12009 in recurrent malignant gliomas: from preclinical to phase I/II studies. *Oligonucleotides.* 2007;17(2):201–212.

40. Dirven CM, van Beusechem VW, Lamfers ML, Grill J, Gerritsen WR, Vandertop WP. Oncolytic adenoviruses for treatment of brain tumours. *Expert Opin Biol Ther.* 2002;2(8):943–952.

41. Zemp FJ, Corredor JC, Lun X, Muruve DA, Forsyth PA. Oncolytic viruses as experimental treatments for malignant gliomas: using a scourge to treat a devil. *Cytokine Growth Factor Rev.* 2010;21(2–3):103–117.

42. Haseley A, Alvarez-Breckenridge C, Chaudhury AR, Kaur B. Advances in oncolytic virus therapy for glioma. *Recent Pat CNS Drug Discov.* 2009;4(1):1–13.

43. Longo SL, Griffith C, Glass A, Shillitoe EJ, Post DE. Development of an oncolytic herpes simplex virus using a tumor-specific HIF-responsive promoter. *Cancer Gene Ther.* 2011;18(2):123–134.

44. Breitbach CJ, Burke J, Jonker D, et al. Intravenous delivery of a multi-mechanistic cancer-targeted oncolytic poxvirus in humans. *Nature.* 2011;477(7362):99–102.

45. Markert JM, Medlock MD, Rabkin SD, et al. Conditionally replicating herpes simplex virus mutant, G207 for the treatment of malignant glioma: results of a phase I trial. *Gene Ther.* 2000;7(10):867–874.

46. Markert JM, Liechty PG, Wang W, et al. Phase Ib trial of mutant herpes simplex virus G207 inoculated pre- and post-tumor resection for recurrent GBM. *Mol Ther.* 2009;17(1):199–207.

47. McKie EA, MacLean AR, Lewis AD, et al. Selective *in vitro* replication of herpes simplex virus type 1 (HSV-1) ICP34.5 null mutants in primary human CNS tumours–evaluation of a potentially effective clinical therapy. *Br J Cancer.* 1996;74(5):745–752.

48. Randazzo BP, Kesari S, Gesser RM, et al. Treatment of experimental intracranial murine melanoma with a neuroattenuated herpes simplex virus 1 mutant. *Virology.* 1995;211(1):94–101.

49. Kesari S, Randazzo BP, Valyi-Nagy T, et al. Therapy of experimental human brain tumors using a neuroattenuated herpes simplex virus mutant. *Lab Invest.* 1995;73(5):636–648.

50. Rampling R, Cruickshank G, Papanastassiou V, et al. Toxicity evaluation of replication-competent herpes simplex virus (ICP 34.5 null mutant 1716) in patients with recurrent malignant glioma. *Gene Ther.* 2000;7(10):859–866.

51. Papanastassiou V, Rampling R, Fraser M, et al. The potential for efficacy of the modified (ICP 34.5(–)) herpes simplex virus HSV1716 following intratumoural injection into human malignant glioma: a proof of principle study. *Gene Ther.* 2002;9(6):398–406.

52. Harrow S, Papanastassiou V, Harland J, et al. HSV1716 injection into the brain adjacent to tumour following surgical resection of high-grade glioma: safety data and long-term survival. *Gene Ther.* 2004;11(22):1648–1658.

53. Bischoff JR, Kirn DH, Williams A, et al. An adenovirus mutant that replicates selectively in p53-deficient human tumor cells. *Science.* 1996;274(5286):373–376.

54. O'Shea CC, Johnson L, Bagus B, et al. Late viral RNA export, rather than p53 inactivation, determines ONYX-015 tumor selectivity. *Cancer Cell.* 2004;6(6):611–623.

55. Chiocca EA, Abbed KM, Tatter S, et al. A phase I open-label, dose-escalation, multi-institutional trial of injection with an E1B-Attenuated adenovirus, ONYX-015, into the peritumoral region of recurrent malignant gliomas, in the adjuvant setting. *Mol Ther.* 2004;10(5):958–966.

56. Strong JE, Tang D, Lee PW. Evidence that the epidermal growth factor receptor on host cells confers reovirus infection efficiency. *Virology.* 1993;197(1):405–411.

57. Forsyth P, Roldán G, George D, et al. A phase I trial of intratumoral administration of reovirus in patients with histologically confirmed recurrent malignant gliomas. *Mol Ther.* 2008;16(3):627–632.

58. Reichard KW, Lorence RM, Cascino CJ, et al. Newcastle disease virus selectively kills human tumor cells. *J Surg Res.* 1992;52(5):448–453.

59. Freeman AI, Zakay-Rones Z, Gomori JM, et al. Phase I/II trial of intravenous NDV-HUJ oncolytic virus in recurrent glioblastoma multiforme. *Mol Ther.* 2006;13(1):221–228.

60. Csatary LK, Bakács T. Use of Newcastle disease virus vaccine (MTH-68/H) in a patient with high-grade glioblastoma. *JAMA.* 1999;281(17):1588–1589.

61. Csatary LK, Gosztonyi G, Szeberenyi J, et al. MTH-68/H oncolytic viral treatment in human high-grade gliomas. *J Neurooncol.* 2004;67(1–2):83–93.

62. Wagner S, Csatary CM, Gosztonyi G, et al. Combined treatment of pediatric high-grade glioma with the oncolytic viral strain MTH-68/H and oral valproic acid. *APMIS.* 2006;114(10):731–743.

63. Laske DW, Youle RJ, Oldfield EH. Tumor regression with regional distribution of the targeted toxin TF-CRM107 in patients with malignant brain tumors. *Nat Med.* 1997;3(12):1362–1368.

64. Dmitrieva N, Yu L, Viapiano M, et al. Chondroitinase ABC I-mediated enhancement of oncolytic virus spread and antitumor efficacy. *Clin Cancer Res.* 2011;17(6):1362–1372.

65. Fulci G, Dmitrieva N, Gianni D, et al. Depletion of peripheral macrophages and brain microglia increases brain tumor titers of oncolytic viruses. *Cancer Res.* 2007;67(19):9398–9406.

66. Fulci G, Breymann L, Gianni D, et al. Cyclophosphamide enhances glioma virotherapy by inhibiting innate immune responses. *Proc Natl Acad Sci USA.* 2006;103(34):12873–12878.

67. Brat DJ, Castellano-Sanchez AA, Hunter SB, et al. Pseudopalisades in glioblastoma are hypoxic, express extracellular matrix proteases, and are formed by an actively migrating cell population. *Cancer Res.* 2004;64(3):920–927.

68. Li Z, Bao S, Wu Q, et al. Hypoxia-inducible factors regulate tumorigenic capacity of glioma stem cells. *Cancer Cell.* 2009;15(6):501–513.

69. Zagzag D, Zhong H, Scalzitti JM, Laughner E, Simons JW, Semenza GL. Expression of hypoxia-inducible factor 1alpha in brain tumors: association with angiogenesis, invasion, and progression. *Cancer.* 2000;88(11):2606–2618.

70. Mohyeldin A, Dalgard CL, Lu H, et al. Survival and invasiveness of astrocytomas promoted by erythropoietin. *J Neurosurg.* 2007;106(2):338–350.

71. Mohyeldin A, Garzón-Muvdi T, Quiñones-Hinojosa A. Oxygen in stem cell biology: a critical component of the stem cell niche. *Cell Stem Cell.* 2010;7(2):150–161.

72. Pipiya T, Sauthoff H, Huang YQ, et al. Hypoxia reduces adenoviral replication in cancer cells by downregulation of viral protein expression. *Gene Ther.* 2005;12(11):911–917.

73. Post DE, Van Meir EG. A novel hypoxia-inducible factor (HIF) activated oncolytic adenovirus for cancer therapy. *Oncogene.* 2003;22(14):2065–2072.

74. Cho WK, Seong YR, Lee YH, et al. Oncolytic effects of adenovirus mutant capable of replicating in hypoxic and normoxic regions of solid tumor. *Mol Ther.* 2004;10(5):938–949.

75. Saito Y, Sunamura M, Motoi F, et al. Oncolytic replication-competent adenovirus suppresses tumor angiogenesis through preserved E1A region. *Cancer Gene Ther.* 2006;13(3):242–252.

76. Mahller YY, Vaikunth SS, Currier MA, et al. Oncolytic HSV and erlotinib inhibit tumor growth and angiogenesis in a novel malignant peripheral nerve sheath tumor xenograft model. *Mol Ther.* 2007;15(2):279–286.

77. Cinatl J Jr, Michaelis M, Driever PH, et al. Multimutated herpes simplex virus g207 is a potent inhibitor of angiogenesis. *Neoplasia.* 2004;6(6):725–735.

78. Hardcastle J, Kurozumi K, Dmitrieva N, et al. Enhanced antitumor efficacy of vasculostatin (Vstat120) expressing oncolytic HSV-1. *Mol Ther.* 2010;18(2):285–294.

79. Alvarez-Breckenridge C, Chiocca EA. A viral strategy to ambush tumors. *Nat Med.* 2011;17(7):784–785.

80. Kottke T, Errington F, Pulido J, et al. Broad antigenic coverage induced by vaccination with virus-based cDNA libraries cures established tumors. *Nat Med.* 2011;17(7):854–859.

81. Mizuno H, Yanoma S, Nishimura G, et al. Therapeutic efficiency of IL-2 gene transduced tumor vaccine for head and neck carcinoma. *Cancer Lett.* 2000;152(2):175–185.

82. Post DE, Sandberg EM, Kyle MM, et al. Targeted cancer gene therapy using a hypoxia inducible factor dependent oncolytic adenovirus armed with interleukin-4. *Cancer Res.* 2007;67(14):6872–6881.

83. Wong RJ, Chan MK, Yu Z, et al. Angiogenesis inhibition by an oncolytic herpes virus expressing interleukin 12. *Clin Cancer Res.* 2004;10(13):4509–4516.

84. Ramesh N, Ge Y, Ennist DL, et al. CG0070, a conditionally replicating granulocyte macrophage colony-stimulating factor–armed oncolytic adenovirus for the treatment of bladder cancer. *Clin Cancer Res.* 2006;12(1):305–313.

85. Kim H, Peng G, Hicks JM, et al. Engineering human tumor-specific cytotoxic T cells to function in a hypoxic environment. *Mol Ther.* 2008;16(3):599–606.

86. Chiocca EA, Aguilar LK, Bell SD, et al. Phase IB study of gene-mediated cytotoxic immunotherapy adjuvant to up-front surgery and intensive timing radiation for malignant glioma. *J Clin Oncol.* 2011;29(27):3611–3619.

87. Bradley JD, Kataoka Y, Advani S, et al. Ionizing radiation improves survival in mice bearing intracranial high-grade gliomas injected with genetically modified herpes simplex virus. *Clin Cancer Res.* 1999;5(6):1517–1522.

88. Lamfers ML, Idema S, Bosscher L, et al. Differential effects of combined Ad5-delta 24RGD and radiation therapy in *in vitro* versus *in vivo* models of malignant glioma. *Clin Cancer Res.* 2007;13(24):7451–7458.

89. Geoerger B, Grill J, Opolon P, et al. Potentiation of radiation therapy by the oncolytic adenovirus dl1520 (ONYX-015) in human malignant glioma xenografts. *Br J Cancer.* 2003;89(3):577–584.

90. Advani SJ, Weichselbaum RR, Chmura SJ. Enhancing radiotherapy with genetically engineered viruses. *J Clin Oncol.* 2007;25(26):4090–4095.

91. Advani SJ, Sibley GS, Song PY, et al. Enhancement of replication of genetically engineered herpes simplex viruses by ionizing radiation: a new paradigm for destruction of therapeutically intractable tumors. *Gene Ther.* 1998;5(2):160–165.

92. Ikeda K, Ichikawa T, Wakimoto H, et al. Oncolytic virus therapy of multiple tumors in the brain requires suppression of innate and elicited antiviral responses. *Nat Med.* 1999;5(8):881–887.

93. Aghi M, Rabkin S, Martuza RL. Effect of chemotherapy-induced DNA repair on oncolytic herpes simplex viral replication. *J Natl Cancer Inst.* 2006;98(1):38–50.

94. Alonso MM, Jiang H, Yokoyama T, et al. Delta-24-RGD in combination with RAD001 induces enhanced anti-glioma effect via autophagic cell death. *Mol Ther.* 2008;16(3):487–493.

95. Otsuki A, Patel A, Kasai K, et al. Histone deacetylase inhibitors augment antitumor efficacy of herpes-based oncolytic viruses. *Mol Ther.* 2008;16(9):1546–1555.

96. Tong RT, Boucher Y, Kozin SV, Winkler F, Hicklin DJ, Jain RK. Vascular normalization by vascular endothelial growth factor receptor 2 blockade induces a pressure gradient across the vasculature and improves drug penetration in tumors. *Cancer Res.* 2004;64(11):3731–3736.

97. Libertini S, Iacuzzo I, Perruolo G, et al. Bevacizumab increases viral distribution in human anaplastic thyroid carcinoma xenografts and enhances the effects of E1A-defective adenovirus dl922–947. *Clin Cancer Res.* 2008;14(20):6505–6514.

98. Zhang W, Fulci G, Buhrman JS, et al. Bevacizumab with angiostatin-armed oHSV increases antiangiogenesis and decreases bevacizumab-induced invasion in U87 glioma. *Mol Ther.* 2012;20(1):37–45.

99. Kendall SE, Najbauer J, Johnston HF, et al. Neural stem cell targeting of glioma is dependent on phosphoinositide 3-kinase signaling. *Stem Cells.* 2008;26(6):1575–1586.

100. Sonabend AM, Ulasov IV, Tyler MA, Rivera AA, Mathis JM, Lesniak MS. Mesenchymal stem cells effectively deliver an oncolytic adenovirus to intracranial glioma. *Stem Cells.* 2008;26(3):831–841.

101. Zhao D, Najbauer J, Garcia E, et al. Neural stem cell tropism to glioma: critical role of tumor hypoxia. *Mol Cancer Res.* 2008;6(12):1819–1829.

demos
MEDICAL

RADIATION
MEDICINE ROUNDS

Immunotherapy for Malignant Gliomas

Richard G. Everson, Elena I. Fomchenko, David S. Foulad, Dominique N. Lisiero, and Linda M. Liau*

UCLA Department of Neurosurgery, David Geffen School of Medicine at UCLA, Los Angeles, CA

■ ABSTRACT

Malignant gliomas invade and infiltrate the surrounding brain, often making complete surgical excision impossible. They are also among the most radiation- and chemotherapy-resistant cancers. As such, innovative treatment approaches are desperately needed. Immunotherapy is a particularly appealing strategy because of the potential ability for immune cells to traffic to and destroy infiltrating tumor cells, which by the time of diagnosis have permeated into normal brain parenchyma far beyond the borders of the tumor recognizable by conventional imaging methods or during surgery. This chapter reviews current strategies for modulating the immune system for the treatment of malignant gliomas.

Keywords: brain tumors, gliomas, immunotherapy, T-cells, dendritic cells, cancer vaccine

■ INTRODUCTION TO IMMUNOTHERAPY

Despite multiple lines of research, the prognosis for malignant glioma patients remains dismal and is characterized by the recurrence of aggressive disease even with application of multiple treatment modalities (1). This is partly due to the diffuse infiltration of glioma cells into the surrounding brain parenchyma at the time of presentation, which is not addressed by existing treatments and requires the ability to specifically target glioma cells far beyond the margin of surgical resection. The goal of immunotherapy is to harness the specificity of the immune system to extinguish these residual cells while sparing normal tissues, and perhaps to do so in a way that generates a long-lasting effect whereby the patient would be immunized against further disease recurrence (2,3). Glioma immunotherapy can be classified into specific and nonspecific, as well as passive or active, approaches (Table 1). Specific immunotherapy targets a defined antigen or set of antigens, whereas nonspecific immunotherapy (i.e., the use of cytokines or other immunomodulating agents) might induce a more broadly targeted response. Their administration can occur via systemic, intrathecal or intratumoral routes, or administration into the tumor resection cavity (4). Immunomodulation can be performed via the use of recombinant cytokines, viral vectors, liposomes, or biopolymer microspheres carrying cytokine-encoding genes, cytokine-secreting cells, or toxin-linked cytokines.

Passive immunotherapy approaches encompass the use of monoclonal antibodies (mAbs) to bolster immune recognition of glioma cells to increase antiglioma response or allow for targeted delivery; and

*Corresponding author, UCLA Department of Neurosurgery, Gonda Building, Room 3357, 695 Charles Young Drive, Los Angeles, CA 90095–1761

E-mail address: LLIAU@mednet.ucla.edu

Radiation Medicine Rounds 3:2 (2012) 289–316.

DOI: 10.5003/2151–4208.3.2.289

adoptive cell transfer therapy, which utilizes the ex vivo expansion and reintroduction of immune effector cells that recognize specific tumor-associated targets (5). *Active immunotherapy* is based on induction or augmentation of individual patients' own immune responses to glioma-specific antigens via immunization or vaccination. Some approaches include the use of DNA, RNA, peptides, and proteins; lysed, whole or cytokine-expressing autologous tumor cell vaccines; antigen-loaded dendritic cells (DCs) (professional antigen-presenting cells); and bacterial vectors or viral particles expressing Ags.

■ IMMUNE MODULATION

In addition to the intrinsic immune-privilege of the brain, gliomas express immunosuppressive cytokines, most notably transforming growth factor-β2 (TGF-β2) and interleukin-10 (IL-10). These mediators promote tumor growth by suppressing T-cell proliferation and the production of immunostimulatory modulators, such as IL-2 and interferon-γ (IFN-γ). Accordingly, attempts have been made to either block immunosuppressive modulators or to induce the expression of immunostimulatory cytokines at the tumor site.

Recombinant cytokines have been used as successful therapeutics in many animal models of cancer. However, the systemic administration of cytokines, such as IFNs, is limited by toxicity (6), and the administration to the tumor site or resection cavity in the central nervous system (CNS) can cause local brain toxicity (7) and poses practical issues (e.g., placement of intracranial catheters) with administration in humans. Thus, there has been the widespread development of local cytokine delivery systems through the use of gene transfer. Many approaches have already been translated to clinical trials including cationic liposomes, adenoviral (Ad) vectors, retroviral vectors, herpes simplex virus type 1 (HSV-1) vectors, and adeno-associated virus (AAV) vectors (8–10). Other clinical approaches include the use of in vitro transfected cells, such as fibroblasts, to secrete cytokines at the peripheral vaccination site (11,12).

IFNs in Enhancing the Immune Response: α, β, and γ

IFNs have an integral role in activating and mediating the immune response. Although IFNs have been well-known as antiviral agents, their antitumor function has also been exploited by researchers. The type I IFNs (IFN-α, IFN-β) are predominantly produced by plasmacytoid DCs (pDCs) in response to viral antigens and other immune-modulating molecules; however, they can be secreted at lower levels by many other cell types (13). Type II IFNs

TABLE 1 Immunotherapy strategies

Type	Description
Immunomodulation	Use of recombinant cytokines or other immune stimulants, directly or via vectors such as cells, liposomes, viruses, biopolymer microspheres to induce nonspecific immune responses
Passive	
Monoclonal antibodies	Specific targeting of cell surface antigen-bearing cells for killing via complement-dependent (CDC) or antibody-dependent (ADCC) mechanisms
Adoptive T-cell transfer	Ex vivo expansion and reintroduction of patient-produced immune effector cells that may be either nonspecific or engineered to recognize specific tumor antigens
Active	
Peptide vaccines	Short peptide epitopes, often conjugated to immunostimulants to generate a targeted antitumor immune response
Autologous tumor vaccines	Reintroduction of irradiated/inactivated tumor cells to generate a nonspecific antitumor immune response
Dendritic cell vaccines	Administration of antigen-presenting DCs with relevant tumor-specific antigens
Bacterial or viral vector vaccines	Delivery of the target antigens in the context of the immunostimulatory environment ("danger signals") provided by bacterial or viral vectors

(IFN-γ) are produced mainly by natural killer (NK) cells, NK T-cells (NKTs), and activated T-cells (cytotoxic T lymphocytes (CTLs), and T_h1 helper cells) (14,15).

Interferon-α

IFN-α increases MHC class I expression on normal cells (16) and tumor cells, including human GBM cells (17), and also enhances the activity of NK cells (18), CTLs (19), B-cells (20) and macrophages (21). IFN-α has been shown to induce apoptosis of tumor cells (21) and stimulate DCs to prime CTLs against tumor antigens (22). The intratumoral induction of IFN-α expression via an Ad vector in a mouse glioma model has shown improved survival especially when combined with the intratumoral delivery of DCs; the antiglioma response was mediated by specific CTL activity against the tumor, and the animals were also protected against tumor rechallenge (23). Multiple phase I/II glioma trials have attempted the subcutaneous administration of IFN-α in combination with a chemotherapeutic agent (e.g., BCNU or TMZ) following surgical debulking and radiation therapy (RT) (24–27) although there was no definitive improvement in survival shown by these trials. A phase III study of 275 patients showed no added benefit of administering systemic IFN-α with BCNU treatment (6). The trial compared BCNU alone versus BCNU with IFN-α in patients who had undergone RT. No significant difference was found between the two groups with regards to time to disease progression or overall survival (OS). Furthermore, the systemic administration of IFN-α had adverse effects including fever, chills, myalgias, and neurological symptoms (6). Due to the inflammatory nature of type I IFNs, higher doses delivered locally to the glioma site led to severe adverse effects in the surrounding brain tissue such as hemorrhagic necrosis (7). One approach to circumvent this toxicity that has been studied in animal models is to attract DCs to the tumor site and stimulate them to produce physiological levels of IFN-α (28) (see section on Flt3L).

Interferon-β

IFN-β has also been shown to have direct antiproliferative (Pro) effects on tumor cells, as well as activating antitumor immunity. For example, the intratumoral administration of the IFN-β gene via liposomes (29) and AAV vectors (30) has been shown to considerably improve survival in mouse glioma models. As with the IFN-α gene therapy, the effects were shown to be dependent on a specific CTL response against the tumor cells; furthermore, the animals were protected from tumor rechallenge, implicating long-term antiglioma immunity (29). Further, the intratumoral coadministration of IFN-β gene therapy with DCs may have an enhanced effect compared to either therapy alone (31). In clinical trials, intravenous delivery of IFN-β did not significantly prolong survival in patients treated with RT (32,33). However, the local expression of IFNs at the tumor site via gene therapy may prove to be more effective and may also avoid the systemic side effects. Liposome-mediated delivery of IFN-β in a pilot trial resulted in antitumor responses and tumor regression in four of five glioma patients (34). In a similar clinical study, phase I trials have tested the delivery of IFN-β–expressing Ad vectors injected in the tumor margins following surgical resection and was associated with inducing tumor apoptosis (7,35).

Interferon-γ

IFN-γ directly stimulates CTLs, NK cells, and macrophages by enhancing activity of these cells and promoting the differentiation of naïve T-cells into effector T-cells (14,36). This cytokine has also been shown to upregulate the expression of MHC class I in glioma cells, thereby increasing their immunogenicity (16,37). Gene transfer of IFN-γ into intracranial gliomas in preclinical models has shown antiglioma immune activation (38,39), including a marked upregulation of MHCII on tumor-infiltrating antigen presenting cells (APCs) (40) and an enhanced recruitment of T-cells (41), as well as inhibition of tumor angiogenesis (42). However, survival results were not as robust as with the use of IFN-α or IFN-β (43). Though IFN-γ is not a likely candidate for clinical trials on its own, a combination with other therapeutic modalities may prove effective (44). A spontaneous glioma canine model showed long-term survival of over 450 days post surgical debulking in a dog treated with Ad IFN-γ gene transfer to the resection margins along with vaccination with glioma cell lysates containing a CpG oligodeoxynucleotide adjuvant (45).

ILs to Activate T-Cells

ILs are a family of cytokines that play a large role in regulating the immune response. Although some ILs (e.g., IL-10) inhibit immune responses, the majority of ILs are known to activate and induce the differentiation and proliferation of several subtypes of immune cells.

Interleukin-2

IL-2 is a cytokine required for the development, function, and proliferation of a variety of T-cells. Of note, it stimulates the growth and differentiation of CTLs (36) and T-helper (T_H) cells (46) in vitro. In a 9L glioma rat model, intracerebral implantation of IL-2-producing glioma cells in combination with peripheral subcutaneous vaccination with irradiated 9L tumor cells had the ability to completely eradicate the tumor and was accompanied by an increase in tumor-specific CTL activity, whereas either therapy alone only prolonged survival (47). However, recent studies with IL-2 (or IL-2 receptor) deficient mice show that general T-cell proliferation in vivo is unaffected by the lack of IL-2, and that it is possible that a primary role of IL-2 may be the proliferation of regulatory T-cells and maintenance of self-tolerance (48–50). Thus, the in vivo transgene expression of IL-2 alone may not be an effective strategy in inducing an antiglioma immune response. Regardless, combinatorial therapies with IL-2 may yield efficacy, such as with intratumoral CTL administration (51) or with strategies that induce tumor apoptosis (52). In the latter trial, treatment of 12 recurrent GBM patients with combined intratumoral gene transfer of IL-2 and HSV-TK (with administration of ganciclovir [GCV]) resulted in tumor responses in half of the patients (including a response in a noninjected distant tumor mass in one patient) with increased plasma Th1 cytokine levels, showing evidence that IL-2 triggered a systemic cytokine cascade and stimulated an immune response to act beyond the direct tumor killing by the activated GCV (52).

Interleukin-12

IL-12 plays an important role in the stimulation of NK cells and in the stimulation and differentiation of T-cells (53,54), including a role in polarizing T-cells toward a IFN-γ producing T_H1 response (55) and a role as a CTL maturation factor in combination with IL-2 (56). IL-12 stimulates the production of IFN-γ (57) and to a lesser extent TNF-α. The systemic and peritumoral administration of IL-12 was found to improve survival in several rodent tumor models. The antitumor effect was dependent on CD4⁺ and CD8⁺ T lymphocytes and IFN-γ (58,59). In an intracranial GL-26 glioma mouse model, local Ad delivery of IL-12 was shown to prolong survival as a result of tumor growth inhibition. Although there was increased $CD4^+$ and $CD8^+$ T-cell infiltration, there was no statistically significant increase in T-cell cytotoxicity shown (60). In an intracranial B16 melanoma mouse model, intratumoral immunization with DCs virally transduced to express IL-12 resulted in a 40% long-term survival of mice (61). Therapies that combine IL-12 with other cytokines or other treatment modalities may prove more effective than the solitary administration of IL-12 (62). For example, the combination of locally delivered IL-12 transgene via PPC polymer with BCNU chemotherapy in a GL261 glioma mouse model resulted in a synergistic increase in survival compared to either therapy alone (63).

Interleukin-4

Although IL-12 promotes the T_H1 response, IL-4 commonly induces the T_H2 response (64), which has important roles in the allergic response and parasite defense. IL-4 is produced mainly by T-cells and regulates the proliferation and differentiation of B-cells (65) and T-cells (66,67), including tumor-infiltrating lymphocytes (68). Mouse gliomas studies comparing IL-2, IL-3, IL-4, IL-6, IL-12, GM-CSF, and IFN-α expressed at a peripheral vaccine site found that IL-4 was the most effective of these cytokines in inducing antiglioma immunity (69,70). The same group has undertaken pilot and phase I studies to evaluate DC vaccines in conjunction with IL-4–expressing fibroblasts delivered at the vaccine site (12,71,72). Another approach is the use of neural stem cells (NSCs) retrovirally transfected ex vivo with IL-4. The injection of these NSCs into established brain tumors led to robust long-term survival in murine and rat gliomas models (73). NSCs were used as the therapeutic vehicle because their extensive distribution throughout the tumor was considered more favorable than with the use of most vectors (70,74). However, obtaining sufficient NSCs for use in clinical applications continues to pose a problematic barrier. To overcome this obstacle, Okada et al. proposed the use of epidermal growth factor receptor (EGFR)-transfected bone marrow stromal cells as a delivery vehicle; these cells adenovirally transfected with IFN-α were able to prolong survival in a mouse gliomas model (75).

Recruitment of DCs with Flt3L

DCs are powerful APCs that are largely exploited by immunotherapeutic strategies. Although normally very scarce in the brain, they can be recruited to the glioma site via the induced expression of fms-like tyrosine kinase 3 ligand(Flt3L). Flt3L induces DC differentiation, proliferation, and activation (76–78). Ad gene-transfer of Flt3L (Ad.Flt3L) to the tumor site has been shown to induce infiltration of DCs into the tumor, resulting in an in situ priming against brain tumor (28,79,80). In addition, an increase in macrophages and T-cells infiltrating the tumor was observed (79). However, intracranial treatment with Ad.Flt3L did not yield a potent antiglioma immune response without the simultaneous administration of an antitumor proapoptotic factor to aid the tumor antigen uptake and priming. The intratumoral delivery of a second adenovirus encoding HSV1-TK (HSV 1 thymidine kinase) in combination with the systemic delivery of GCV has been found to be a promising tumor-killing strategy in combination with the immunostimulatory Flt3L (81) (Figure 1). The TK-induced apoptosis of tumor cells exposes tumor antigens whereas releasing inflammatory signals, such as HMGB1, has been shown to be integral in activating the antiglioma immunity by DCs (81,82). It has been shown that, of the strategies to pulse DCs in vitro, the coincubation of DCs with apoptotic glioma cells markedly improves antigen presentation (83); the same is shown to occur in vivo. However, an advantage of stimulating DCs with tumor antigen in vivo instead of ex vivo is that DCs encounter the tumor antigen in their natural environment and other cofactors will be readily available (43).

In a variety of syngeneic mice and rat glioma models of the aforementioned studies, a 60% to 80% long-term survival (documented beyond 175 days) resulted from the combined Flt3L+TK therapy, where each individual therapy and other evaluated therapies failed (43,81,84). This significant improvement of survival contrasts with the lack of prolonged survival in the same glioma model where TK therapy was combined with the Ad gene transfer of IL-12 instead of Flt3L (85). Further, Ad.TK+Flt3L toxicity is shown to be very minimal and similar to controls, and behavior deficits due to the tumor itself have been shown to resolve with treatment. In addition, rechallenge of tumor to the contralateral brain hemisphere in the treated long-term survivors did not result in tumor formation in the majority of rechallenged animals (86), confirming long-term antiglioma immunity by these animals and the ability to combat multifocal and recurrent disease. Tumor regression with this therapeutic modality was also shown in a spontaneous canine glioblastoma model with results which have led to clinical trials in glioblastoma-bearing dogs (87–89). Human phase I clinical trials with this

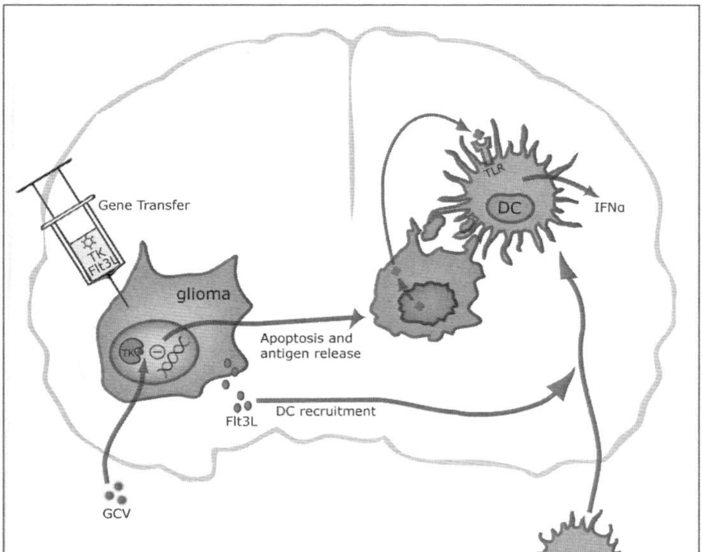

FIGURE 1 Dendritic cell recruitment by Flt3L. This strategy uses viral vectors to insert genes to reengineer the brain tumor microenvironment in favor of immune stimulation. In this example, the tumor area is induced to express cytokine Flt3L and the conditionally cytotoxic HSV-1 thymidine kinase (TK). The Flt3L recruits dendritic cells (DCs) to the tumor site. The viral TK halts DNA replication in the presence of systemically administered ganciclovir (GCV), which induces tumor cell apoptosis. The dying tumor cells release antigens that act on the dendritic cell (e.g., HMGB1 acting on the TLR2). The DCs uptake and process other tumor antigens and present them to T-cells, generating an antiglioma immunological response.

dual-gene Ad transfer to the glioma margins after surgical resection are currently underway.

Blocking TGF-β

TGF-β plays multiple roles in tumor progression including powerful immune suppression (90,91), promoting invasiveness, and inducing angiogenesis (92). Most notably, TGF-β inhibits T-cell proliferation and inhibits the cytotoxic activity of T-cells and NK cells (93). In particular, the TGF-β2 isoform is strongly expressed by malignant gliomas (94,95). An antisense TGF-β2 peptide inhibitor AP12009 has been developed to partially reduce TGF-β2 expression by GBM cells and to thus reduce gliomas cell proliferation (96). A phase I/II trial of 24 recurrent glioma patients of the intratumoral administration of AP12009 via catheter showed increased survival relative to historical controls and a complete remission in 2 patients with anaplastic astrocytoma; although the overall results of the treatment (median survival for GBM patients: 44 weeks) were not substantially different from standard therapies (96,97), AP12009 has moved to phase III clinical trials (98). Since tumor expression of TGF-β2 has been shown to inversely correlate with DC vaccine efficacy in clinical trials (99), a combinatorial approach with tumor vaccine modalities may yield more favorable results.

Anti-CTLA Antibodies

One of the hallmark features seen in patients with malignant glioma is systemic immunosuppression which is believed to be due to reduced T-cell function (100,101). T-cell activation not only requires the binding of an antigen-MHC complex from an APC to a T-cell bearing the cognate T-cell receptor but also depends on the molecular context of costimulatory signaling molecules which either enhance or repress the T-cell response. Of those, CD28 and CTLA-4 competitively interact with the B7–1 and B7–2 ligands located on the APC, with antagonistic effects: CD28 enhances T-cell activation and IL-2 production whereas CTLA-4 antagonizes T-cell activation by interfering with IL-2 secretion and IL-2 receptor expression and activating pathways that lead to T-cell anergy and/or programmed cell death (102,103). On the basis of these findings, mAbs against CTLA-4 have been developed. In experimental models of glioma, treatment with anti-CTLA-4 antibodies led to a decreased T_{reg} fraction, increased overall T-cell counts, T-cell Pro response, and conferred a survival benefit to treatment groups (104,105). Fully human antibodies against CTLA-4, ipilimumab (MDX-010), and tremelimumab (CP-675,206), have been developed and have been tested in clinical trials of cancers other than glioma where meaningful clinical responses have been documented, as well as their potential to enhance other forms of immunotherapy (106,107). Such strategies are currently of interest for the treatment of malignant gliomas (108), and a large randomized clinical trial of ipilimumab for newly diagnosed glioblastoma is currently being undertaken by the Radiation Therapy Oncology Group (RTOG).

■ PASSIVE IMMUNOTHERAPY

mAbs

Mechanisms of mAb action include disruption of cell signaling (109,110), direct opsonization of glioma cells and immune effector activation (111,112), and induction of cellular cytotoxicity via complement-dependent (CDC) or antibody-dependent (ADCC) mechanisms via secretion of TNF-α, IFN-γ, perforins, and granzymes (113–116). mAbs can be targeted toward glioma-specific sAgs, matrix proteins or ligand-receptor pairs essential in glioma cell signaling (112,117). In order to be effective, the Ag need to be abundant (>10^5 molecules/cell) (118), stably expressed, minimally toxic, immune enhancing, and specific to glioma cells. mAbs have been used against EGFR/EGFRvIII, VEGFR, Her2/neu, NCAM (119), IL-13Rα2, EphA2 (120), HGF/SF (121), VEGF, tenascin-C (122), chondroitin sulfate, Trp1/2, tyrosinase, gp100, and surviving (123). Difficulties associated with multiple mAb administration include generation of human anti-mouse immunogenicity, toxicity, allergic reactions, and the inability to cross the blood–brain barrier (BBB). While the former are reduced/prevented by the use of chimeric or humanized antibodies or mice engineered to produce fully human antibodies with an added benefit of prolonged mAb half-life and enhanced CDC/ADCC (112), crossing the BBB requires reduced-size Abs (Fab fragments, Fv domains, single-chain Abs from other animals) (124–126), developing diabodies/minibodies with multivalent construct-improved retention to enhance intratumor delivery and distribution throughout the tumor (127–129), or bypassing the BBB by using transnasal and convection-enhanced delivery (CED) approaches (130–134).

Adoptive Cell Transfer

Adoptive cell transfer involves the harvesting and ex vivo expansion of immune effector cells; their activation and/or target-specific programming; and their reintroduction back to the patient (Figure 2). The idea for the adoptive transfer of potent antitumor effectors cells stems from the observation that the degree of lymphocytic infiltrate into tumors was positively correlated with survival (135–138). The interpretation was that the patients' immune systems were recognizing the tumors and mounting an immune response. Subsequent studies involved the adoptive transfer of autologous leukocytes intracranially to patients with recurrent GBM (139–142). Although these studies demonstrated the safety of infusing autologous leukocytes into the tumor resection cavity, the efficacy of using leukocytes was limited.

In preclinical or clinical studies, the use of leukocytes, NK cells, γδ T-cells, activated T-cells, tumor-infiltrating lymphocytes antigen-specific T-cells, or genetically modified T-cells have been evaluated. These approaches offer the advantage of circumventing deficits of antitumor effector cell populations in the host by providing optimal conditions for the culture and expansion of these cells in vitro, in the absence of tumor-derived immunosuppressive factors in vivo.

LAK Cells

NK cells are effective cytotoxic lymphocytes against a broad range of tumors and virus-infected tumor cells (143). Furthermore, some genetic experiments in mice reveal that absence of NK cells results in spontaneous tumor development and induced primary oncogenesis (144). Lymphokine activated killer (LAK) cells is the name given to populations of white blood cells that become activated against tumors when stimulated with cytokines. LAK cells are cytotoxic to tumors in vitro and exhibit their effect in a non-MHC restricted manner. Clinical trials treating glioblastoma patients with LAKs administered intracerebrally into the operative cavity or directly into the lesion have included over 200 patients. Combining all reports in the literature, there were 5 complete responses and 13 partial responses in a total of 118 evaluable patients. Correlation between the clinical results and radiological response has not been significant (3,143). In some trials, median survival for vaccinated GBM patients was higher than that observed for control groups. For a recent trial involving newly diagnosed GBM, median OS was 20.5 months, with 75% of

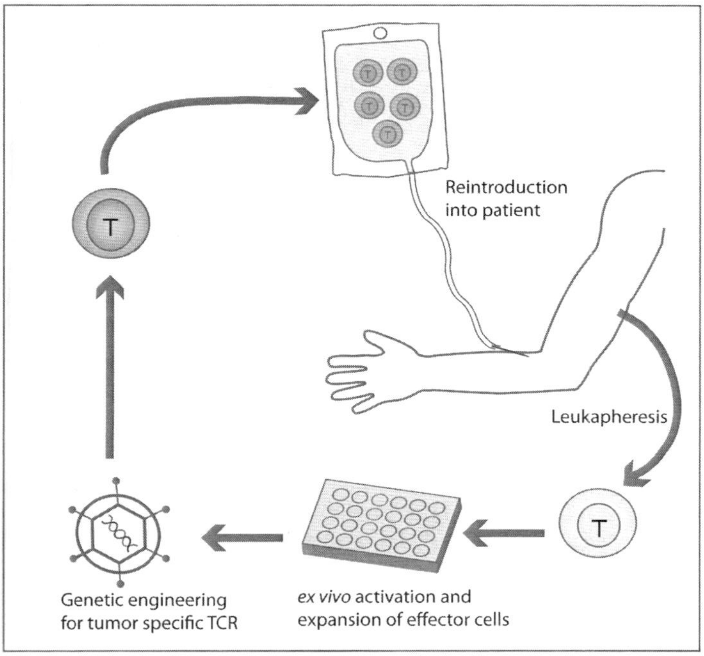

FIGURE 2 Adoptive transfer of genetically engineered T-cells. Lymphocytes are obtained from patients via leukapheresis, activated, and placed into culture for ex vivo expansion. Lymphocytes are then transduced (with retroviral mediators) to express T-cell receptors (TCRs) for the target tumor antigen. The now activated, specific, cytotoxic T lymphocytes (CTLs) are then reintroduced into the patient.

patients alive at 1 year. In this study, a positive correlation was demonstrated between the number of LAK cells injected and survival as well as a negative correlation between corticosteroid therapy and survival (145). Most of these trials were conducted in the 1980s and early 1990s in the pretemozolomide era. The modest survival benefit of LAK cell therapy compared to temozolomide has limited the enthusiasm to pursue these cells as immunotherapy strategies for glioblastoma. However, recent advances in the field of NK cell biology have caused renewed interest in NK cell–based immunotherapy for cancer.

γδ T-Cells

γδ T-cells are a subset of T-lymphocytes, which express T-cell receptors (TCRs) that consist of one γ-chain and one δ-chain. Unlike conventional αβ T-cells that recognize only specific peptide antigens presented in the context of a MHC molecule, γδ T-cells recognize a broader range of antigens in a MHC-independent fashion. Lamb and colleagues showed that these cells expanded in the presence of low doses of IL-2 and had the ability to recognize and kill glioma cells in vitro, while not harming normal astrocytes (146). Human γδ T-cells, when implanted into nude mice, showed immunological efficacy against U251 xenografts (147,148).

To date, no clinical experience with the adoptive transfer of γδ T-cells is available. One of the major limitations in the past has been the inability to generate sufficient numbers of γδ T-cells that retain their broad antitumor activity without becoming exhausted or anergic from overstimulation. However, recent studies indicate that these limitations can be overcome. Phase I/II trials have demonstrated the feasibility of stimulating and expanding γδ T-cells in vivo through the use of aminobisphosphonates in patients with non-Hodgkin's lymphoma, multiple myeloma, and metastatic prostate cancer (149,150).

Allogeneic Mixed Lymphocyte Reactive T-Cells

Another adoptive cell transfer therapy strategy for malignant gliomas was pioneered by Kruse et al. Lymphocytes derived from histoincompatible allogeneic human blood donors were combined with irradiated patient-derived lymphocytes (151,152). The mixed lymphocyte reaction sensitized the allogeneic donor lymphocytes against patient MHC. These alloreactive T-cells are then expanded ex vivo with IL-2 and subsequently injected into the tumor resection cavity. These cells then react against glioma cells which express MHC while sparing normal CNS component-cells, which do not express MHC. Long-term survivorship was observed in a few patients with grade III astrocytoma (51). Early concerns that these allospecific CTLs would indiscriminately kill non-tumorous host brain cells and induce autoimmunity were not borne out. Thus, a larger dose-escalation phase I study using this technique for recurrent malignant gliomas is currently underway to expand and confirm the safety/toxicity of this therapeutic modality.

Genetically Engineered T-Cells

Gene transfer allows the rapid generation of large numbers of antigen-specific T-cells for adoptive T-cell immunotherapy. Whereas endogenous tumor antigen-specific T-cells may have low-affinity TCRs limiting their cytotoxic activity, these cells can be generated with high-affinity α/β TCRs or chimeric antigen receptors (CARs). However, to date, lack of specific antigens and limited persistence of adoptively transferred cells remain significant technical hurdles. Strategies employing TCRs are additionally HLA-type restricted, which may further limit the feasibility of bringing them to clinic.

TCRs

At present, no clinical study with genetically engineered α/β TCR T-cells has yet been conducted in brain tumor patients. Preclinical models have used antigen specific T-cells to target antigens that were upregulated in response to pharmacologic treatment with demethylating agents (153). Adoptive transfer of engineered T-cells has been shown to be clinically feasible in other cancers including metastatic melanoma, which may share common antigens with GBM, with some patients demonstrating complete responses (154–156).

CARs

CARs are generated by joining the variable regions of an antibody with the transmembrane- and cytoplasmic-signaling domains derived from the TCR ζ-chain and costimulatory molecules such as CD28 CD134, and CD137. T-cells engineered with such CARs can target antigens in an HLA-unrestricted manner and exhibit the cytotoxic activity of T-cells. The extracellular binding domain is, however, ligand specific for antigens expressed on the cell surface of tumor cells. Because CARs provide T-cell activation in a non-MHC–restricted manner, they are immune to some of the major mechanisms by which tumors avoid MHC-restricted T-cell recognition, such as downregulation of HLA class I molecules and defects in antigen processing. CARs have been generated for some glioma-specific antigens, including IL-13Rα2, HER2, and EGFRvIII. T-cells expressing these GBM-specific CARs had potent antitumor activity in preclinical animal models (157–162). In addition, a study with T-cells expressing HER2-specific CARs showed that these cells had potent antitumor activity against HER2-positive, CD133-positive glioma stem cells, which were chemo- and radiotherapy resistant (162). Phase I clinical studies with T-cells expressing IL-13R α2-specific CARs is currently underway.

ACTIVE IMMUNOTHERAPY

Active immunotherapy approaches attempt to induce long-lasting T-cell immunity in glioma patients and can be accomplished by in vivo vaccination. Successful vaccine design requires host generation of T lymphocytes or antibodies to target Ags, an absence of side effects, biological stability, and the ability to generate immunologic memory. Several strategies of glioma vaccination have been used, as detailed below. Strategies to improve the various approaches often rely on potentially toxic but efficacious adjuvants used to augment antigen immunogenicity, reduce specific toxicities, improve delivery to the site of antigen presentation (e.g., mannose), enhance APCs or costimulatory molecules, and/or selectively promote specific types of immune response (e.g., IL-12 to select for T_H1 response; Table 2) (170,171).

Peptide-Based Vaccines

Peptide-based vaccines represent a relatively simple, inexpensive, and potentially safe method to induce glioma-specific immune responses via the action of APCs that process the peptides and present them to cytotoxic or helper T lymphocytes. Peptide vaccines are often conjugated to a carrier protein such as keyhole limpet cyanin (KLH), which can activate APCs, induce a strong $CD4^+$ helper T lymphocyte response, and increase peptide half-life (172).

EGFRvIII

EGFRvIII is a glioma-specific tumor antigen derived from aberrant splicing of EGFR via deletion of exons 2–7 with the loss of extracellular domain and exons 1–8 fusion with the addition of a novel glycine residue. This results in a constitutively activated form of EGFR (EGFRvIII) (173) implicated in dysregulated cell growth, invasion, survival, malignant transformation of glioma cells, and enhanced angiogenesis in approximately 40% of glioblastomas (174,175). EGFRvIII expression is characterized by poor prognosis (176); however, it also predicts the lack of self-tolerance. Preclinical trials for EGFRvIII-targeted vaccination included subcutaneous or intracerebral transplantation of NIH3T3 or melanoma cells overexpressing EGFRvIII into mice or rats immunized with KLH-conjugated EGFRvIII-containing peptides in IFA adjuvant pre- or posttumor transplantation (177–179), and showed induction of $CD8^+$ T lymphocyte-mediated, NK-mediated, and/or humoral immune responses, resulting in reduced tumor incidence, tumor regression, variably improved survival, and generation of immune memory. These effects were found to be further augmented by the use of GM-CSF.

Initial phase I clinical trials using six intradermal injections of KLH-conjugated EGFRvIII peptide and GM-CSF focused on patients diagnosed with ovarian and prostate cancers and showed promising safety profiles (180). These trials were later reproduced in a phase I Vaccine for Intra-Cranial Tumors I trial (VICTORI), where 16 patients diagnosed with WHO grade III/IV gliomas were administered three vaccine injections at 2-week intervals, starting 2 weeks after completion of surgical treatment and RT (181,182). All patients responded to KLH, and approximately 62% responded to the EGFRvIII peptide and developed humoral B-cell and cellular T-cell proliferative responses without profound toxicity, as only NCI grade I/II injection site local reactions were observed. These trial data were followed up with a Complementary Trial of Immunotherapy Vaccine Against Tumor-Specific EGFRvIII (ACTIVATE) phase II trial in which 23 patients with newly diagnosed $EGFRvIII^+$ glioblastomas were treated with surgery, radiation, and temozolomide, and administered EGFRvIII-conjugate vaccine using the above schedule (181,183,184). ACTIVATE showed progression-free survival (PFS) of 64 weeks and median OS of 126 weeks, which represented a more than 2.5-fold increase compared to historical controls. If tumors recurred, they no longer showed EGFRvIII expression, indicating relative inhibition of $EGFRvIII^+$

TABLE 2 Immune adjuvants

Adjuvant	Description	Intended Use
Incomplete Freund's (IFA)	Water, oil	Delayed Ag release, enhanced macrophage uptake
Complete Freund's (CFA)	Water, oil, killed mycobacterium	As above, + induce costimulation in macrophages
Freund's with MDP (FAM?)	Above+ muramyldipeptide (MDP)	Similar to CFA
Aluminum hydroxide	Gel	Similar to IFA
Alum/pertussis	Gel + killed bordetella	Similar to CFA
Immune stimulation complexes (ISCOMs)	Viral protein matrix with Quil A	Ag delivery to cytosol, induction of cytotoxic T-cells
Granulocyte/macrophage colony-stimulating factor (GM-CSF)	Secreted protein	Induces hematopoietic stem cell differentiation into granulocytes and monocytes which further differentiate into macrophages and dendritic cells
Pathogen-associated molecular patterns (PAMPs), including LPS, flagellin, LTA, HSP, dsRNA, imiquimod, unmethylated CpG oligonucleotides	Immunostimulatory agents (small molecular motifs) acting on APCs and effector T-cells via pattern recognition receptors (e.g., TLR3)	Identify as nonself and helping elicit innate immune responses via cell signaling, induction of proinflammatory mediators and antitumor cytokines, enhancing Ag presentation (163)
CpG oligonucleotides (CpG ODNs)	Oligonucleotide containing CpG motifs	Strong immunostimulation activity, select for T_H1 phenotype
Poly-ICLC (Hiltonol™)	dsRNA molecule used to induce IFN expression; immune modulation at high doses via IFN-dependent and IFN-independent pathways	Induces cytokine expression and activation of macrophages, NK cells, T-cells at high doses; low-dose administration results in TLR3-mediated DC activation, activation of T and NK cells, and cytokine/IFN induction resulting in antiviral and antiproliferative responses (164–169)
Imiquimod (Aldara™)	Topical immune modifier	Activates immune cells through the toll-like receptor 7 (TLR7), commonly involved in pathogen recognition to secrete cytokines IFN-α IL-6 and TNF-α

glioma cells, or possible downregulation of EGFRvIII. ACTIVATE participants developed CD8+ IFN-γ-expressing EGFRvIII-specific CTLs, anti-KLH, and anti-EGFRvIII antibodies, and minimal toxicity (185). As the standard treatment regimen for glioma patients has been amended to include surgery, RT, and six cycles of neoadjuvant temozolomide since the start of this trial, 21 more patients newly diagnosed with glioblastomas were included into the ACTIVATE II trial and treated with EGFRvIII vaccine (now called CDX-110) administered throughout the six cycles of temozolomide therapy on day 21 of the 28-day cycle in an effort to target hypothetically recovered immune cells, as most chemotherapies induce profound lyphodepletion (181,186–192). This trial is being followed up with a randomized multicenter phase II/III trial comparing standard treatments with or without CDX-110 vaccination (193).

Other Peptide Vaccines

A recent phase I study in 12 HLA-A24+ patients with progressing or recurrent GBMs investigated the safety and tolerability of 14 candidate peptides (EGFR, EZH2, Lck, MRP3, PAP, PSA, PSMA, PTH-rP, SART2/3). The numbers of cytotoxic T-cells and induction of peptide-specific IgG to at least four peptides were used as a measure of a positive immunologic response. This study showed dose-dependent immune system activation without significant toxicity other than injection site reactions, partial responses in 2 of 12 patients (15 months PFS), no change in 5 patients, and disease progression in 5, with OS of 2.3 months in all patients (194). An older phase I study evaluating 25 peptide vaccines (SART1/2/3, cyclophilin B, LCK, ART1/4, MRP3, EZH2, EGFR, HER2, PSCA, PTH-rP, WHSC2, UBE2V, HNRPL) in HLA-A24$^+$ or HLA-A2$^+$ patients with advanced malignant gliomas indicated safety, low toxicity (only redness and swelling at the injection site), and induction of cellular and humoral immune responses to at least one peptide observed in 67% and 52% patients, respectively, with high levels of peptide-specific IgG in CSF within the glioma cavity (195). Clinically, 5 of 21 patients showed partial response, 8 patients had stable disease, and 8 patients showed glioma progression; median OS was 622 days. Further clinical trials using this platform are underway.

■ AUTOLOGOUS TUMOR VACCINES

Irradiated, killed, or otherwise inactivated tumor cells or proteins derived from tumor cell lysates are often used as cancer vaccines. Such agents are often combined with adjuvant immunostimulants. Sloan et al. showed the ability of an autologous glioma cell vaccine administered with GM-CSF to induce cell-mediated immunologic responses in 19 patients with recurrent glioblastomas (196). Patients had been previously treated with surgery, RT and had failed chemotherapy. Coadministration of autologous glioma cell vaccine and activated T-lymphocytes was found to be feasible and safe. A study by Parney et al. showed that the use of irradiated autologous glioma cells expressing B7–2 and GM-CSF in three patients resulted in the induction of an inflammatory response with only minor toxicity. In this case, the immunogenicity of glioma cells was increased with transduction of B7–2/CD86, a proinflammatory costimulant for the generation of effector T-cells from glioma-specific naïve T-cells (197). Further studies of patients vaccinated with irradiated autologous glioma cells mixed with IL-4 expressing fibroblasts by Okada et al. showed activation of CD4$^+$ and CD8$^+$ lymphocytes (12). Another study by Moviglia et al. reported the use of autologous glioma-B cell hybridomas in 12 patients with recurrent glioblastomas initially treated with debulking surgery, showing minimal toxicity and the ability to act synergistically with mixed leukocyte cultures (198). A study of nine recurrent malignant glioma patients by Clavreul et al. reported on the feasibility of using autologous glioma cell vaccines and GM-CSF delivered by a subcutaneous programmable pump (199). Of the five patients who completed the protocol, three demonstrated a greater than expected survival of 62, 42, and 88 weeks, respectively. Two patients appeared to develop delayed-type hypersensitivity.

■ HEAT SHOCK PROTEIN (HSP) VACCINES

HSPs are stress-inducible chaperone proteins that are immunogenic, highly expressed in glioma cells, and have been implicated in glioma progression and resistance to therapy; due to their nature, HSPs are normally bound to improperly folded, misassembled or untransported proteins, which may represent products of glioma-associated genetic alterations or altered glioma microenvironment (200,201). Experimental evidence shows that APCs recognize tumor cell-derived, antigen-bound HSPs via specific receptors and present antigens on MHC I molecules triggering CD8$^+$ T lymphocyte responses (202), causing up-regulation of MHC II, expression of costimulatory molecules (B7–1, B7–1, CD40), and cytokine (GM-CSF, TNFα, IL-1β, IL-6, IL-12) and chemokine (NO, MCP-1, MIP-1, RANTES) released from APCs (203–207). As HSPs are bound to different tumor-associated antigens, immune specificity in this case is due to the ability to create polyvalent strong noncovalent bonds between glioma-specific Ag and HSPs and internalization by HSP-specific receptors (204).

An autologous peptide HSP vaccine termed "oncophage" (vitespen, HSP-Pc96) has been tested in clinical trials for patients with sarcoma, melanoma, pancreatic, colorectal, and renal cancers (204). Autologous Hsp-Ag complexes isolated from resected glioma specimens are now being tested as a vaccine in patients with recurrent malignant gliomas. HSP vaccine benefits include safety, minor side effects, specificity, no need for identification and isolation of immunogenic Ags, and theoretically lower chances of immune evasion. However, problematic areas include "dilution" of HSP-bound Ags with normal cell antigen, insufficient isolation of Hsp-Ag complexes dependent on glioma size and handling given the large amount of autologous glioma tissue (up to 15 g) is required for vaccine generation, and the possibility of rapid glioma progression during vaccine generation time (204).

■ BACTERIAL AND VIRAL VECTOR VACCINES

The use of live, attenuated bacteria and viruses as vaccine vectors has also been considered for active immunotherapies against gliomas. The signals provided by these pathogens can be exploited to attract and activate APCs, deliver tumor-associated antigens, and induce CTL-mediated immunity (208). In this approach, target antigens are presented in an environment with the bacterial- or viral-derived costimulatory "danger signals" involved in generating an effective immune response.

Bacterial Vaccines

Bacterial vaccine vectors have been used to deliver tumor-associated antigens while strongly stimulating both innate and adaptive immunity that can be directed toward cancer cells (209). For example, attenuated recombinant forms of the intracellular bacteria *Listeria monocytogenes* have been used to induce tumor rejection, an approach that is dependent on and mediated by vaccine-induced, tumor-specific CD8⁺ and CD4⁺ T-cells (210). Due to its unique life cycle, in which it escapes from phagolysosomes to the cell cytosol and directly transfers to other cells, *L. monocytogenes* expresses antigens that are presented by both MHC class I and II to CD8⁺ and CD4⁺ T-cells, respectively (209,211). The bacteria have also been shown to activate TLRs on APCs (212) and internal pattern recognition molecules (213). In a rat intracranial tumor model, Liau et al. demonstrated that immunization with recombinant *L. monocytogenes* bacteria expressing the pseudotumor antigen, lymphocytic choriomeningitis virus nucleoprotein (LCMV-NP), resulted in the rejection of gliomas that expressed the antigen. Additionally, when the rats were rechallenged with tumor cells not expressing the antigen, these tumors were also rejected, an immunity that is attributed to epitope spreading, a concept which may be exploited by immunotherapy for enhanced antitumor responses (214). Other strains of *L. monocytogenes* have been shown to target angiogenesis and tumor vasculature in multiple cancer models, including gliomas, by targeting such proteins as VEGFR2 (215–217). A recent phase I clinical trial for cervical cancer using an *L. monocytogenes* vaccine (Lm-LLO-E7 strain which expresses the tumor antigen E7) revealed that this strategy has a favorable safety profile and potential efficacy (218).

Another bacterial vaccine vector *Salmonella typhimurium* has also been used to express tumor antigens (including VEGFR2 (219) and survivin) (220,221), as well as to deliver immune-modulating cytokines such as CCL21 (208). A phase I clinical trial of an attenuated *S. typhimurium* (VNP20009) genetically modified to increase safety and reduce toxicity administered intravenously to patients with metastatic melanoma showed it to be safe with evidence of bacteria colonizing the tumor. Yet, the antitumor efficacy that was seen in animal models (222,223) was not observed in the trial (224). Another clinical trial that employed the intratumoral injection of a similar strain also showed safety, yet lacked efficacy (209,225). However, the approaches used by these clinical trials relied on direct tumor killing and did not include the expression of tumor antigens by the bacteria to orchestrate an antitumor immune response; accordingly, the lack of efficacy may not extend to a vaccine strategy. Nevertheless, the clinical trials demonstrated encouraging safety profiles for the use of bacteria in vaccines.

Viral Vector Vaccines

In addition, viral-based vaccines have also been developed against glioma for clinical trials using virus-infected autologous glioma cells (226). A nonrandomized pilot trial that administered a vaccine prepared by infecting glioblastoma patients' own tumor cells in vitro with Newcastle disease virus (a live attenuated oncolytic viral strain) to mount antitumor immune response showed that the approach was safe and feasible, and there was a significant improvement of survival with demonstrated antitumor immune responses; the median OS was 100 weeks in vaccinated patients versus 49 weeks in controls (227). Vaccines using an attenuated oncolytic Edmonston strain of the measles virus have also shown antitumor activity. A strain that has been engineered to express human carcinoembryonic antigen has entered phase I clinical trials (228). A trial for ovarian cancer showed intraperitoneal injections to be safe and to prolong survival compared to historic controls (229); a trial for recurrent glioblastoma patients is ongoing, and preliminary results have shown no significant toxicity with vaccine injections in the glioma resection cavities or within the tumor (228,230).

■ DC VACCINES

DCs Pulsed With Autologous Antigens

Brain tumor-specific or tumor-associated antigens for pulsing DC-based vaccines can be obtained from several sources. A common source is derived from autologous tumor cells obtained from surgical resection (231). This method theoretically allows for tumor targeting even if specific antigens are unknown, if tumors fail to express well-characterized or HLA-matched antigens, or if broad targeting is desired through multiple antigens. However, antigenic material derived from autologous tumor cells is heterogeneous in nature and makes monitoring the resulting immune response a much more complex task. Furthermore, if not enough tumor is obtained from surgical resection, preparing patient-specific tumor lysates may not be feasible.

Antitumor immunity has been induced with DCs pulsed with autologous tumor-eluted peptides (99,232,233), tumor lysates (234–239), and tumor-derived RNA (240,241) (Figure 3). In the case of acid-eluted peptides from autologous tumor samples, surgical tissue is used to establish glioma cell lines in vitro. These passaged lines are subsequently exposed to a citrate phosphate buffer (pH = 3.2) to gently dissociate peptides from the surface of MHC I. From there, the peptides are concentrated through silica columns and are then exposed to monocyte-derived DCs overnight (233). These peptide-pulsed DCs are tested for contamination before they are transferred to patients to stimulate an immune response (233). Clinical trials reported by Liau et al. and Yu et al. demonstrated the feasibility and safety of this methodology (99,232,233). Yu et al. detected intratumoral memory T-cells ($CD45RO^+$) in certain patients that underwent reoperation demonstrating the bioactivity of this particular vaccine (233). Liau et al. demonstrated that increased T-cell infiltration was positively correlated with clinical survival, but inversely correlated with TGF-β2 expression in the tumor (99). This result highlights the potential impact of an immunosuppressive tumor environment during the course of a DC vaccination. In the future, utilization of TGF-β2 expression as a prognostic marker may be useful to identify tumor subtypes differentially responsive to DC-based therapies.

In addition to acid-eluted autologous tumor peptides, DCs pulsed with autologous tumor lysate have also been tested for safety and feasibility.

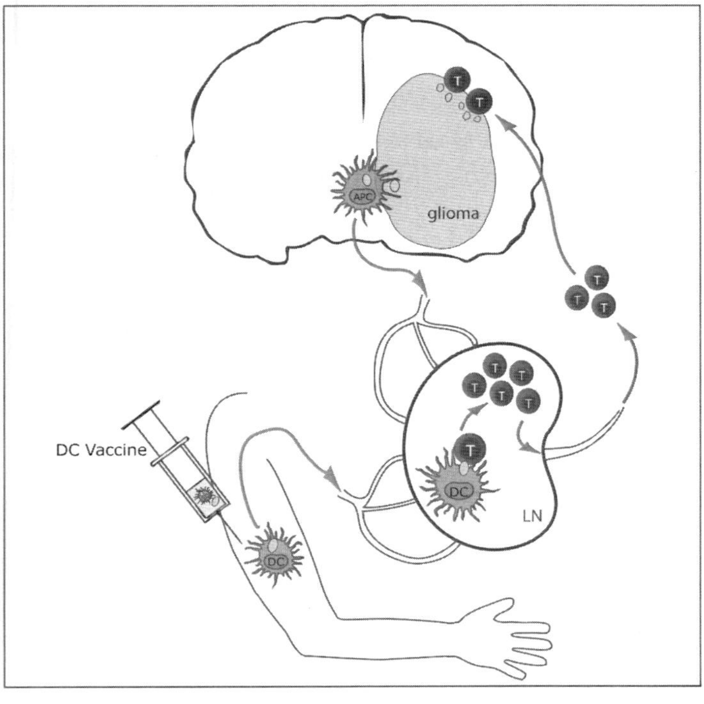

FIGURE 3 Dendritic cell-based vaccination. Dendritic cells (DCs) are activated and introduced to tumor antigens either by a peripheral DC vaccination approach or by immune-stimulatory molecules delivered to the tumor via gene therapy. Activated DCs migrate to the lymph node to present tumor antigens to T-cells. This induces T-cell activation and clonal cytotoxic T-lymphocyte (CTL) expansion. The activated CTLs leave the lymph nodes to attack the tumor.

Tumor lysate is obtained by first mincing and digesting autologous tumor tissue. This is followed by 3 to 6 freeze–thaw cycles, in which the cell-free supernatant results in a mixture of peptides derived from both the cell surface and the cell interior (236). By increasing the antigenic material available, utilization of tumor lysate has the ability to widen the adaptive immune response. Several phase I trials have been conducted to test the safety and feasibility of tumor lysate-pulsed DCs. Various groups have shown results of prolonged clinical PFS and OS) (234–239). Prins et al. recently reported the utilization of microarray gene expression analysis of patient tumor samples in order to characterize whether specific glioblastoma genetic signatures could correlate with clinical outcome (236). Analysis of patient tumor samples resulted in three previously described hierarchical clusters, proneural (PN), proliferative (Pro), and mesenchymal (Mes). Typically, glioblastoma patients that are stratified within the Mes group have a worse prognosis than those in the PN group. However, the Mes group is associated with an increase in many inflammatory/immune-associated genes in comparison to the PN and Pro groups. Bearing this in mind, patients in this DC vaccine trial showed significantly extended survival if they were associated with the Mes gene expression signature in comparison to tumors collected concurrently with the same signature and not having received the DC vaccine. This was not observed in the case of the PN or Pro molecular subgroups. Furthermore, increased intratumoral infiltration of $CD3^+$ and $CD8^+$ lymphocytes in DC vaccine patients, a known positive prognostic indicator, was also correlated with a favorable response in the Mes subgroup. Currently, the exact molecular mechanisms responsible for differential treatment responsiveness to immunotherapies in the various glioblastoma subgroups are unknown, but will be very interesting to follow.

DCs Pulsed with Synthetic Peptide Antigens

In order to focus the antigenic response, DCs pulsed with known tumor-associated antigens have also been tested. These tumor-associated antigens have included the mutated form of the EGFR (EGFRvIII), as well as the IL-13 receptor α2 (IL-13α2), ephrin A2 (EphA2), YKL-40, and gp100 (192,242). DCs pulsed with these peptides were able to induce specific responses in patients as measured by in vitro proliferation assays and measurement of tetramer-positive $CD8^+$ T-cells. Although these studies did not demonstrate significantly increased OS, their ability to induce antigen-specific responses may warrant further investigation.

In the trial utilizing DCs pulsed with EGFRvIII peptide, it turned out that many tumors displayed heterogeneous or absent EGFRvIII expression (192), which may have limited the efficacy of this approach. Furthermore, many gliomas are known to express very low levels of the melanoma-associated antigen, gp100, which could account for the lack of efficacy of gp100-pulsed DC vaccines for malignant gliomas (242). Stratifying patients to receive an appropriately matched cocktail of peptides based upon actual expression of tumor-associated antigens may increase the relative efficacy of peptide-pulsed DC vaccines. If expression of these antigens is absent, then autologous tumor lysate-pulsed DCs may be a more appropriate choice.

DC vaccines have shown promise in multiple phase I and phase II clinical trials around the world. Although it was initially hypothesized that autologous tumor lysate preparations could induce severe autoimmune reactions in the CNS, no major adverse events related to experimental allergic encephalitis have been reported. Furthermore, these vaccines have been shown to induce antigen-specific immune responses, potentiate immune cell infiltration into the tumor, and increase OS. In the future, further molecular characterizations of tumors will undoubtedly allow for more custom-tailored, personalized DC vaccines for glioblastoma patients to generate more potent antitumor immunity.

■ MONITORING RESPONSES TO IMMUNOTHERAPY

Monitoring immune responses is essential to evaluate treatment efficacy and mechanism of action, assess the overall immunologic state of a patient, determine clinical and prognostic correlates, compare to other vaccine trials via standardization, and apply immune readouts as prognostic markers for newly treated patients. Immunotherapy responses can be measured by a variety of cell and molecular techniques, as well as by the use of imaging modalities discussed below. However, monitoring immunotherapy responses is complicated by glioma heterogeneity, tumor location, and multiple comorbid conditions in glioma patients, who often exhibit poor or suppressed immune function. Concomitant use of steroids (e.g., dexamethasone to reduce brain edema) or chemotherapeutic agents (e.g., temozolomide, lomustine) likewise have unknown immune-related effects.

Immunologic Monitoring Studies

Previously, immunotherapy responses were measured by standard proliferation, cytotoxicity, and cytokine release assays, which could not accurately quantify the numbers of cells in a given population. These were replaced with immunosorbent assays (ELISA, ELISPOT), tetramer assays, and cytokine flow cytometry that have been shown to have a more measurable prognostic value (104,243–246), and are currently commonly used in immunotherapy clinical trials for malignant gliomas to measure glioma-specific T-cells in peripheral blood samples, detect T-cells specific for a given peptide-MHC complex, assess cytokine expression, or evaluate CTL activity (233,239,247). Detailed descriptions of cell and molecular methods for immune monitoring in clinical trials are provided in Table 3. Of note, it is still unclear whether any of these in vitro measurements correlate with immunotherapeutic efficacy or if they carry true prognostic/predictive significance. Moreover, many of the current immune assays require impractical and expensive equipment and systematic controls, which make them less widely available in the routine clinical setting.

Imaging of Immune Responses

Standard imaging approaches such as conventional MRI cannot differentiate between glioma recurrence, the effects of RT and/or chemotherapy, or pseudoprogression (the initial subacute response to Tx resulting in mass effect that tends to occur <2 months posttreatment) (248,249). Pseudoprogression, commonly located in the periventricular white matter with frail blood supply (250–252), is exacerbated by increased RT doses, repeated exposure, hyperfractionation, brachytherapy, or additional chemotherapy, while radiation necrosis results in endothelial thickening, hyalinization, gliosis, edema, necrosis, and glioma cell infiltration that could alter imaging results. The use of immunotherapy is likely to further complicate differentiating between the above conditions due to the likely increase in contrast-enhancing and T2/FLAIR signals due to immune-related inflammatory responses (248,253). Diffusion weighted-MRI (DWI) using changes in diffusion coefficients may be more successful at differentiating glioma recurrence from such treatment effects (250,251,254,255), while a combination of DWI with multivoxel 3D proton-based MR spectroscopy may add further diagnostic specificity (256–261). PET scanning is likewise being developed to differentiate between glioma recurrence versus treatment effect, and the incorporation of new radioactive tracers (i.e., DOPA or FLT) may be useful for monitoring of immunotherapy responses in the future (252,262–264).

■ USE OF COMBINATION APPROACHES FOR GLIOMA TREATMENT

Chemotherapy and Immunotherapy

Chemotherapy can cause a generalized immunosuppression and was previously deemed incompatible with immunotherapy (265). However, more recently, preclinical trials have shown some evidence that chemotherapy and the immune system may be synergistic in some cases. Chemotherapy may affect the microenvironment surrounding tumor cells and minimize immune suppression (266), reduce the activity of or eliminate T_{regs} (189,267), enhance glioma cell immunogenicity by up-regulating tumor antigens and MHC expression (268–270), or more readily allow phagocytosis and presentation of tumor antigens to immune effector cells by APCs (265). Clinical trial data from other cancers indicate that antibody production can inhibit DNA repair and topoisomeraze functions while chemosensitizing chemoresistant-glioma cells; the exact mechanisms are unknown and the synergy of the above treatments is thought to depend on treatment timing and scheduling (271,272). Yet, chemotherapy combined with active immunization with DCs or autologous glioma lysates in glioblastoma patients resulted in postvaccination chemotherapy sensitivity (273), while chemotherapy-induced lymphodepletion followed by adoptive T-cell transfer combined with IL-2 have shown positive antitumor responses in children with recurrent gliomas (274–276).

Radiotherapy and Immunotherapy

Immunologic modulation can act as an adjunct to local RT. RT increases tumor cell peptide expression,

TABLE 3 Immune monitoring assays

Assay	Advantages	Disadvantages
Lymphoproliferative assay Measure proliferation 72–100 hours post incubation of PBMCs/T-cells with irradiated autologous APCs and Ag stimulation	Can use unprocessed peripheral blood samples	In vitro—culture conditions will alter results May reflect patient's immunosuppression Is not representative of heterogeneous proliferation indices in T-cell subpopulations
Cytotoxicity assay Measurement of expression and target release upon mixing of PBMCs/T-cells with labeled Ag	May reflect in vivo antitumor activity	In vitro—culture conditions will alter results and differ from the in vivo state Nonautologous targets used for stimulation; results may not be applicable to a given tumor Measures direct cytotoxicity only
DTH Measurement of induration and/or erythema 48–72 hours after an intradermal Ag injection	Convenient and easy Correlates with T-cell proliferation	Ag amounts vary Response may not be Ag specific Subjective, no cutoff for positive response Marker of lesser immunosuppression and better performance
Cr release assay Measure cell lysis by Cr release after preincubation of target-cells with Cr and addition of effector T-cells	Quantitative Sensitive	Not based on single-cell analysis Positive results differ depending on Cr uptake Wide range (minutes to hours) of when lysis may occur Ineffective for evaluation of slow-acting or drawn-out effects
ELISA/multiplex flow cytometry Cytokine detection in the supernatant of PBMCs preincubated with Ag; can measure secreted proteins, Ag or Ab-secreting cells	Easy to perform Reliable, sensitive, specific	Not based on single-cell analysis Positive results differ Measures in vitro cytokine release, not in vivo activity
ELISPOT Identifies single cells secreting cytokine of interest, determines precursor frequency upon T-cell incubation with microtiter plate coated with cytokine-specific Ab	Reliable, sensitive, specific; qualitative and quantitative Rapid detection of Ag-specific T-cells Rapid data processing and availability Large-scale studies possible	
Peptide MHC tetramer assay Detection of Ag-specific T-cells upon incubation with fluorescently labeled MHC tetramer	Correlates with T-cell avidity May provide similar results to cytotoxicity assays Can select and use Ag-specific T-cells for further study	Requires identification and knowledge of tumor Ag Positive T-cells may not cause target-cell destruction Only MHC I tetramers used Does not differentiate between memory and naïve T-cells
Multiparameter flow cytometry Ab-mediated detection of surface and intracellular Ag following T-cell prestimulation, fixation, and permeabilization	Possible to analyze multiple cell populations simultaneously	Cannot use cells for further functional studies

including MHC, cytokines (IL-1,6, TNFα, TGFβ), chemokines (CXCL16, SDF-1), adhesion molecules (E-selectin, ICAM-1, VCAM-1), and stress ligands (Hsp70, NKG2D) (266,277–280), many of which are involved in immune cell recruitment (266,281). Additionally, RT causes translocation of phagocytosis signals such as CRT-ERp57 to the cell membrane, helps DCs recognize and engulf dying tumor cells, and stimulates cytotoxic CD8⁺ T-cell responses (282). RT-exposed tumor cells release inflammatory mediators from dying tumor cells that interact with toll-like receptors on tumor-resident immature DCs to induce specific T-cell responses, as well as signals that promote DC antigen processing and cross-presentation (283,284). Moreover, studies show that RT responses may activate NK cells, while CTLs become reactive to survivin overexpressed by affected tumor cells post RT (280). Furthermore, RT enhances tumor antigen uptake and presentation by DCs, promotes DC migration into draining lymph nodes to induce efficient T-cell priming when combined with DC activation, and can be further enhanced by immunotherapy (Hsp administration) (285). RT dose and administration regimen directly correlate with tumor control and the presence of reactive T-cells; however, high RT doses may increase the presence of T_{regs} and counter the effects of immunotherapy (286,287).

Studies show that abscopal effects—post-RT reduction in tumor growth outside the treatment field—may be mediated by the immune system and may be due to increased inflammatory mediators, DC activation, and diversification of the immune response (288,289). Indeed, RT has been shown to induce Fas expression, susceptibility to T-cell killing, T-cell responses to tumor antigens not associated with vaccines, and abscopal tumor regression proportional to tumor immunogenicity and the ability of RT to release high antigen load from tumor cells (280).

CONCLUSIONS AND FUTURE DIRECTIONS

Conventional surgical, radiation, and chemotherapy approaches for malignant gliomas, though improved, have not cured this deadly disease. Immunotherapy approaches hold promise of specific, nontoxic, diverse and potentially lasting eradication of tumor cells. These could, in principle, be tailored to specific patients based on their immune status, glioma antigen expression profiles, tumor microenvironment, and/or the presence of comorbid conditions. In combination with classical treatment approaches and logically incorporated into appropriate treatment regimens, immunotherapy will likely be part of the clinical armamentarium against brain cancer.

REFERENCES

1. Stupp R, Mason WP, van den Bent MJ, et al.; European Organisation for Research and Treatment of Cancer Brain Tumor and Radiotherapy Groups; National Cancer Institute of Canada Clinical Trials Group. Radiotherapy plus concomitant and adjuvant temozolomide for glioblastoma. *N Engl J Med*. 2005;352(10):987–996.
2. Mitchell DA, Sampson JH. Toward effective immunotherapy for the treatment of malignant brain tumors. *Neurotherapeutics*. 2009;6(3):527–538.
3. Vauleon E, Avril T, Collet B, Mosser J, Quillien V. Overview of cellular immunotherapy for patients with glioblastoma. *Clin Dev Immunol*. 2010;2010 pii: 689171. Epub 2010 Oct 4.
4. Rosenberg SA. Progress in human tumour immunology and immunotherapy. *Nature*. 2001;411(6835):380–384.
5. Engelhardt B, Ransohoff RM. The ins and outs of T-lymphocyte trafficking to the CNS: anatomical sites and molecular mechanisms. *Trends Immunol*. 2005;26(9):485–495.
6. Buckner JC, Schomberg PJ, McGinnis WL, et al. A phase III study of radiation therapy plus carmustine with or without recombinant interferon-alpha in the treatment of patients with newly diagnosed high-grade glioma. *Cancer*. 2001;92(2):420–433.
7. Chiocca EA, Smith KM, McKinney B, et al. A phase I trial of Ad.hIFN-beta gene therapy for glioma. *Mol Ther*. 2008;16(3):618–626.
8. Kamimura K, Suda T, Zhang G, Liu D. Advances in Gene Delivery Systems. *Pharmaceut Med*. 2011;25(5):293–306.
9. Rainov NG, Heidecke V. Clinical development of experimental virus-mediated gene therapy for malignant glioma. *Anticancer Agents Med Chem*. 2011;11(8):739–747.
10. Castro MG, Candolfi M, Kroeger K, et al. Gene therapy and targeted toxins for glioma. *Curr Gene Ther*. 2011;11(3):155–180.
11. Sobol RE, Fakhrai H, Shawler D, et al. Interleukin-2 gene therapy in a patient with glioblastoma. *Gene Ther*. 1995;2(2):164–167.
12. Okada H, Lieberman FS, Walter KA, et al. Autologous glioma cell vaccine admixed with interleukin-4 gene transfected fibroblasts in the treatment of patients with malignant gliomas. *J Transl Med*. 2007;5:67.
13. Hervas-Stubbs S, Perez-Gracia JL, Rouzaut A, Sanmamed MF, Le Bon A, Melero I. Direct effects of type I

interferons on cells of the immune system. *Clin Cancer Res.* 2011;17(9):2619–2627.

14. Schoenborn JR, Wilson CB. Regulation of interferon-gamma during innate and adaptive immune responses. *Adv Immunol.* 2007;96:41–101.
15. Platanias LC. Mechanisms of type-I- and type-II-interferon-mediated signalling. *Nat Rev Immunol.* 2005;5(5):375–386.
16. Isaacs A, Lindenmann J. Virus interference. I. The interferon. By A. Isaacs and J. Lindenmann, 1957. *J Interferon Res.* 1987;7(5):429–438.
17. Yang I, Kremen TJ, Giovannone AJ, et al. Modulation of major histocompatibility complex Class I molecules and major histocompatibility complex-bound immunogenic peptides induced by interferon-alpha and interferon-gamma treatment of human glioblastoma multiforme. *J Neurosurg.* 2004;100(2):310–319.
18. Herberman RB, Reynolds CW, Ortaldo JR. Mechanism of cytotoxicity by natural killer (NK) cells. *Annu Rev Immunol.* 1986;4:651–680.
19. Lindahl P, Leary P, Gresser I. Enhancement by interferon of the specific cytotoxicity of sensitized lymphocytes. *Proc Natl Acad Sci USA.* 1972;69(3):721–725.
20. Morikawa K, Kubagawa H, Suzuki T, Cooper MD. Recombinant interferon-alpha, -beta, and -gamma enhance the proliferative response of human B cells. *J Immunol.* 1987;139(3):761–766.
21. Kemp TJ, Elzey BD, Griffith TS. Plasmacytoid dendritic cell-derived IFN-alpha induces TNF-related apoptosis-inducing ligand/Apo-2L-mediated antitumor activity by human monocytes following CpG oligodeoxynucleotide stimulation. *J Immunol.* 2003;171(1):212–218.
22. Tosi D, Valenti R, Cova A, et al. Role of cross-talk between IFN-alpha-induced monocyte-derived dendritic cells and NK cells in priming CD8+ T cell responses against human tumor antigens. *J Immunol.* 2004;172(9):5363–5370.
23. Tsugawa T, Kuwashima N, Sato H, et al. Sequential delivery of interferon-alpha gene and DCs to intracranial gliomas promotes an effective antitumor response. *Gene Ther.* 2004;11(21):1551–1558.
24. Rajkumar SV, Buckner JC, Schomberg PJ, Cascino TL, Burch PA, Dinapoli RP. Phase I evaluation of radiation combined with recombinant interferon alpha-2a and BCNU for patients with high-grade glioma. *Int J Radiat Oncol Biol Phys.* 1998;40(2):297–302.
25. Olson JJ, McKenzie E, Skurski-Martin M, Zhang Z, Brat D, Phuphanich S. Phase I analysis of BCNU-impregnated biodegradable polymer wafers followed by systemic interferon alfa-2b in adults with recurrent glioblastoma multiforme. *J Neurooncol.* 2008;90(3):293–299.
26. Buckner JC, Brown LD, Kugler JW, et al. Phase II evaluation of recombinant interferon alpha and BCNU in recurrent glioma. *J Neurosurg.* 1995;82(3):430–435.
27. Groves MD, Puduvalli VK, Gilbert MR, et al. Two phase II trials of temozolomide with interferon-alpha2b (pegylated and non-pegylated) in patients with recurrent glioblastoma multiforme. *Br J Cancer.* 2009;101(4):615–620.
28. Curtin JF, King GD, Barcia C, et al. Fms-like tyrosine kinase 3 ligand recruits plasmacytoid dendritic cells to the brain. *J Immunol.* 2006;176(6):3566–3577.
29. Natsume A, Tsujimura K, Mizuno M, Takahashi T, Yoshida J. IFN-beta gene therapy induces systemic antitumor immunity against malignant glioma. *J Neurooncol.* 2000;47(2):117–124.
30. Yoshida J, Mizuno M, Nakahara N, Colosi P. Antitumor effect of an adeno-associated virus vector containing the human interferon-beta gene on experimental intracranial human glioma. *Jpn J Cancer Res.* 2002;93(2):223–228.
31. Nakahara N, Pollack IF, Storkus WJ, Wakabayashi T, Yoshida J, Okada H. Effective induction of antiglioma cytotoxic T cells by coadministration of interferon-beta gene vector and dendritic cells. *Cancer Gene Ther.* 2003;10(7):549–558.
32. Yoshida J, Kajita Y, Wakabayashi T, Sugita K. Long-term follow-up results of 175 patients with malignant glioma: importance of radical tumour resection and postoperative adjuvant therapy with interferon, ACNU and radiation. *Acta Neurochir (Wien).* 1994;127(1–2):55–59.
33. Colman H, Berkey BA, Maor MH, et al.; Radiation Therapy Oncology Group. Phase II Radiation Therapy Oncology Group trial of conventional radiation therapy followed by treatment with recombinant interferon-beta for supratentorial glioblastoma: results of RTOG 9710. *Int J Radiat Oncol Biol Phys.* 2006;66(3):818–824.
34. Yoshida J, Mizuno M, Fujii M, et al. Human gene therapy for malignant gliomas (glioblastoma multiforme and anaplastic astrocytoma) by *in vivo* transduction with human interferon beta gene using cationic liposomes. *Hum Gene Ther.* 2004;15(1):77–86.
35. Eck SL, Alavi JB, Judy K, et al. Treatment of recurrent or progressive malignant glioma with a recombinant adenovirus expressing human interferon-beta (H5.010CMVhIFN-beta): a phase I trial. *Hum Gene Ther.* 2001;12(1):97–113.
36. Maraskovsky E, Chen WF, Shortman K. IL-2 and IFN-gamma are two necessary lymphokines in the development of cytolytic T cells. *J Immunol.* 1989;143(4):1210–1214.
37. Wu A, Wiesner S, Xiao J, et al. Expression of MHC I and NK ligands on human CD133+ glioma cells: possible targets of immunotherapy. *J Neurooncol.* 2007;83(2):121–131.
38. Saleh M, Jonas NK, Wiegmans A, Stylli SS. The treatment of established intracranial tumors by in situ retroviral IFN-gamma transfer. *Gene Ther.* 2000;7(20):1715–1724.
39. Wu A, Oh S, Ericson K, et al. Transposon-based interferon gamma gene transfer overcomes limitations of episomal plasmid for immunogene therapy of glioblastoma. *Cancer Gene Ther.* 2007;14(6):550–560.
40. Dutta T, Spence A, Lampson LA. Robust ability of IFN-gamma to upregulate class II MHC antigen expression in tumor bearing rat brains. *J Neurooncol.* 2003;64(1–2):31–44.
41. Phillips LM, Lampson LA. Site-specific control of T cell traffic in the brain: T cell entry to brainstem vs.

hippocampus after local injection of IFN-gamma. *J Neuroimmunol.* 1999;96(2):218–227.

42. Fathallah-Shaykh HM, Zhao LJ, Kafrouni AI, Smith GM, Forman J. Gene transfer of IFN-gamma into established brain tumors represses growth by antiangiogenesis. *J Immunol.* 2000;164(1):217–222.
43. Curtin JF, King GD, Candolfi M, et al. Combining cytotoxic and immune-mediated gene therapy to treat brain tumors. *Curr Top Med Chem.* 2005;5(12):1151–1170.
44. Ehtesham M, Samoto K, Kabos P, et al. Treatment of intracranial glioma with in situ interferon-gamma and tumor necrosis factor-alpha gene transfer. *Cancer Gene Ther.* 2002;9(11):925–934.
45. Pluhar GE, Grogan PT, Seiler C, et al. Anti-tumor immune response correlates with neurological symptoms in a dog with spontaneous astrocytoma treated by gene and vaccine therapy. *Vaccine.* 2010;28(19):3371–3378.
46. Chang JF, Thomas CA 3rd, Kung JT. Mitogen-induced IL-2 production and proliferation at defined stages of T helper cell development. *J Immunol.* 1991;147(3):860–866.
47. Iwadate Y, Yamaura A, Sato Y, Sakiyama S, Tagawa M. Induction of immunity in peripheral tissues combined with intracerebral transplantation of interleukin-2-producing cells eliminates established brain tumors. *Cancer Res.* 2001;61(24):8769–8774.
48. Furtado GC, Curotto de Lafaille MA, Kutchukhidze N, Lafaille JJ. Interleukin 2 signaling is required for CD4(+) regulatory T cell function. *J Exp Med.* 2002;196(6):851–857.
49. Almeida AR, Legrand N, Papiernik M, Freitas AA. Homeostasis of peripheral CD4+ T cells: IL-2R alpha and IL-2 shape a population of regulatory cells that controls CD4+ T cell numbers. *J Immunol.* 2002;169(9):4850–4860.
50. Malek TR. The main function of IL-2 is to promote the development of T regulatory cells. *J Leukoc Biol.* 2003;74(6):961–965.
51. Kruse CA, Cepeda L, Owens B, Johnson SD, Stears J, Lillehei KO. Treatment of recurrent glioma with intracavitary alloreactive cytotoxic T lymphocytes and interleukin-2. *Cancer Immunol Immunother.* 1997;45(2):77–87.
52. Colombo F, Barzon L, Franchin E, et al. Combined HSV-TK/IL-2 gene therapy in patients with recurrent glioblastoma multiforme: biological and clinical results. *Cancer Gene Ther.* 2005;12(10):835–848.
53. Kobayashi M, Fitz L, Ryan M, et al. Identification and purification of natural killer cell stimulatory factor (NKSF), a cytokine with multiple biologic effects on human lymphocytes. *J Exp Med.* 1989;170(3):827–845.
54. Gately MK, Desai BB, Wolitzky AG, et al. Regulation of human lymphocyte proliferation by a heterodimeric cytokine, IL-12 (cytotoxic lymphocyte maturation factor). *J Immunol.* 1991;147(3):874–882.
55. Zou JP, Yamamoto N, Fujii T, et al. Systemic administration of rIL-12 induces complete tumor regression and protective immunity: response is correlated with a striking reversal of suppressed IFN-gamma production by anti-tumor T cells. *Int Immunol.* 1995;7(7):1135–1145.
56. Stern AS, Podlaski FJ, Hulmes JD, et al. Purification to homogeneity and partial characterization of cytotoxic lymphocyte maturation factor from human B-lymphoblastoid cells. *Proc Natl Acad Sci USA.* 1990;87(17):6808–6812.
57. Chan SH, Kobayashi M, Santoli D, Perussia B, Trinchieri G. Mechanisms of IFN-gamma induction by natural killer cell stimulatory factor (NKSF/IL-12). Role of transcription and mRNA stability in the synergistic interaction between NKSF and IL-2. *J Immunol.* 1992;148(1):92–98.
58. Brunda MJ, Luistro L, Warrier RR, et al. Antitumor and antimetastatic activity of interleukin 12 against murine tumors. *J Exp Med.* 1993;178(4):1223–1230.
59. Nastala CL, Edington HD, McKinney TG, et al. Recombinant IL-12 administration induces tumor regression in association with IFN-gamma production. *J Immunol.* 1994;153(4):1697–1706.
60. Liu Y, Ehtesham M, Samoto K, et al. In situ adenoviral interleukin 12 gene transfer confers potent and long-lasting cytotoxic immunity in glioma. *Cancer Gene Ther.* 2002;9(1):9–15.
61. Yamanaka R, Zullo SA, Ramsey J, et al. Marked enhancement of antitumor immune responses in mouse brain tumor models by genetically modified dendritic cells producing Semliki Forest virus-mediated interleukin-12. *J Neurosurg.* 2002;97(3):611–618.
62. Parker JN, Meleth S, Hughes KB, Gillespie GY, Whitley RJ, Markert JM. Enhanced inhibition of syngeneic murine tumors by combinatorial therapy with genetically engineered HSV-1 expressing CCL2 and IL-12. *Cancer Gene Ther.* 2005;12(4):359–368.
63. Sonabend AM, Velicu S, Ulasov IV, et al. A safety and efficacy study of local delivery of interleukin-12 transgene by PPC polymer in a model of experimental glioma. *Anticancer Drugs.* 2008;19(2):133–142.
64. Ebner S, Hofer S, Nguyen VA, et al. A novel role for IL-3: human monocytes cultured in the presence of IL-3 and IL-4 differentiate into dendritic cells that produce less IL-12 and shift Th cell responses toward a Th2 cytokine pattern. *J Immunol.* 2002;168(12):6199–6207.
65. Stack RM, Lenschow DJ, Gray GS, Bluestone JA, Fitch FW. IL-4 treatment of small splenic B cells induces costimulatory molecules B7–1 and B7–2. *J Immunol.* 1994;152(12):5723–5733.
66. Löhning M, Richter A, Stamm T, et al. Establishment of memory for IL-10 expression in developing T helper 2 cells requires repetitive IL-4 costimulation and does not impair proliferation. *Proc Natl Acad Sci USA.* 2003;100(21):12307–12312.
67. Hu-Li, J., et al., *B cell stimulatory factor 1 (interleukin 4) is a potent costimulant for normal resting T lymphocytes.* J Exp Med, 1987. 165(1): p. 157–72.
68. Kawakami Y, Rosenberg SA, Lotze MT. Interleukin 4 promotes the growth of tumor-infiltrating lymphocytes cytotoxic for human autologous melanoma. *J Exp Med.* 1988;168(6):2183–2191.
69. Okada H, Villa L, Attanucci J, et al. Cytokine gene therapy of gliomas: effective induction of therapeutic

immunity to intracranial tumors by peripheral immunization with interleukin-4 transduced glioma cells. *Gene Ther.* 2001;8(15):1157–1166.

70. Okada H, Pollack IF. Cytokine gene therapy for malignant glioma. *Expert Opin Biol Ther.* 2004;4(10):1609–1620.

71. Okada H, Pollack IF, Lieberman F, et al. Gene therapy of malignant gliomas: a pilot study of vaccination with irradiated autologous glioma and dendritic cells admixed with IL-4 transduced fibroblasts to elicit an immune response. *Hum Gene Ther.* 2001;12(5):575–595.

72. Okada H, Lieberman FS, Edington HD, et al. Autologous glioma cell vaccine admixed with interleukin-4 gene transfected fibroblasts in the treatment of recurrent glioblastoma: preliminary observations in a patient with a favorable response to therapy. *J Neurooncol.* 2003;64(1–2):13–20.

73. Benedetti S, Pirola B, Pollo B, et al. Gene therapy of experimental brain tumors using neural progenitor cells. *Nat Med.* 2000;6(4):447–450.

74. Ehtesham M, Black KL, Yu JS. Recent progress in immunotherapy for malignant glioma: treatment strategies and results from clinical trials. *Cancer Control.* 2004;11(3):192–207.

75. Sato H, Kuwashima N, Sakaida T, et al. Epidermal growth factor receptor-transfected bone marrow stromal cells exhibit enhanced migratory response and therapeutic potential against murine brain tumors. *Cancer Gene Ther.* 2005;12(9):757–768.

76. Maraskovsky E, Brasel K, Teepe M, et al. Dramatic increase in the numbers of functionally mature dendritic cells in Flt3 ligand-treated mice: multiple dendritic cell subpopulations identified. *J Exp Med.* 1996;184(5):1953–1962.

77. Saunders D, Lucas K, Ismaili J, et al. Dendritic cell development in culture from thymic precursor cells in the absence of granulocyte/macrophage colony-stimulating factor. *J Exp Med.* 1996;184(6):2185–2196.

78. Lyman SD, James L, Johnson L, et al. Cloning of the human homologue of the murine flt3 ligand: a growth factor for early hematopoietic progenitor cells. *Blood.* 1994;83(10):2795–2801.

79. Ali S, Curtin JF, Zirger JM, et al. Inflammatory and anti-glioma effects of an adenovirus expressing human soluble Fms-like tyrosine kinase 3 ligand (hsFlt3L): treatment with hsFlt3L inhibits intracranial glioma progression. *Mol Ther.* 2004;10(6):1071–1084.

80. King GD, Muhammad AK, Larocque D, et al. Combined Flt3L/TK gene therapy induces immunological surveillance which mediates an immune response against a surrogate brain tumor neoantigen. *Mol Ther.* 2011;19(10):1793–1801.

81. Candolfi M, Yagiz K, Foulad D, et al. Release of HMGB1 in response to proapoptotic glioma killing strategies: efficacy and neurotoxicity. *Clin Cancer Res.* 2009;15(13):4401–4414.

82. Curtin JF, Liu N, Candolfi M, et al. HMGB1 mediates endogenous TLR2 activation and brain tumor regression. *PLoS Med.* 2009;6(1):e10.

83. Parajuli P, Mathupala S, Sloan AE. Systematic comparison of dendritic cell-based immunotherapeutic strategies for malignant gliomas: *in vitro* induction of cytolytic and natural killer-like T cells. *Neurosurgery.* 2004;55(5):1194–1204.

84. Muhammad AK, Puntel M, Candolfi M, et al. Study of the efficacy, biodistribution, and safety profile of therapeutic gutless adenovirus vectors as a prelude to a phase I clinical trial for glioblastoma. *Clin Pharmacol Ther.* 2010;88(2):204–213.

85. Ali S, King GD, Curtin JF, et al. Combined immunostimulation and conditional cytotoxic gene therapy provide long-term survival in a large glioma model. *Cancer Res.* 2005;65(16):7194–7204.

86. King GD, Muhammad AK, Curtin JF, et al. Flt3L and TK gene therapy eradicate multifocal glioma in a syngeneic glioblastoma model. *Neuro-oncology.* 2008;10(1):19–31.

87. Candolfi M, Curtin JF, Nichols WS, et al. Intracranial glioblastoma models in preclinical neuro-oncology: neuropathological characterization and tumor progression. *J Neurooncol.* 2007;85(2):133–148.

88. Candolfi M, Kroeger KM, Pluhar GE, et al. Adenoviral-mediated gene transfer into the canine brain in vivo. *Neurosurgery.* 2007;60(1):167–77; discussion 178.

89. Xiong W, Candolfi M, Liu C, et al. Human Flt3L generates dendritic cells from canine peripheral blood precursors: implications for a dog glioma clinical trial. *PLoS ONE.* 2010;5(6):e11074.

90. Jennings MT, Pietenpol JA. The role of transforming growth factor beta in glioma progression. *J Neurooncol.* 1998;36(2):123–140.

91. Wojtowicz-Praga S. Reversal of tumor-induced immunosuppression by TGF-beta inhibitors. *Invest New Drugs.* 2003;21(1):21–32.

92. Akhurst RJ, Derynck R. TGF-beta signaling in cancer–a double-edged sword. *Trends Cell Biol.* 2001;11(11):S44–S51.

93. Weller M, Fontana A. The failure of current immunotherapy for malignant glioma. Tumor-derived TGF-beta, T-cell apoptosis, and the immune privilege of the brain. *Brain Res Brain Res Rev.* 1995;21(2):128–151.

94. Kjellman C, Olofsson SP, Hansson O, et al. Expression of TGF-beta isoforms, TGF-beta receptors, and SMAD molecules at different stages of human glioma. *Int J Cancer.* 2000;89(3):251–258.

95. Tada T, Yabu K, Kobayashi S. Detection of active form of transforming growth factor-beta in cerebrospinal fluid of patients with glioma. *Jpn J Cancer Res.* 1993;84(5):544–548.

96. Hau P, Jachimczak P, Schlingensiepen R, et al. Inhibition of TGF-beta2 with AP 12009 in recurrent malignant gliomas: from preclinical to phase I/II studies. *Oligonucleotides.* 2007;17(2):201–212.

97. Johnson LA, Sampson JH. Immunotherapy approaches for malignant glioma from 2007 to 2009. *Curr Neurol Neurosci Rep.* 2010;10(4):259–266.

98. Rolle CE, Sengupta S, Lesniak MS. Challenges in clinical design of immunotherapy trials for malignant glioma. *Neurosurg Clin N Am*. 2010;21(1):201–214.

99. Liau LM, Prins RM, Kiertscher SM, et al. Dendritic cell vaccination in glioblastoma patients induces systemic and intracranial T-cell responses modulated by the local central nervous system tumor microenvironment. *Clin Cancer Res*. 2005;11(15):5515–5525.

100. Albesiano, E., J.E. Han, and M. Lim, *Mechanisms of local immunoresistance in glioma*. Neurosurg Clin N Am, 2010. 21(1): p. 17–29.

101. Waziri A. Glioblastoma-derived mechanisms of systemic immunosuppression. *Neurosurg Clin N Am*. 2010;21(1):31–42.

102. Walunas TL, Lenschow DJ, Bakker CY, et al. CTLA-4 can function as a negative regulator of T cell activation. *Immunity*. 1994;1(5):405–413.

103. Krummel MF, Allison JP. CD28 and CTLA-4 have opposing effects on the response of T cells to stimulation. *J Exp Med*. 1995;182(2):459–465.

104. Fecci PE, Mitchell DA, Whitesides JF, et al. Increased regulatory T-cell fraction amidst a diminished CD4 compartment explains cellular immune defects in patients with malignant glioma. *Cancer Res*. 2006;66(6):3294–3302.

105. Fecci PE, Ochiai H, Mitchell DA, et al. Systemic CTLA-4 blockade ameliorates glioma-induced changes to the CD4+ T cell compartment without affecting regulatory T-cell function. *Clin Cancer Res*. 2007;13(7):2158–2167.

106. Ascierto PA, Marincola FM, Ribas A. Anti-CTLA4 monoclonal antibodies: the past and the future in clinical application. *J Transl Med*. 2011;9:196.

107. Callahan MK, Wolchok JD, Allison JP. Anti-CTLA-4 antibody therapy: immune monitoring during clinical development of a novel immunotherapy. *Semin Oncol*. 2010;37(5):473–484.

108. Humphries W, Wei J, Sampson JH, Heimberger AB. The role of tregs in glioma-mediated immunosuppression: potential target for intervention. *Neurosurg Clin N Am*. 2010;21(1):125–137.

109. Cragg MS, French RR, Glennie MJ. Signaling antibodies in cancer therapy. *Curr Opin Immunol*. 1999;11(5):541–547.

110. Glennie MJ. Signalling antibodies for the treatment of neoplastic disease. *Dis Markers*. 2000;16(1–2):63.

111. Nadler LM, Stashenko P, Hardy R, et al. Serotherapy of a patient with a monoclonal antibody directed against a human lymphoma-associated antigen. *Cancer Res*. 1980;40(9):3147–3154.

112. Weiner LM, Surana R, Wang S. Monoclonal antibodies: versatile platforms for cancer immunotherapy. *Nat Rev Immunol*. 2010;10(5):317–327.

113. Eisenthal A, Cameron RB, Rosenberg SA. Induction of antibody-dependent cellular cytotoxicity *in vivo* by IFN-alpha and its antitumor efficacy against established B16 melanoma liver metastases when combined with specific anti-B16 monoclonal antibody. *J Immunol*. 1990;144(11):4463–4471.

114. Eisenthal A, McIntosh JK. Effect of recombinant human tumor necrosis factor alpha on the induction of antibody-dependent cellular cytotoxicity in the treatment of established B16 melanoma liver nodules. *Cancer Immunol Immunother*. 1990;31(4):243–249.

115. Shiloni E, Eisenthal A, Sachs D, Rosenberg SA. Antibody-dependent cellular cytotoxicity mediated by murine lymphocytes activated in recombinant interleukin 2. *J Immunol*. 1987;138(6):1992–1998.

116. Bleeker WK, Lammerts van Bueren JJ, van Ojik HH, et al. Dual mode of action of a human anti-epidermal growth factor receptor monoclonal antibody for cancer therapy. *J Immunol*. 2004;173(7):4699–4707.

117. Wu TN, Lin KH, Chang YJ, et al. Avidity of CD1d-ligand-receptor ternary complex contributes to T-helper 1 (Th1) polarization and anticancer efficacy. *Proc Natl Acad Sci USA*. 2011;108(42):17275–17280.

118. Wikstrand CJ, Cokgor I, Sampson JH, Bigner DD. Monoclonal antibody therapy of human gliomas: current status and future approaches. *Cancer Metastasis Rev*. 1999;18(4):451–464.

119. Hopkins K, Papanastassiou V, Kemshead JT. The treatment of patients with recurrent malignant gliomas with intratumoral radioimmunoconjugates. *Recent Results Cancer Res*. 1996;141:159–175.

120. Wykosky J, Gibo DM, Stanton C, Debinski W. EphA2 as a novel molecular marker and target in glioblastoma multiforme. *Mol Cancer Res*. 2005;3(10):541–551.

121. Prasad G, Wang H, Hill DL, Zhang R. Recent advances in experimental molecular therapeutics for malignant gliomas. *Curr Med Chem Anticancer Agents*. 2004;4(4):347–361.

122. Bourdon MA, Wikstrand CJ, Furthmayr H, Matthews TJ, Bigner DD. Human glioma-mesenchymal extracellular matrix antigen defined by monoclonal antibody. *Cancer Res*. 1983;43(6):2796–2805.

123. Prins RM, Liau LM. Cellular immunity and immunotherapy of brain tumors. *Front Biosci*. 2004;9:3124–3136.

124. Omidfar K, Rasaee MJ, Kashanian S, Paknejad M, Bathaie Z. Studies of thermostability in Camelus bactrianus (Bactrian camel) single-domain antibody specific for the mutant epidermal-growth-factor receptor expressed by Pichia. *Biotechnol Appl Biochem*. 2007;46(Pt 1):41–49.

125. Omidfar K, Rasaee MJ, Modjtahedi H, et al. Production and characterization of a new antibody specific for the mutant EGF receptor, EGFRvIII, in Camelus bactrianus. *Tumour Biol*. 2004;25(4):179–187.

126. Omidfar K, Rasaee MJ, Modjtahedi H, Forouzandeh M, Taghikhani M, Golmakani N. Production of a novel camel single-domain antibody specific for the type III mutant EGFR. *Tumour Biol*. 2004;25(5–6):296–305.

127. Adams GP, Weiner LM. Intracellular single-chain Fv antibodies–a knockout punch for neoplastic cells? *Gynecol Oncol*. 1995;59(1):6–7.

128. Schaedel O, Reiter Y. Antibodies and their fragments as anti-cancer agents. *Curr Pharm Des*. 2006;12(3):363–378.

129. Scott AM, Lee FT, Tebbutt N, et al. A phase I clinical trial with monoclonal antibody ch806 targeting transitional state and mutant epidermal growth factor receptors. *Proc Natl Acad Sci USA*. 2007;104(10):4071–4076.

130. Bobo RH, Laske DW, Akbasak A, Morrison PF, Dedrick RL, Oldfield EH. Convection-enhanced delivery of macromolecules in the brain. *Proc Natl Acad Sci USA*. 1994;91(6):2076–2080.

131. Morrison PF, Laske DW, Bobo H, Oldfield EH, Dedrick RL. High-flow microinfusion: tissue penetration and pharmacodynamics. *Am J Physiol*. 1994;266(1 Pt 2):R292–R305.

132. Sampson JH, Reardon DA, Friedman AH, et al. Sustained radiographic and clinical response in patient with bifrontal recurrent glioblastoma multiforme with intracerebral infusion of the recombinant targeted toxin TP-38: case study. *Neuro-oncology*. 2005;7(1):90–96.

133. Vogelbaum MA, Sampson JH, Kunwar S, et al. Convection-enhanced delivery of cintredekin besudotox (interleukin-13-PE38QQR) followed by radiation therapy with and without temozolomide in newly diagnosed malignant gliomas: phase 1 study of final safety results. *Neurosurgery*. 2007;61(5):1031–7; discussion 1037.

134. Rand RW, Kreitman RJ, Patronas N, Varricchio F, Pastan I, Puri RK. Intratumoral administration of recombinant circularly permuted interleukin-4-Pseudomonas exotoxin in patients with high-grade glioma. *Clin Cancer Res*. 2000;6(6):2157–2165.

135. Ridley A, Cavanagh JB. Lymphocytic infiltration in gliomas: evidence of possible host resistance. *Brain*. 1971;94(1):117–124.

136. Brooks WH, Markesbery WR, Gupta GD, Roszman TL. Relationship of lymphocyte invasion and survival of brain tumor patients. *Ann Neurol*. 1978;4(3):219–224.

137. Palma L, Di Lorenzo N, Guidetti B. Lymphocytic infiltrates in primary glioblastomas and recidivous gliomas. Incidence, fate, and relevance to prognosis in 228 operated cases. *J Neurosurg*. 1978;49(6):854–861.

138. Safdari H, Hochberg FH, Richardson EP Jr. Prognostic value of round cell (lymphocyte) infiltration in malignant gliomas. *Surg Neurol*. 1985;23(3):221–226.

139. Young H, Kaplan A, Regelson W. Immunotherapy with autologous white cell infusions ("lymphocytes") in the treatment of recurrrent glioblastoma multiforme: a preliminary report. *Cancer*. 1977;40(3):1037–1044.

140. Steinbok P, Thomas JP, Grossman L, Dolman CL. Intratumoral autologous mononuclear cells in the treatment of recurrent glioblastoma multiforme. A phase 1 (toxicity) study. *J Neurooncol*. 1984;2(2):147–151.

141. Vaquero J, Martínez R, Oya S, et al. Intratumoural injection of autologous lymphocytes plus human lymphoblastoid interferon for the treatment of glioblastoma. *Acta Neurochir (Wien)*. 1989;98(1–2):35–41.

142. Vaquero J, Martínez R, Ramiro J, Salazar FG, Barbolla L, Regidor C. Immunotherapy of glioblastoma with intratumoural administration of autologous lymphocytes and human lymphoblastoid interferon. A further clinical study. *Acta Neurochir (Wien)*. 1991;109(1–2):42–45.

143. Ogbomo H, Cinatl J Jr, Mody CH, Forsyth PA. Immunotherapy in gliomas: limitations and potential of natural killer (NK) cell therapy. *Trends Mol Med*. 2011;17(8):433–441.

144. Hayakawa Y, Smyth MJ. Innate immune recognition and suppression of tumors. *Adv Cancer Res*. 2006;95:293–322.

145. Dillman RO, Duma CM, Ellis RA, et al. Intralesional lymphokine-activated killer cells as adjuvant therapy for primary glioblastoma. *J Immunother*. 2009;32(9):914–919.

146. Lamb LS Jr. Gammadelta T cells as immune effectors against high-grade gliomas. *Immunol Res*. 2009;45(1):85–95.

147. Bryant NL, Gillespie GY, Lopez RD, et al. Preclinical evaluation of ex vivo expanded/activated ?d T cells for immunotherapy of glioblastoma multiforme. *J Neurooncol*. 2011;101(2):179–188.

148. Bryant NL, Suarez-Cuervo C, Gillespie GY, et al. Characterization and immunotherapeutic potential of gammadelta T-cells in patients with glioblastoma. *Neuro-oncology*. 2009;11(4):357–367.

149. Wilhelm M, Kunzmann V, Eckstein S, et al. Gammadelta T cells for immune therapy of patients with lymphoid malignancies. *Blood*. 2003;102(1):200–206.

150. Dieli F, Vermijlen D, Fulfaro F, et al. Targeting human {gamma}delta} T cells with zoledronate and interleukin-2 for immunotherapy of hormone-refractory prostate cancer. *Cancer Res*. 2007;67(15):7450–7457.

151. Hofman FM, Stathopoulos A, Kruse CA, Chen TC, Schijns VE. Immunotherapy of malignant gliomas using autologous and allogeneic tissue cells. *Anticancer Agents Med Chem*. 2010;10(6):462–470.

152. Kruse CA, Schiltz PM, Bellgrau D, Kong Q, Kleinschmidt-DeMasters BK. Intracranial administrations of single or multiple source allogeneic cytotoxic T lymphocytes: chronic therapy for primary brain tumors. *J Neurooncol*. 1994;19(2):161–168.

153. Natsume A, Wakabayashi T, Tsujimura K, et al. The DNA demethylating agent 5-aza-2'-deoxycytidine activates NY-ESO-1 antigenicity in orthotopic human glioma. *Int J Cancer*. 2008;122(11):2542–2553.

154. Robbins PF, Morgan RA, Feldman SA, et al. Tumor regression in patients with metastatic synovial cell sarcoma and melanoma using genetically engineered lymphocytes reactive with NY-ESO-1. *J Clin Oncol*. 2011;29(7):917–924.

155. Morgan RA, Dudley ME, Wunderlich JR, et al. Cancer regression in patients after transfer of genetically engineered lymphocytes. *Science*. 2006;314(5796):126–129.

156. Johnson LA, Morgan RA, Dudley ME, et al. Gene therapy with human and mouse T-cell receptors mediates cancer regression and targets normal tissues expressing cognate antigen. *Blood*. 2009;114(3):535–546.

157. Kahlon KS, Brown C, Cooper LJ, Raubitschek A, Forman SJ, Jensen MC. Specific recognition and killing of glioblastoma multiforme by interleukin 13-zetakine redirected cytolytic T cells. *Cancer Res*. 2004;64(24):9160–9166.

158. Wu AH, Xiao J, Anker L, et al. Identification of EGFRvIII-derived CTL epitopes restricted by HLA A0201 for dendritic cell based immunotherapy of gliomas. *J Neurooncol.* 2006;76(1):23–30.

159. Ahmed N, Ratnayake M, Savoldo B, et al. Regression of experimental medulloblastoma following transfer of HER2-specific T cells. *Cancer Res.* 2007;67(12):5957–5964.

160. Stastny MJ, Brown CE, Ruel C, Jensen MC. Medulloblastomas expressing IL13Ralpha2 are targets for IL13-zetakine+ cytolytic T cells. *J Pediatr Hematol Oncol.* 2007;29(10):669–677.

161. Bullain SS, Sahin A, Szentirmai O, et al. Genetically engineered T cells to target EGFRvIII expressing glioblastoma. *J Neurooncol.* 2009;94(3):373–382.

162. Ahmed N, Salsman VS, Kew Y, et al. HER2-specific T cells target primary glioblastoma stem cells and induce regression of autologous experimental tumors. *Clin Cancer Res.* 2010;16(2):474–485.

163. Carpentier A, Laigle-Donadey F, Zohar S, et al. Phase 1 trial of a CpG oligodeoxynucleotide for patients with recurrent glioblastoma. *Neuro-oncology.* 2006;8(1):60–66.

164. Dick RS, Hubbell HR. Sensitivities of human glioma cell lines to interferons and double-stranded RNAs individually and in synergistic combinations. *J Neurooncol.* 1987;5(4):331–338.

165. Strayer DR, Weisband J, Carter WA, Black P, Nidzgorski F, Cook AW. Growth of astrocytomas in the human tumor clonogenic assay and sensitivity to mismatched dsRNA and interferons. *Am J Clin Oncol.* 1987;10(4):281–284.

166. Black PL, Hartmann D, Pennington R, et al. Effect of tumor burden and route of administration on the immunotherapeutic properties of polyinosinic-polycytidylic acid stabilized with poly-L-lysine in carboxymethyl cellulose [Poly(I,C)-LC]. *Int J Immunopharmacol.* 1992;14(8):1341–1353.

167. Matsumoto M, Seya T. TLR3: interferon induction by double-stranded RNA including poly(I:C). *Adv Drug Deliv Rev.* 2008;60(7):805–812.

168. Kim H, Yang E, Lee J, et al. Double-stranded RNA mediates interferon regulatory factor 3 activation and interleukin-6 production by engaging Toll-like receptor 3 in human brain astrocytes. *Immunology.* 2008;124(4):480–488.

169. Salazar AM, Levy HB, Ondra S, et al. Long-term treatment of malignant gliomas with intramuscularly administered polyinosinic-polycytidylic acid stabilized with polylysine and carboxymethylcellulose: an open pilot study. *Neurosurgery.* 1996;38(6):1096–103; discussion 1103.

170. Butowski N. Immunostimulants for malignant gliomas. *Neurosurg Clin N Am.* 2010;21(1):53–65.

171. Meng Y, Carpentier AF, Chen L, et al. Successful combination of local CpG-ODN and radiotherapy in malignant glioma. *Int J Cancer.* 2005;116(6):992–997.

172. Harris JR, Markl J. Keyhole limpet hemocyanin (KLH): a biomedical review. *Micron.* 1999;30(6):597–623.

173. Fernandes H, Cohen S, Bishayee S. Glycosylation-induced conformational modification positively regulates receptor-receptor association: a study with an aberrant epidermal growth factor receptor (EGFRvIII/DeltaEGFR) expressed in cancer cells. *J Biol Chem.* 2001;276(7):5375–5383.

174. Humphrey PA, Wong AJ, Vogelstein B, et al. Anti-synthetic peptide antibody reacting at the fusion junction of deletion-mutant epidermal growth factor receptors in human glioblastoma. *Proc Natl Acad Sci USA.* 1990;87(11):4207–4211.

175. Wong AJ, Ruppert JM, Bigner SH, et al. Structural alterations of the epidermal growth factor receptor gene in human gliomas. *Proc Natl Acad Sci USA.* 1992;89(7):2965–2969.

176. Heimberger AB, Hlatky R, Suki D, et al. Prognostic effect of epidermal growth factor receptor and EGFRvIII in glioblastoma multiforme patients. *Clin Cancer Res.* 2005;11(4):1462–1466.

177. Moscatello DK, Ramirez G, Wong AJ. A naturally occurring mutant human epidermal growth factor receptor as a target for peptide vaccine immunotherapy of tumors. *Cancer Res.* 1997;57(8):1419–1424.

178. Heimberger AB, Crotty LE, Archer GE, et al. Epidermal growth factor receptor VIII peptide vaccination is efficacious against established intracerebral tumors. *Clin Cancer Res.* 2003;9(11):4247–4254.

179. Ciesielski MJ, Kazim AL, Barth RF, Fenstermaker RA. Cellular antitumor immune response to a branched lysine multiple antigenic peptide containing epitopes of a common tumor-specific antigen in a rat glioma model. *Cancer Immunol Immunother.* 2005;54(2):107–119.

180. Li G, Wong AJ. EGF receptor variant III as a target antigen for tumor immunotherapy. *Expert Rev Vaccines.* 2008;7(7):977–985.

181. Sampson JH, Archer GE, Mitchell DA, Heimberger AB, Bigner DD. Tumor-specific immunotherapy targeting the EGFRvIII mutation in patients with malignant glioma. *Semin Immunol.* 2008;20(5):267–275.

182. Archer, G.E., et al., *Dendritic cell vaccine for intracranial tumors I (DC Victori trial).* Neuro-Oncology, 2004. **6**(4): p. 341–341.

183. Heimberger, A.B., et al., *Tumor-specific peptide vaccination in newly-diagnosed patients with GBM.* Journal of Clinical Oncology, 2006. 24(18): p. 107s-107s.

184. Sampson, J.H., Aldape, K., Gilbert, S., et al. . *Temozolomide as a vaccine adjuvant in GBM.* in *ASCO Annual Meeting Proceedings Part 1.* 2007. J Clin Oncol.

185. Schmittling RJ, Archer GE, Mitchell DA, et al. Detection of humoral response in patients with glioblastoma receiving EGFRvIII-KLH vaccines. *J Immunol Methods.* 2008;339(1):74–81.

186. Emens LA, Reilly RT, Jaffee EM. Cancer vaccines in combination with multimodality therapy. *Cancer Treat Res.* 2005;123:227–245.

187. Sampson, J.H., Archer, G.E., Bigner, D.D., et al. *Effect of EGFRvIII-targeted vaccine (CDX-110) on immune response*

and TTP when given with simultaneous standard and continuous temozolomide in patients with GBM [abstract]. 2008. J Clin Oncol.

188. Sampson, J.H., *Temozolomide enhances efficacy of EGFRvIII vaccine (CDX-110) in patients with newly-diagnosed GBM.* Journal of Neurosurgery, 2008. 108(4): p. A885-A885.

189. Sampson JH, Aldape KD, Archer GE, et al. Greater chemotherapy-induced lymphopenia enhances tumor-specific immune responses that eliminate EGFRvIII-expressing tumor cells in patients with glioblastoma. *Neuro-oncology.* 2011;13(3):324–333.

190. Sampson JH, Heimberger AB, Archer GE, et al. Immunologic escape after prolonged progression-free survival with epidermal growth factor receptor variant III peptide vaccination in patients with newly diagnosed glioblastoma. *J Clin Oncol.* 2010;28(31):4722–4729.

191. Archer GE, Sampson JH, McLendon RE, et al. Intrathecal busulfan treatment of human neoplastic meningitis in athymic nude rats. *J Neurooncol.* 1999;44(3):233–241.

192. Sampson JH, Archer GE, Mitchell DA, et al. An epidermal growth factor receptor variant III-targeted vaccine is safe and immunogenic in patients with glioblastoma multiforme. *Mol Cancer Ther.* 2009;8(10):2773–2779.

193. Sonabend AM, Dana K, Lesniak MS. Targeting epidermal growth factor receptor variant III: a novel strategy for the therapy of malignant glioma. *Expert Rev Anticancer Ther.* 2007;7(12 Suppl):S45–S50.

194. Terasaki M, Shibui S, Narita Y, et al. Phase I trial of a personalized peptide vaccine for patients positive for human leukocyte antigen–A24 with recurrent or progressive glioblastoma multiforme. *J Clin Oncol.* 2011;29(3):337–344.

195. Yajima N, Yamanaka R, Mine T, et al. Immunologic evaluation of personalized peptide vaccination for patients with advanced malignant glioma. *Clin Cancer Res.* 2005;11(16):5900–5911.

196. Sloan AE, Dansey R, Zamorano L, et al. Adoptive immunotherapy in patients with recurrent malignant glioma: preliminary results of using autologous whole-tumor vaccine plus granulocyte-macrophage colony-stimulating factor and adoptive transfer of anti-CD3-activated lymphocytes. *Neurosurg Focus.* 2000;9(6):e9.

197. Parney IF, Chang LJ, Farr-Jones MA, Hao C, Smylie M, Petruk KC. Technical hurdles in a pilot clinical trial of combined B7–2 and GM-CSF immunogene therapy for glioblastomas and melanomas. *J Neurooncol.* 2006;78(1):71–80.

198. Moviglia GA, Carrizo AG, Varela G, et al. Preliminary report on tumor stem cell/B cell hybridoma vaccine for recurrent glioblastoma multiforme. *Hematol Oncol Stem Cell Ther.* 2008;1(1):3–13.

199. Clavreul A, Piard N, Tanguy JY, et al. Autologous tumor cell vaccination plus infusion of GM-CSF by a programmable pump in the treatment of recurrent malignant gliomas. *J Clin Neurosci.* 2010;17(7):842–848.

200. Park HG, Han SI, Oh SY, Kang HS. Cellular responses to mild heat stress. *Cell Mol Life Sci.* 2005;62(1):10–23.

201. Graner MW, Bigner DD. Therapeutic aspects of chaperones/heat-shock proteins in neuro-oncology. *Expert Rev Anticancer Ther.* 2006;6(5):679–695.

202. Yamanaka R. Cell- and peptide-based immunotherapeutic approaches for glioma. *Trends Mol Med.* 2008;14(5):228–235.

203. Srivastava PK. Peptide-binding heat shock proteins in the endoplasmic reticulum: role in immune response to cancer and in antigen presentation. *Adv Cancer Res.* 1993;62:153–177.

204. Yang I, Fang S, Parsa AT. Heat shock proteins in glioblastomas. *Neurosurg Clin N Am.* 2010;21(1):111–123.

205. Blachere NE, Li Z, Chandawarkar RY, et al. Heat shock protein-peptide complexes, reconstituted *in vitro,* elicit peptide-specific cytotoxic T lymphocyte response and tumor immunity. *J Exp Med.* 1997;186(8):1315–1322.

206. Suto R, Srivastava PK. A mechanism for the specific immunogenicity of heat shock protein-chaperoned peptides. *Science.* 1995;269(5230):1585–1588.

207. Basu S, Binder RJ, Suto R, Anderson KM, Srivastava PK. Necrotic but not apoptotic cell death releases heat shock proteins, which deliver a partial maturation signal to dendritic cells and activate the NF-kappa B pathway. *Int Immunol.* 2000;12(11):1539–1546.

208. Loeffler M, Le'Negrate G, Krajewska M, Reed JC. Salmonella typhimurium engineered to produce CCL21 inhibit tumor growth. *Cancer Immunol Immunother.* 2009;58(5):769–775.

209. Shahabi V, Maciag PC, Rivera S, Wallecha A. Live, attenuated strains of Listeria and Salmonella as vaccine vectors in cancer treatment. *Bioeng Bugs.* 2010;1(4):235–243.

210. Weiskirch LM, Pan ZK, Paterson Y. The tumor recall response of antitumor immunity primed by a live, recombinant Listeria monocytogenes vaccine comprises multiple effector mechanisms. *Clin Immunol.* 2001;98(3):346–357.

211. Tilney LG, Portnoy DA. Actin filaments and the growth, movement, and spread of the intracellular bacterial parasite, Listeria monocytogenes. *J Cell Biol.* 1989;109(4 Pt 1):1597–1608.

212. Barton GM, Medzhitov R. Toll-like receptors and their ligands. *Curr Top Microbiol Immunol.* 2002;270:81–92.

213. Ulevitch RJ. Therapeutics targeting the innate immune system. *Nat Rev Immunol.* 2004;4(7):512–520.

214. Liau LM, Jensen ER, Kremen TJ, et al. Tumor immunity within the central nervous system stimulated by recombinant Listeria monocytogenes vaccination. *Cancer Res.* 2002;62(8):2287–2293.

215. Feng K, Zhao H, Chen J, Yao D, Jiang X, Zhou W. Anti-angiogenesis effect on glioma of attenuated Salmonella typhimurium vaccine strain with flk-1 gene. *J Huazhong Univ Sci Technol Med Sci.* 2004;24(4):389–391.

216. Seavey MM, Maciag PC, Al-Rawi N, Sewell D, Paterson Y. An anti-vascular endothelial growth factor receptor 2/fetal liver kinase-1 Listeria monocytogenes anti-angiogenesis cancer vaccine for the treatment of primary and

metastatic Her-2/neu+ breast tumors in a mouse model. *J Immunol.* 2009;182(9):5537–5546.

217. Maciag PC, Seavey MM, Pan ZK, Ferrone S, Paterson Y. Cancer immunotherapy targeting the high molecular weight melanoma-associated antigen protein results in a broad antitumor response and reduction of pericytes in the tumor vasculature. *Cancer Res.* 2008;68(19):8066–8075.

218. Maciag PC, Radulovic S, Rothman J. The first clinical use of a live-attenuated Listeria monocytogenes vaccine: a Phase I safety study of Lm-LLO-E7 in patients with advanced carcinoma of the cervix. *Vaccine.* 2009;27(30):3975–3983.

219. Xiang R, Luo Y, Niethammer AG, Reisfeld RA. Oral DNA vaccines target the tumor vasculature and microenvironment and suppress tumor growth and metastasis. *Immunol Rev.* 2008;222:117–128.

220. Fest S, Huebener N, Bleeke M, et al. Survivin minigene DNA vaccination is effective against neuroblastoma. *Int J Cancer.* 2009;125(1):104–114.

221. Xiong G, Husseiny MI, Song L, et al. Novel cancer vaccine based on genes of Salmonella pathogenicity island 2. *Int J Cancer.* 2010;126(11):2622–2634.

222. Rosenberg SA, Spiess PJ, Kleiner DE. Antitumor effects in mice of the intravenous injection of attenuated Salmonella typhimurium. *J Immunother.* 2002;25(3):218–225.

223. Clairmont C, Lee KC, Pike J, et al. Biodistribution and genetic stability of the novel antitumor agent VNP20009, a genetically modified strain of Salmonella typhimurium. *J Infect Dis.* 2000;181(6):1996–2002.

224. Toso JF, Gill VJ, Hwu P, et al. Phase I study of the intravenous administration of attenuated Salmonella typhimurium to patients with metastatic melanoma. *J Clin Oncol.* 2002;20(1):142–152.

225. Cunningham C, Nemunaitis J. A phase I trial of genetically modified Salmonella typhimurium expressing cytosine deaminase (TAPET-CD, VNP20029) administered by intratumoral injection in combination with 5-fluorocytosine for patients with advanced or metastatic cancer. Protocol no: CL-017. Version: April 9, 2001. *Hum Gene Ther.* 2001;12(12):1594–1596.

226. Schneider T, Gerhards R, Kirches E, Firsching R. Preliminary results of active specific immunization with modified tumor cell vaccine in glioblastoma multiforme. *J Neurooncol.* 2001;53(1):39–46.

227. Steiner HH, Bonsanto MM, Beckhove P, et al. Antitumor vaccination of patients with glioblastoma multiforme: a pilot study to assess feasibility, safety, and clinical benefit. *J Clin Oncol.* 2004;22(21):4272–4281.

228. Msaouel P, Dispenzieri A, Galanis E. Clinical testing of engineered oncolytic measles virus strains in the treatment of cancer: an overview. *Curr Opin Mol Ther.* 2009;11(1):43–53.

229. Galanis E, Hartmann LC, Cliby WA, et al. Phase I trial of intraperitoneal administration of an oncolytic measles virus strain engineered to express carcinoembryonic antigen for recurrent ovarian cancer. *Cancer Res.* 2010;70(3):875–882.

230. Myers R, Harvey M, Kaufmann TJ, et al. Toxicology study of repeat intracerebral administration of a measles virus derivative producing carcinoembryonic antigen in rhesus macaques in support of a phase I/II clinical trial for patients with recurrent gliomas. *Hum Gene Ther.* 2008;19(7):690–698.

231. Walker, P.R., et al., *Harnessing T-cell immunity to target brain tumors.*, in *CNS Cancer: Models, Markers, Prognostic Factors, Targets, and Therapeutic Approaches.*, E.G. Van Meir, Editor 2009, Humana Press. p. 1165–1217.

232. Liau LM, Black KL, Martin NA, et al. Treatment of a patient by vaccination with autologous dendritic cells pulsed with allogeneic major histocompatibility complex class I-matched tumor peptides. Case Report. *Neurosurg Focus.* 2000;9(6):e8.

233. Yu JS, Wheeler CJ, Zeltzer PM, et al. Vaccination of malignant glioma patients with peptide-pulsed dendritic cells elicits systemic cytotoxicity and intracranial T-cell infiltration. *Cancer Res.* 2001;61(3):842–847.

234. Ardon H, Van Gool S, Lopes IS, et al. Integration of autologous dendritic cell-based immunotherapy in the primary treatment for patients with newly diagnosed glioblastoma multiforme: a pilot study. *J Neurooncol.* 2010;99(2):261–272.

235. De Vleeschouwer S, Fieuws S, Rutkowski S, et al. Postoperative adjuvant dendritic cell-based immunotherapy in patients with relapsed glioblastoma multiforme. *Clin Cancer Res.* 2008;14(10):3098–3104.

236. Prins RM, Soto H, Konkankit V, et al. Gene expression profile correlates with T-cell infiltration and relative survival in glioblastoma patients vaccinated with dendritic cell immunotherapy. *Clin Cancer Res.* 2011;17(6):1603–1615.

237. Yamanaka R, Abe T, Yajima N, et al. Vaccination of recurrent glioma patients with tumour lysate-pulsed dendritic cells elicits immune responses: results of a clinical phase I/II trial. *Br J Cancer.* 2003;89(7):1172–1179.

238. Yamanaka R, Homma J, Yajima N, et al. Clinical evaluation of dendritic cell vaccination for patients with recurrent glioma: results of a clinical phase I/II trial. *Clin Cancer Res.* 2005;11(11):4160–4167.

239. Yu JS, Liu G, Ying H, Yong WH, Black KL, Wheeler CJ. Vaccination with tumor lysate-pulsed dendritic cells elicits antigen-specific, cytotoxic T-cells in patients with malignant glioma. *Cancer Res.* 2004;64(14):4973–4979.

240. Caruso DA, Orme LM, Neale AM, et al. Results of a phase 1 study utilizing monocyte-derived dendritic cells pulsed with tumor RNA in children and young adults with brain cancer. *Neuro-oncology.* 2004;6(3):236–246.

241. Kobayashi T, Yamanaka R, Homma J, et al. Tumor mRNA-loaded dendritic cells elicit tumor-specific CD8(+) cytotoxic T cells in patients with malignant glioma. *Cancer Immunol Immunother.* 2003;52(10):632–637.

242. Okada H, Kalinski P, Ueda R, et al. Induction of CD8+ T-cell responses against novel glioma-associated antigen peptides and clinical activity by vaccinations with {alpha}-type 1 polarized dendritic cells and polyinosinic-polycytidylic acid stabilized by lysine and carboxymethylcellulose

in patients with recurrent malignant glioma. *J Clin Oncol.* 2011;29(3):330–336.

243. Galon J, Costes A, Sanchez-Cabo F, et al. Type, density, and location of immune cells within human colorectal tumors predict clinical outcome. *Science.* 2006;313(5795):1960–1964.

244. Korangy F, Ormandy LA, Bleck JS, et al. Spontaneous tumor-specific humoral and cellular immune responses to NY-ESO-1 in hepatocellular carcinoma. *Clin Cancer Res.* 2004;10(13):4332–4341.

245. Janetzki S, Panageas KS, Ben-Porat L, et al.; Elispot Proficiency Panel of the CVC Immune Assay Working Group. Results and harmonization guidelines from two large-scale international Elispot proficiency panels conducted by the Cancer Vaccine Consortium (CVC/SVI). *Cancer Immunol Immunother.* 2008;57(3):303–315.

246. Klinman DM, Nutman TB. ELISPOT assay to detect cytokine-secreting murine and human cells. *Curr Protoc Immunol.* 2001;Chapter 6:Unit 6.19.

247. Brunner KT, Mauel J, Cerottini JC, Chapuis B. Quantitative assay of the lytic action of immune lymphoid cells on 51-Cr-labelled allogeneic target cells *in vitro*; inhibition by isoantibody and by drugs. *Immunology.* 1968;14(2):181–196.

248. Brandsma D, Stalpers L, Taal W, Sminia P, van den Bent MJ. Clinical features, mechanisms, and management of pseudoprogression in malignant gliomas. *Lancet Oncol.* 2008;9(5):453–461.

249. Chamberlain MC, Glantz MJ, Chalmers L, Van Horn A, Sloan AE. Early necrosis following concurrent Temodar and radiotherapy in patients with glioblastoma. *J Neurooncol.* 2007;82(1):81–83.

250. Zeng QS, Li CF, Liu H, Zhen JH, Feng DC. Distinction between recurrent glioma and radiation injury using magnetic resonance spectroscopy in combination with diffusion-weighted imaging. *Int J Radiat Oncol Biol Phys.* 2007;68(1):151–158.

251. Smith JS, Cha S, Mayo MC, et al. Serial diffusion-weighted magnetic resonance imaging in cases of glioma: distinguishing tumor recurrence from postresection injury. *J Neurosurg.* 2005;103(3):428–438.

252. Rachinger W, Goetz C, Pöpperl G, et al. Positron emission tomography with O-(2-[18F]fluoroethyl)-l-tyrosine versus magnetic resonance imaging in the diagnosis of recurrent gliomas. *Neurosurgery.* 2005;57(3):505–11; discussion 505.

253. Brandes AA, Tosoni A, Cavallo G, et al.; GICNO. Temozolomide 3 weeks on and 1 week off as first-line therapy for recurrent glioblastoma: phase II study from gruppo italiano cooperativo di neuro-oncologia (GICNO). *Br J Cancer.* 2006;95(9):1155–1160.

254. Verma R, Zacharaki EI, Ou Y, et al. Multiparametric tissue characterization of brain neoplasms and their recurrence using pattern classification of MR images. *Acad Radiol.* 2008;15(8):966–977.

255. Asao C, Korogi Y, Kitajima M, et al. Diffusion-weighted imaging of radiation-induced brain injury for differentiation from tumor recurrence. *AJNR Am J Neuroradiol.* 2005;26(6):1455–1460.

256. Rock JP, Scarpace L, Hearshen D, et al. Associations among magnetic resonance spectroscopy, apparent diffusion coefficients, and image-guided histopathology with special attention to radiation necrosis. *Neurosurgery.* 2004;54(5):1111–7; discussion 1117.

257. Weybright P, Sundgren PC, Maly P, et al. Differentiation between brain tumor recurrence and radiation injury using MR spectroscopy. *AJR Am J Roentgenol.* 2005;185(6):1471–1476.

258. Zeng QS, Li CF, Zhang K, Liu H, Kang XS, Zhen JH. Multivoxel 3D proton MR spectroscopy in the distinction of recurrent glioma from radiation injury. *J Neurooncol.* 2007;84(1):63–69.

259. McKnight TR, von dem Bussche MH, Vigneron DB, et al. Histopathological validation of a three-dimensional magnetic resonance spectroscopy index as a predictor of tumor presence. *J Neurosurg.* 2002;97(4):794–802.

260. Yang I, Huh NG, Smith ZA, Han SJ, Parsa AT. Distinguishing glioma recurrence from treatment effect after radiochemotherapy and immunotherapy. *Neurosurg Clin N Am.* 2010;21(1):181–186.

261. Hein PA, Eskey CJ, Dunn JF, Hug EB. Diffusion-weighted imaging in the follow-up of treated high-grade gliomas: tumor recurrence versus radiation injury. *AJNR Am J Neuroradiol.* 2004;25(2):201–209.

262. Wong TZ, van der Westhuizen GJ, Coleman RE. Positron emission tomography imaging of brain tumors. *Neuroimaging Clin N Am.* 2002;12(4):615–626.

263. Ricci PE, Karis JP, Heiserman JE, Fram EK, Bice AN, Drayer BP. Differentiating recurrent tumor from radiation necrosis: time for re-evaluation of positron emission tomography? *AJNR Am J Neuroradiol.* 1998;19(3):407–413.

264. Tsuyuguchi N, Takami T, Sunada I, et al. Methionine positron emission tomography for differentiation of recurrent brain tumor and radiation necrosis after stereotactic radiosurgery–in malignant glioma. *Ann Nucl Med.* 2004;18(4):291–296.

265. Frazier JL, Han JE, Lim M, Olivi A. Immunotherapy combined with chemotherapy in the treatment of tumors. *Neurosurg Clin N Am.* 2010;21(1):187–194.

266. Zhang B, Bowerman NA, Salama JK, et al. Induced sensitization of tumor stroma leads to eradication of established cancer by T cells. *J Exp Med.* 2007;204(1):49–55.

267. Liu JY, Wu Y, Zhang XS, et al. Single administration of low dose cyclophosphamide augments the antitumor effect of dendritic cell vaccine. *Cancer Immunol Immunother.* 2007;56(10):1597–1604.

268. Casares N, Pequignot MO, Tesniere A, et al. Caspase-dependent immunogenicity of doxorubicin-induced tumor cell death. *J Exp Med.* 2005;202(12):1691–1701.

269. Park SD, Kim CH, Kim CK, et al. Cross-priming by temozolomide enhances antitumor immunity of dendritic cell vaccination in murine brain tumor model. *Vaccine.* 2007;25(17):3485–3491.

270. Chaichana K, Parker S, Olivi A, Quiñones-Hinojosa A. A proposed classification system that projects outcomes based on preoperative variables for adult patients with glioblastoma multiforme. *J Neurosurg.* 2010;112(5):997–1004.

271. Marty M, Cognetti F, Maraninchi D, et al. Randomized phase II trial of the efficacy and safety of trastuzumab combined with docetaxel in patients with human epidermal growth factor receptor 2-positive metastatic breast cancer administered as first-line treatment: the M77001 study group. *J Clin Oncol.* 2005;23(19):4265–4274.

272. Smith I, Procter M, Gelber RD, et al.; HERA study team. 2-year follow-up of trastuzumab after adjuvant chemotherapy in HER2-positive breast cancer: a randomised controlled trial. *Lancet.* 2007;369(9555):29–36.

273. Wheeler CJ, Das A, Liu G, Yu JS, Black KL. Clinical responsiveness of glioblastoma multiforme to chemotherapy after vaccination. *Clin Cancer Res.* 2004;10(16):5316–5326.

274. Peres E, Wood GW, Poulik J, et al. High-dose chemotherapy and adoptive immunotherapy in the treatment of recurrent pediatric brain tumors. *Neuropediatrics.* 2008;39(3):151–156.

275. Appay V, Voelter V, Rufer N, et al. Combination of transient lymphodepletion with busulfan and fludarabine and peptide vaccination in a phase I clinical trial for patients with advanced melanoma. *J Immunother.* 2007;30(2):240–250.

276. Dudley ME, Wunderlich JR, Yang JC, et al. Adoptive cell transfer therapy following non-myeloablative but lymphodepleting chemotherapy for the treatment of patients with refractory metastatic melanoma. *J Clin Oncol.* 2005;23(10):2346–2357.

277. Reits EA, Hodge JW, Herberts CA, et al. Radiation modulates the peptide repertoire, enhances MHC class I expression, and induces successful antitumor immunotherapy. *J Exp Med.* 2006;203(5):1259–1271.

278. Shiao SL, Coussens LM. The tumor-immune microenvironment and response to radiation therapy. *J Mammary Gland Biol Neoplasia.* 2010;15(4):411–421.

279. Meng, Y., et al., *Radiation-inducible Immunotherapy for Cancer: Senescent Tumor Cells as a Cancer Vaccine.* Mol Ther, 2012.

280. Shiao SL, Ganesan AP, Rugo HS, Coussens LM. Immune microenvironments in solid tumors: new targets for therapy. *Genes Dev.* 2011;25(24):2559–2572.

281. Demaria S, Ng B, Devitt ML, et al. Ionizing radiation inhibition of distant untreated tumors (abscopal effect) is immune mediated. *Int J Radiat Oncol Biol Phys.* 2004;58(3):862–870.

282. Obeid M, Panaretakis T, Joza N, et al. Calreticulin exposure is required for the immunogenicity of gamma-irradiation and UVC light-induced apoptosis. *Cell Death Differ.* 2007;14(10):1848–1850.

283. Apetoh L, Ghiringhelli F, Tesniere A, et al. Toll-like receptor 4-dependent contribution of the immune system to anticancer chemotherapy and radiotherapy. *Nat Med.* 2007;13(9):1050–1059.

284. Ghiringhelli F, Apetoh L, Tesniere A, et al. Activation of the NLRP3 inflammasome in dendritic cells induces IL-1beta-dependent adaptive immunity against tumors. *Nat Med.* 2009;15(10):1170–1178.

285. Fadul CE, Fisher JL, Hampton TH, et al. Immune response in patients with newly diagnosed glioblastoma multiforme treated with intranodal autologous tumor lysate-dendritic cell vaccination after radiation chemotherapy. *J Immunother.* 2011;34(4):382–389.

286. Schaue D, Ratikan JA, Iwamoto KS, McBride WH. Maximizing tumor immunity with fractionated radiation. *Int J Radiat Oncol Biol Phys.* 2012;83(4):1306–1310.

287. Chiocca EA, Aguilar LK, Bell SD, et al. Phase IB study of gene-mediated cytotoxic immunotherapy adjuvant to up-front surgery and intensive timing radiation for malignant glioma. *J Clin Oncol.* 2011;29(27):3611–3619.

288. Dewan MZ, Galloway AE, Kawashima N, et al. Fractionated but not single-dose radiotherapy induces an immune-mediated abscopal effect when combined with anti-CTLA-4 antibody. *Clin Cancer Res.* 2009;15(17):5379–5388.

289. Hodge JW, Sharp HJ, Gameiro SR. Abscopal regression of antigen disparate tumors by antigen cascade after systemic tumor vaccination in combination with local tumor radiation. *Cancer Biother Radiopharm.* 2012;27(1):12–22.

demos MEDICAL

RADIATION MEDICINE ROUNDS

The Role of Advanced Radiation Modalities in the Treatment of Gliomas

Aashish D. Bhatt, Jay S. Loeffler, and Helen A. Shih*

Department of Radiation Oncology, Massachusetts General Hospital, Boston, MA; Harvard Medical School, Boston, MA

ABSTRACT

Malignant gliomas account for more than two-thirds of all adult primary malignant brain tumors diagnosed every year in the United States. Significant advancements have been achieved in treatment modalities of surgery, chemotherapy, and radiotherapy. However, the median survival times remain just over a year for glioblastoma and less than 5 years for anaplastic gliomas. Several different radiotherapeutic approaches have been investigated in the context of management of gliomas. In this chapter, we attempt to enumerate the role of advanced radiotherapy techniques and to summarize the pertinent clinical data. Despite the limited survival, enthusiasm to explore novel treatment strategies remains high with the ultimate goal of prolonging survival, improving the quality of patient lives, and minimizing toxicity.

Keywords: brachytherapy, hypofractionated stereotactic radiotherapy, intensity modulated radiotherapy, malignant gliomas, particle therapy, proton therapy, radioimmunotherapy, stereotactic radiosurgery

INTRODUCTION

Malignant gliomas represent a challenging tumor type to treat and carry a poor overall survival. Historically, surgery followed by radiotherapy (RT) has been the main stay of treatment. Postoperative conventional RT delivered at 2 Gy per fraction using three-dimensional techniques is the most widely used approach and is the standard of care. Rapid advances in imaging and improvements in radiation delivery techniques have led to several studies reevaluating the role of the radiation oncologist to improve survival. Stereotactic radiosurgery (SRS), hypofractionated stereotactic RT (HFSRT), intensity modulated RT (IMRT), brachytherapy, radioimmunotherapy (RIT), and particle therapy have emerged as means of delivering a higher dose of radiation more conformally to the target while achieving maximal sparing of the surrounding normal brain and critical structures. With the identification of several molecular pathways and development of new targeted therapies, the role of conventional and advanced RT modalities in combination with these is also being reassessed.

*Corresponding author, Chief of Service, Central Nervous System and Eye Services, Department of Radiation Oncology, Massachusetts General Hospital, 30 Fruit Street, Boston, MA 02114.

E-mail address: hshih@partners.org

Radiation Medicine Rounds 3:2 (2012) 317–338.

DOI: 10.5003/2151–4208.3.2.317

STEREOTACTIC RADIOSURGERY (SRS)

SRS is a technique of delivering a high dose of radiation very conformally to a target, usually in a single fraction. Stereotaxis refers to localization of a target in a 3-D space. Several different treatment delivery techniques exist including Linac-based, Gamma Knife, CyberKnife, and charged-particles (protons, carbon ions) radiosurgery. It involves a high degree of precision and accuracy of <1 to 1.5 mm using either frame-based or frameless approaches (1–3). The radiation dose fall-off is also rapid such that sparing of the surrounding normal structures can be safely achieved. The definition of SRS is allowed by some to include up to 3 to 5 fractions. Fractionated stereotactic RT (FSRT) or HFSRT includes several fractions (usually >3–5) with the use of stereotaxis for localization. The typical per fraction dose with FSRT is 1.8–2 Gy/fraction whereas that with HFSRT is >2 Gy.

The conformality of SRS depends on the size and shape of the target and the diameter of the collimator. Single or multiple isocenters can be used to achieve the desired conformality. Collimation is achieved using either circular collimators or micro-multileaf collimators (mMLCs). With careful planning, Linac-based plans can achieve a high-degree of conformity similar to the Gamma Knife (4), Cyber Knife (5), and proton therapy (6,7). The ideal radiosurgery team is a multi-disciplinary arrangement including a radiation oncologist, neurosurgeon, physicist, radiation therapists, and nurses. Stringent quality assurance is required prior to treatment delivery.

RATIONALE FOR SRS

External beam RT has been shown to have a dose response (8,9). Studies have shown that most recurrences (>90%) occur at or immediately adjacent to the primary site (10,11). It was thus felt that addition of SRS might minimize recurrence rates and potentially improve survival. Studies of dose escalation up to 90 Gy have been conducted with mixed results. A study from the Massachusetts General Hospital (MGH) (12) using accelerated fractionation proton/photon irradiation to 90 cobalt Gy equivalent (Gy [RBE], 1 proton Gy = 1.1 Gy) showed decreased local recurrences but at the cost of increased radiation necrosis whereas two studies from University or Michigan to the dose levels of 70 to 80 Gy (13) or 90 Gy (14) using conventional techniques had 91% patients failing locally.

Biologically, SRS produces higher than predicted tumor control rates based on *in vitro* and *in vivo* killing of tumor cells (15). It has been proposed that at high doses of radiation, the vascular endothelium becomes an additional important target. Radiation-induced apoptosis of the endothelial cells potentially become apparent after high doses (16). SRS is believed to elicit endothelial damage by induction of an inflammatory response with fibroblastic proliferation, hyalinization, and scarring of vessels (17,18).

TARGET DELINEATION, TECHNIQUE, AND DOSE

A contrast-enhanced MRI with T1, T2, and FLAIR sequences is necessary to delineate the target in conventional RT. This is clearly the most important initial step in treatment planning. In contrast to conventional RT, the radiosurgical target volume is defined by any residual T1-enhancement postoperatively or at the time of recurrence. Set-up error for SRS is usually in the submillimeter range for all delivery techniques (1–3). Prescribed dose depends on target size and location. The Radiation Therapy Oncology Group (RTOG) study 90–05 was a radiosurgery study designed to determine the maximum tolerated dose (MTD) by target volume (19). Patients with recurrent malignant gliomas and brain metastases were stratified according to the maximum diameter of tumor enhancement and dose-limiting neurotoxicity was assessed for different radiosurgical dose levels. The MTD was not reached for tumors less than 2 cm but dose escalation was stopped at 24 Gy. Tolerable dose for tumors 2 to 3 cm was defined at 18 Gy and for 3 to 4 cm was 15 Gy. In a study of brain metastases with lesions ≤2 cm, Shehata et al. (20) noted that SRS doses >20 Gy resulted in no additional benefit to tumor local control and were associated with a greater rate of complication. In our opinion and also of others (21), a dose of 18 to 20 Gy could be considered adequate and safe for both primary and metastatic lesions measuring ≤2 cm.

Proton SRS (PSRS) can be performed by adjusting the depth and width of the Bragg peak to match the target's dimensions in the brain. Most commonly, two to three stationary intersecting beams each with its own custom-shaped collimator, often referred to as the aperture, are used to conform to the target. Compensators are interposed in the beam path to compensate for skull curvature and brain tissue inhomogeneity.

■ RESULTS

Early institutional prospective studies from 1990 evaluating the role of SRS given as a boost after conventional external beam RT (EBRT) showed encouraging results. Loeffler et al. (22) treated 37 patients (23 with glioblastoma [GBM]) with an SRS boost (median dose – 12 Gy) after conventional RT to 59.4 Gy. After a median follow-up of 19 months, only 9 of 37 (24%) patients had died. Six patients (all GBM) died of recurrent tumor, whereas death was attributable to complications of treatment in two cases and intercurrent disease in one. Four patients with recurrent tumor failed at the margins of the radiosurgical treatment volume, whereas two patients progressed locally. A multi-institutional retrospective series in 115 patients by Sarkaria et al. (23) also seem to suggest a benefit to incorporating SRS into the initial management treatment scheme when patient survival was compared to the RTOG recursive partitioning analysis classes (24).

A counter point was suggested by some that the benefit seen with SRS could be due to a selection bias rather than a genuine treatment effect. Irish et al. (25) conducted a retrospective study on 101 consecutive patients evaluating them to be eligible for SRS or not at completion of EBRT. They found 27% eligibility for SRS and a median survival of 23.4 months in this group despite none actually receiving an SRS boost. The median survival in the remaining 73% ineligible patients was only 8.6 months. Curran et al. (26) performed a similar study evaluating 778 patients treated on RTOG 83–02 trial of HFRT with carmustine (BCNU) chemotherapy. Eighty-nine patients (11.9%) were identified as potentially SRS-eligible. The median survival times (MSTs) and 18-month survival rates of the 89 eligible and 643 ineligible patients were 14.4 versus 11.7 months and 40% versus 27%, respectively (P =.047). They concluded that this advantage is due to selection of a subgroup with good Karnofsky performance status (KPS). Both the above studies showed a similar trend with improved median survival in patients eligible for SRS.

There was thus much enthusiasm about the potential benefit of SRS in addition to conventional RT and the need for a phase III trial. RTOG 93–05 (27) was conducted to prospectively evaluate the role of SRS in patients with newly diagnosed GBM. This trial is the first and only randomized trial to-date evaluating SRS and randomized 203 patients of which there were 186 evaluable. After initial surgery, SRS was administered to the postoperative residual (≤4 cm) without any additional margins, before conventional EBRT to a dose of 60 Gy. This was a different strategy to the institutional trials where the decision to incorporate SRS was determined on scanning after the completion of external beam therapy. Patients who progressed during external beam radiation were excluded from a SRS boost. All patients in RTOG 93–05 received concurrent adjuvant BCNU after RT was completed. SRS dose was determined based on tumor size per RTOG 90–05 (19) recommendations (15–24 Gy). Patients were stratified based on age (±50) and KPS (±80). Primary end point was survival.

Results showed a median survival of 13.5 months in the SRS group versus 13.6 months in the control group. Local failure was a component of failure in 92.5% cases and was defined as recurrent/persistent tumor located within 2 cm of the enhancing edge of the postoperative lesion. A comparison of the SRS technique did not show any difference with median survival being 14 months (Linac-based) versus 12.1 months (Gamma Knife) (P = .71). Quality of life deterioration and cognitive decline as compared to baseline were comparable in both arms. Of note, in the subset of patients with local failure only there was a nonsignificant difference favoring the SRS group (67% vs. 58%). The number of patients undergoing surgery for salvage was also similar. An analysis from patients undergoing either a partial or a total resection at reoperation reveals that the incidence of necrosis in the surgical specimen without evidence of residual tumor was 4% (1/25) in the standard arm versus 20% (4/20) in the SRS arm. Small patient numbers limit interpretation of these results. Of note, the experimental arm had an 18% rate of "unacceptable deviation" in quality control. RTOG 93–05 thus failed to show a benefit to adding SRS prior to conventional RT. Even subgroup analyses failed to identify any specific group benefitting from SRS. It should be noted that this study does not address the efficacy of SRS as a boost (post EBRT) or its use in the recurrence setting.

Kondziolka et al. (28) in a study of 64 patients with GBM evaluated the role of SRS in the adjuvant setting. The study involved the use of SRS 5 to 8 months after the initial diagnosis and after EBRT and chemotherapy was completed. The median survival from initial diagnosis was 26 months and from after the SRS was 21 months. The 2-year survival rate was encouraging at 51%. They also reported a median survival of 30 months in patients who underwent SRS at the time of tumor progression.

PATIENT SELECTION FOR SRS

Patients suitable for SRS usually include those with residual or recurrent tumors ≤4 cm, not in the brainstem, >5 mm from the optic apparatus, no subependymal spread, and KPS>60. Patients with larger tumors and in proximity to eloquent areas may be suitable for a HFSRT approach. These criteria are based upon safety and not efficacy as the existing data is insufficient to guide a population of patients that would clearly benefit from this treatment.

TOXICITY

The use of SRS boost has been associated with a variable risk of toxicity in some studies with increased rates of radionecrosis and need for reoperation (22,29). In RTOG 93–05, there were four grade 3 late toxicities in the SRS arm, all in patients who received a 15 Gy SRS boost. There were no grade 4 or 5 toxicities related to fractionated RT or SRS. Of the 59 patients who underwent surgery as salvage therapy, 3 (3/31) in arm 1 had documented necrosis only in the operative specimen and all others had active tumor. In the SRS arm, 7 patients (7/28) had necrosis only and the remaining had active tumor.

A summary of some of the studies on the use of SRS in the initial management of malignant gliomas is presented in Table 1.

REIRRADIATION

Since the majority of the patients with malignant gliomas fail or progress, salvage therapy is often administered. Surgery is possible only in a select subgroup of patients and carries a substantial risk for morbidity (35,36). Retreating patients with malignant gliomas is a radiotherapeutic challenge and is usually offered to a select group of good performance status patients. The choice is driven by individual patient factors, including repeat surgical excision, size and location of the recurrent disease, performance status, and expected life expectancy. There are no prospective randomized trials defining the standard for RT treatment in the recurrence setting. Several single-arm and institutional experiences have been reported but definitive conclusions cannot be drawn from these studies due to variable inclusion criteria and selection bias. To understand the prognosis of this patient population and options for alternative therapy, systemic chemotherapy provides only a modest survival benefit in the recurrent setting with median survival ranging from 4 to 8 months (37–40).

A variety of techniques have been used in the salvage setting including SRS, HFSRT, IMRT, and brachytherapy (Figure 1). SRS is clearly the most convenient of all of these options since it is usually done in a single outpatient visit, is noninvasive and is generally well tolerated. However, SRS can be limited

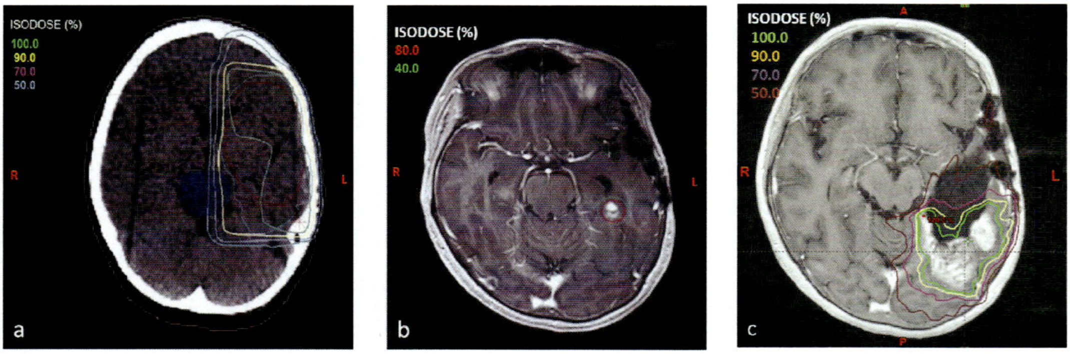

FIGURE 1 Serial images of a 63-year-old female patient who was diagnosed with a left parietotemporal GBM and underwent a gross tumor resection (GTR) of a 4.8 × 3.5 cm lesion. She then received adjuvant 3-D conformal conventional RT to 60 Gy (1a) with temozolomide. Serial follow-up MRI scans revealed no disease progression until 22 months later when she was found to have a new 1.2 cm lesion in the left temporal lobe. She received salvage Linac-based radiosurgery using a cone-based technique to a dose of 20 Gy in a single fraction. Follow-up MRI scan revealed progression of her left temporal lobe lesion which now measured 6.1 × 3.8 cm. She underwent reoperation with a subtotal resection 8 months after the salvage SRS which confirmed GBM recurrence. Four Gliadel wafers were placed at the time of salvage surgery. She then received repeat salvage radiosurgery to a dose of 12 Gy using a RapidArc-based technique.

TABLE 1 Studies of SRS in the initial management of malignant gliomas

Author (Year)	Loeffler et al. (1992) (22)	Mehta et al. (1994) (29)	Gannett et al. (1995) (30)	Sarkaria et al. (1995) (23)	Shrieve et al. (1999) (31)	Nwokedi et al. (2002) (32)	Prisco et al. (2002) (33)	Souhami et al. (2004) (27)	Smith et al. (2008) (34)
Study type*	P	P	P	R, multi-institutional	R	RMP; Arm 1: EBRT alone, Arm 2: EBRT + SRS	RMP; Arm 1: EBRT alone, Arm 2: EBRT + SRS	RCT phase III: Arm 1: no SRS, Arm 2: SRS	P
n	37	31	30	115	78	64 (Arm 1: 33, Arm 2: 31)	32 (Arm 1: 17, Arm 2: 15)	203 (186 evaluable)	Std risk: 19; high risk: 8
Median age	51	57	54	NR (53% were <50 yr)	51	50.4	51	Arm 1: 55.5, Arm 2: 56.4 (mean)	Std risk: 52; high risk: 67.5
Histology	G3: 14; G4: 23	G4: 31	G3: 10; Mixed-3; G4: 17	G3: 19; G4: 96	G4: 78	G4: 64	G3: 2; G4: 30	G4: 203	G4: 27
Surgery	Surg: 20; Bx: 17	–	GTR: 9; STR: 18; Bx: 3	GTR: 3; STR: 61; Bx: 51	–	Surg: 45; Bx: 19	Surg: 28; Bx: 4	–	–
Median target vol (cc)	4.8	17.4	24	10	9.4	18.5	15	3 (both arms)	34.6 (mean)
Previous EBRT (Gy) (median)	59.4	54	59.4	NR (54–60)	59.4	59.7	60 (53–66)	SRS first, then EBRT: 60	SRS first, then EBRT to 60 Gy
EBRT and SRS time (wks)	2–4	2–4	4 (upto 8 wk)	NR	–	6	5	1	2 wk
SRS modality	LBRS	LBRS	LBRS	LBRS	LBRS	GKRS	LBRS	LBRS (47); GKRS (32)	GKRS
Median SRS dose (range) (Gy)	12–15 (10–25)	12–18.6 (10–30)	10 (5–18)	12 (6–20)	12 (6–24)	17.1 (10–28)	10 (8–12.5)	15–24	12 (50% IDL)
Chemotherapy	None	–	–	10%	–	Arm 1: 42%; Arm 2: 65%	28%	BCNU: 100%	Gliadel wafers: 100%
Median follow-up (mos)	19	3–43	30 (12–45)	22.7	40.8 (25.5–79.4)	17.5	NR (10.5–67.9)	61	–
Median survival (mos)	Gr 4: 26; Gr 3: not reached	10.5	G4: 13; G3: 28	24	19.9	Arm 1: 13; Arm 2: 25	Arm 1: 11.6; Arm 2: 21.4	Arm 1: 13.6; Arm 2: 13.5	SR: 19; HR: 8.25
Overall survival (OS)	–	2 yr: 28%	1 yr: G3: 65%; G4: 43%	2 yr: 45%	2 yr: 35.9%	1 yr: 67% 2 yr: 40%	–	2yr Arm 1: 19%, Arm 2: 21%; 3yr Arm 1: 13%, Arm 2: 9%	2 yr: SR: 33%; HR: 0%

Abbreviations: NR = not reported, Gy = gray, cc = cubic centimeters, wks = weeks, mos = months, yr = year, OS = overall survival, G = grade of tumor; G3 = grade 3, G4 = grade 4, SRS = stereotactic radiosurgery, LBRS = linear accelerator-based radiosurgery, GKRS = Gamma knife-based radiosurgery, *study type: RCT = randomized control trial, P = prospective, R = retrospective, RMP = retrospective matched pair study, Surg = surgery, Bx = biopsy, GTR = gross total resection, STR = subtotal resection.

TABLE 2 Studies of SRS in the management of recurrent gliomas

Author (Year)	Chamberlain et al. (1994) (42)	Hall et al. (1995) (43)	Shrieve et al. (1995) (41)	Selch et al. (1998) (44)	Sanghavi et al. (1999) (45)	Larson et al. (2002) (46)	Sarkar et al. (2002) (47)	Combs et al. (2005) (48)	Mahajan et al. (2005) (49)	Hsieh et al. (2005) (50)	Patel et al. (2009) (51)	Pouratian et al. (2009) (52)
Study type*	P	P	R	R	R	P	R	R	R, CCS	R	R	R
n	20	35	B: 32; SRS-86	18	30	26	18 (21 tumors)	32 (36 tumors)	41	Initial: 25; Rec: 26	SRS-26; FSRT: 10	Initial: 22; Rec: 26
Median age (yrs)	34	48	B-45; SRS-46	52	52	G3: 44; G4: 53	43	56	54	59	GBM:57; MT: 39	60.1
Histology	G3: 10; G4: 5; others: 5	G3: 9; G4: 26	G4: 118	G3: 6; G4: 12	G3: 8; G4: 22	G3: 12; G4: 14	ODG: G1: 1; G2: 1; G3: 8; G4: 7	G4: 32	G4: 41	G4: 51	GBM: 31; MT: 5	GBM: 48
Median target volume (cc)	17	28	B: 29; SRS: 10.1	G3: 19.6; G4: 22.6	7.2	G3: 2.7; G4: 8	8.2	10	4.7	13.6	SRS: 10.4; FSRT: 51.1	Initial: 13.4; Rec: 21.3
Previous EBRT median (Gy)	59.7	60	–	60	59.4	–	54.9 (17 patients)	54	60	60	50–60	60
SRS modality	LBRS	GKRS	LBRS	LBRS	LBRS	GKRS	GKRS	LBRS	LBRS	GKRS	LBRS	GKRS
Median SRS dose (range) (Gy)	13.4 (12–15.7)	20 (7.5–40)	SRS: 13(6–20); B: 50	27: 55	12: 18.75	G3: 16.5–55; G4: 15–50	Margin: 15; Max: 32	15(10–20)	–	12 Gy (50% IDL)	SRS: 18; FSRT: 36 in 6 no	6(3–15)
Salvage chemo	50%	83%	NR	NR	33%	100%	NR	0%	NR	73%	100%	21%
Median F/U (mos)	8	NR	B: 43.3; SRS: 17.5	7.5	70	NR	24 (min)	10	21	21	NR	9.5
Median survival after SRS (mos)	7	6.5	B: 11.5; SRS: 10.2	G3: 8; G4: 7	8	G3: 17; G4: 9.5	ODG: 28; Mixed: 8	10	11	Initial: 16.7; Rec: 10	SRS: 8.4 FSRT: 7.5	OS: 9.5; Initial: 10.0; Rec: 9.4

*Study type: P = prospective, R = retrospective.

Abbreviations: CCS = case control study, EBRT = external beam radiation therapy, SRS = stereotactic radiosurgery, B = brachytherapy, G = grade of tumor (according to WHO classification), ODG = oligodendrogliomas, cc = cubic centimeters, Gy = Gray, mos = months, yrs = years, min = minimum, max = maximum, LBRS = linear accelerator based radiosurgery, GKRS = Gamma knife-based radiosurgery, MT = malignant transformation, Rec = Recurrence.

by the size and location of the recurrence such that a fractionated approach may be more safely feasible. Despite this, the median and overall survival results have been dismal. A summary of the pertinent studies has been tabulated in Table 2.

In a retrospective comparison of the efficacy of SRS versus brachytherapy in the treatment of recurrent GBM, Shrieve et al. (41) evaluated 32 patients treated with interstitial brachytherapy and 86 treated with SRS. The patient characteristics were similar in both groups. Those patients treated with SRS had a median tumor volume of 10.1 cm^3 and received a median peripheral tumor dose of 13 Gy. Patients treated with brachytherapy had a median tumor volume of 29 cm^3. Median dose to the periphery of the tumor volume was 50 Gy delivered at a median dose rate of 43 cGy/hour. Twenty-one patients (24%) treated with SRS were alive at a median follow-up of 17.5 months. Median actuarial survival, measured from the time of treatment for recurrence, for all patients treated with SRS was 10.2 months, with survivals of 12 and 24 months being 45% and 19%, respectively. A younger age and a smaller tumor volume were predictive of better outcome. The tumor dose, the interval from initial diagnosis, and the need for reoperation were not predictive of outcome after SRS. Five patients (16%) treated with brachytherapy were alive at a median follow-up of 43.3 months. The median actuarial survival for all patients treated with brachytherapy was 11.5 months. Survivals of 12 and 24 months were 44% and 17%, respectively. The age of the patient (but not tumor volume, interval from initial diagnosis, or tumor dose) was predictive of outcome in these patients. A comparison of the results between patients treated with SRS and brachytherapy indicated a similar survival rate. Nineteen patients (22%) required reoperation after SRS, compared with 14 (44%) in the brachytherapy group. The actuarial risk for reoperation was 33% at 12 months and 48% at 24 months after SRS, compared with 54% and 65%, respectively, after brachytherapy (P = .195). Those patients undergoing reoperation after brachytherapy survived longer than similar patients not undergoing reoperation. The outcome after SRS was independent of a need for reoperation. In the absence of confirmatory phase III trials, such retrospective comparison suggests that the treatment of recurrent GBM with SRS can result in a survival rate similar to that obtained with interstitial high-activity ^{125}I implantation with less morbidity. SRS is also usually accomplished as an outpatient procedure and many of the risks involved with brachytherapy do not apply to SRS (for example, infection, hemorrhage, exposure of personnel to radiation).

■ HYPOFRACTIONATED STEREOTACTIC RT (HFSRT)

Hypofractionated SRS is a method of delivering focal stereotactic radiation in a fractionated and often hypofractionated scheme. HFSRT is advantageous in treating recurrent previously irradiated tumors particularly when they are located in an eloquent area where it would not be safe to administer SRS. Fractionation allows for potentially reduced normal tissue toxicity by allowing repair to occur between fractions. This approach has also been studied in the initial management and in the recurrence settings both as a sole modality and in combination with chemotherapy. A summary of studies using HFSRT is shown in Table 3.

Hulshof et al. (53) compared three different RT fractionation schemes; 33 × 2, 8 × 5 and 4 × 7 Gy. The 4 × 7 Gy conformal radiation was given to poor-prognosis patients whereas more favorable patients received the conventionally fractionated scheme up to 66 Gy. Median survival was 7, 5.6, and 6.6 months for the 33 × 2, 8 × 5, and 4 × 7 Gy, respectively. In general, patients in the hypofractionation group had far worse prognostic factors compared to patients treated with the conventional scheme. The period of neurological improvement or stabilization was similar between the 4 × 7 and 33 × 2 Gy groups. They concluded that the shorter scheme is well tolerated, convenient for the patient, and provides equal palliation without negative effects on survival compared with conventional fractionation.

Studies evaluating incorporating a hypofractionated stereotactic boost have also been conducted. RTOG 00–23 (54) was a phase II study of 76 patients with histologically confirmed GBM and postoperative enhancing tumor plus tumor cavity diameter <60 mm. In this study, patients received 50 Gy (2 Gy/fraction) postoperatively and then four treatments of 5 or 7 Gy (tumor size dependent) once per week during weeks 3 to 6 of EBRT. BCNU was also given as per RTOG 93–05. The MST was 12.5 months. No survival difference was seen when compared with the RTOG historical database. Subset analysis revealed a trend toward improved outcome for GTR patients suggesting that patients with minimal disease burden may benefit most from this form of accelerated RT.

TABLE 3 Studies of HFSRT in the initial or recurrent management of malignant gliomas

Author (Year)	Laing et al. (1993) (65)	Cardinale et al. (1998) (66)	Nieder et al. (1999) (67)	Lederman et al. (2000) (68)	Baumert et al. (2003) (56)	Grosu et al. (2005) (57)	Ernst-Stecken et al. (2007) (69)	Schwer et al. (2008) (70)	Fokas et al. (2009) (71)	Henke et al. (2009) (72)	Fogh et al. (2010) (73)
Study type/arm	P; HFSRT (Rec)	P; EBRT+HFSRT (boost) (init.)	P; HFSRT only (init.)	P; HFSRT (Rec)	P; EBRT+HFSRT (boost) (init.)	P; Group 1: FSRT; Group 2: HFSRT+TMZ (Rec)	P; HFSRT only (Rec)	P; HFSRT SRS+gefitinib	R; HFSRT only (Rec)	R; HFSRT only (Rec)	R; HFSRT only (Rec)
n	22	12	19	88	17	Group 1: 15; Group 2: 29	15	15	53	31	147
Median age (yrs)	34	43	57	56.2	51	50	49	47	53	50	53
Histology	G1, G2: 3; G3: 7; G4: 12	G3: 3; G4: 9	G3: 5; G4: 14	G4: 88	G3: 2; G4: 15	G3: 9; G4: 35	G3: 4; G4: 11	GBM: 11; AA: 4	GBM: 53	G3: 2; G4: 29	GBM: 105; AA: 42
Surgery	Bx: 3; STR: 6	Bx: 2; STR: 10	Bx: 10; STR: 9	–	GTR: 15; STR: 2	–	None	Bx: 1; GTR: 7; PR: 7	Bx: 1; STR: 13; GTR: 39	Bx: 2; GTR: 22; STR: 7	Bx: 7; GTR: 41; STR: 99
Median target vol (range) (cc)	25	15.9	20.4	32.7	75	15	22.4	41.3	35.01	52.7	22
Previous EBRT (Gy)	55	44	None	60	54–60	60	57.75	60	54	59	60
EBRT to HFSRT time (wks)	20 mos	FSRT given on wks 3,4,5 of EBRT	–	–	2	16 mos	10 mos	11.9	–	18 mos	–
HFSRT modality	LB–SRT	LB–SRT	LB–SRT	LB–SRT	LB–SRT	LB–SRT	LB–SRT	LB–SRT	LB–SRT	LB–SRT	LB–SRT
Median HFSRT dose (range) (Gy)	Variable 5 Gy × 4 upto 5 Gy × 10	12 Gy × 3	5 Gy × 5; 6 Gy × 5; 7 Gy × 5	6 Gy × 4	4 Gy × 5; 5 Gy × 2	5 Gy × 6	7 Gy × 5	Variable 6 Gy × 3 upto 12 Gy × 3	30 Gy	20 Gy	3.5 Gy fractions to 35 Gy
Chemo at Rec	36%	100%	None	47%	None	29 pts: TMZ	53%	Gefitinib	47%	77%	33%
Median F/U (mos)	7	26	–	–	25	–	9	7	8	–	21
Median survival (mos)	G3: 9; G4: 11	G3: 33; G4: 16	7	7	20	Group 1: 6; Group 2: 11	–	10.3	9	10.2	G3: 10; G4: 11
Overall survival (OS)	–	–	1 yr: 32%	1 yr: 17%; 2 yr: 3.4%	2 yr: 42%	–	6 mos: 85%; 1yr: 43%	6mos: 63%; 1yr: 40%	1yr: 3%; 2yr: 45%	6mos: 72%; 1yr: 43%	–

NR = not reported, Gy = gray, cc = cubic centimeters, wks = weeks, mos = months, yr = year, OS = overall survival, G = grade of tumor, G1 = grade 1, G2 = grade 2, G3 = grade 3,
Abbreviations: G4 = grade 4, GBM = glioblastoma multiforme, AA = anaplastic astrocytoma, TMZ = temozolomide, Bx = biopsy, GTR = gross total resection, STR = subtotal resection, LB-SRT = LINAC-based stereotactic RT, Init. = Initial, Rec = Recurrence.

The European Organization for Research and Treatment for Cancer (EORTC) and the Medical Research Council (MRC) started a joint phase III trial (EORTC 22972–26991/MRC BR10) evaluating a HFSRT boost of four 5 Gy fractions after EBRT, but this trial had to be closed in 2001 due to poor accrual. Results on 25 patients enrolled did, however, reveal the toxicity to be low (55). The phase II study leading to this study had earlier shown encouraging median survival of 20 months in 17 patients which was significantly better than historical controls (56).

Biologic imaging has also been incorporated into the treatment planning strategy. In a prospective nonrandomized single-institution trial of 44 patients with recurrent HGG treated with HFSRT (5 Gy × 6 in 6 days), Grosu et al. (57) defined the gross tumor volume was by C^{11}-methionine positron emission tomography (MET-PET) or I^{123}-alpha-methyl-tyrosine (IMT) single-photon computed emission tomography (SPECT)/computed tomography (CT)/MRI fusion in 82% of the patients, and by CT/T1+gadolinium-MRI image fusion in 18% of the patients. Treatment planning based on PET(SPECT)/CT/MRI imaging was associated with improved survival in comparison to treatment planning using CT/MRI alone with MSTs of 9 months versus 5 months ($P = .03$).

Malignant gliomas are innately hypoxic tumors with strong endogenous expression of hypoxia-inducible factor-1 (HIF-1), vascular endothelial growth factor (VEGF), and VEGF receptors and consequently demonstrate vigorous angiogenesis (58–61). Bevacizumab, a humanized monoclonal antibody to VEGF, has been used alone or in combination with irinotecan in recurrent malignant gliomas (62,63). In a prospective study, Gutin et al. (64) treated 25 patients with recurrent gliomas (GBM-20; Anaplastic-5) to a total dose of 30 Gy in 5 fractions given over 2.5 weeks. Median dose of prior RT was 59.4 Gy and median time from prior RT to FSRT was 15 months. Three patients discontinued treatment because of grade 3 central nervous system intratumoral hemorrhage, wound dehiscence, and bowel perforation. Other nonhematologic and hematologic toxicities were transient and no radiation necrosis was seen. For the GBM cohort, overall response rate was 50%, 6-month progression-free survival was 65%; median overall survival was 12.5 months, and 1-year survival was 54%. The authors concluded that bevacizumab with HFSRT is safe and well tolerated, and that this regimen is active in recurrent malignant glioma.

INTENSITY MODULATED RT (IMRT)

A critical aspect of RT planning is to spare the surrounding normal structures while simultaneously delivering the prescription dose to the tumor. In case of gliomas, proximity to several radiosensitive tissues, including the eyes, lacrimal glands, optic apparatus, cochlea, and brainstem, can be a limiting factor as damage to these areas can cause severe morbidity. Any effort to decrease the treatment toxicity might result in compromised target coverage with conventional therapy. IMRT is a more sophisticated approach to delivering conformal RT. It is now becoming increasingly used in several disease sites such as head and neck, prostate, lung, brain, and pediatric malignancies. It relies on an inverse-planning system, which optimizes delivery of non-uniform beam fluences from multiple directions to allow the intended dose to reach the target with maximal sparing of high doses to normal tissues. The treatment system involves use of multi-leaf collimators that divide each beam into many small beamlets, which are each modulated such that the overall beam intensity patterns achieve the desired target coverage and critical tissue sparing (74).

There are no prospective studies comparing IMRT to conventional RT for the treatment of gliomas; however, it is generally felt that IMRT has the potential to decrease RT-related toxicity. Several comparison studies have consistently shown that IMRT allows for improvement in target dose conformity and reduction in the maximum doses to organs at risk, while achieving comparable target coverage in several other disease sites (75–79). Improved clinical outcomes such as reduction in auditory toxicity in pediatric medulloblastoma patients treated with IMRT as compared with conventional RT have also been reported (80).

For gliomas, retrospective dosimetric analyses have presented the potential benefits of IMRT (74,81). Narayana et al. (81) noted that regardless of tumor location, IMRT resulted in a decreased maximum dose as compared to standard 3-D based planning to the spinal cord, optic nerves, and eye by 16%, 7%, and 15%, respectively, owing to its improved dose conformality. The mean brainstem dose was decreased by 7%. However, IMRT did not significantly improve target coverage compared with 3-D planning. IMRT also did not result in an increased dose to the normal brain. The authors concluded that it is unlikely that IMRT would improve local control in HGG without further dose escalation compared with conventional RT; however, it might result in decreased late toxicities associated with RT. In another similar dosimetric comparison study, IMRT allowed for improved target conformity, better critical tissue sparing, without increasing integral dose and the volume of normal brain tissue exposed to low doses of radiation (74).

Another advantage to IMRT is the ability to administer a simultaneous integrated boost (SIB-IMRT) to the high-risk area and/or residual tumor, thus allowing for hypofractionation (accelerated hypofractionated IMRT). This can potentially be achieved with no additional excess radiation to the surrounding tissues due to the inverse-planning technique. Several investigators have studied this approach with or without concurrent chemotherapy. A comparison study of FSRT versus IMRT with an integrated boost showed that while the dose coverage of the planning target volume (PTV) was slightly higher with FSRT, the conformity to the integrated boost volume shape was improved by IMRT (82).

In a retrospective study, Panet-Raymond et al. (83) reported on 35 patients with GBM who received 40 Gy to the PTV and 60 Gy to the gross tumor volume (GTV) with an IMRT–concomitant boost technique, delivered in 20 fractions. Only one patient showed grade 3 to 4 toxicity. The total RT treatment time was effectively reduced by 2 weeks as conventional RT is delivered in 6 weeks. In a prospective trial of 25 patients with GBM (84), IMRT was used to deliver 60 Gy in 20 daily fractions of 3 Gy to the GTV, whereas the PTV received a minimum of 40 Gy in 20 fractions of 2 Gy each at its periphery. Toxicity was acceptable but improvement in survival was not observed.

A phase I dose-escalation study performed to define the MTD of accelerated IMRT (with the simultaneous integrated boost technique) with concurrent and adjuvant temozolomide (TMZ) found that a dose of 65 Gy in 25 fractions is well tolerated (85).

SIB-IMRT has also led to the evaluation of significantly higher doses per fraction of up to 6 Gy. In a dose-escalation study of 16 patients, Chen et al. (86) found that 60 Gy IMRT delivered in 6 Gy fractions within 2 weeks with concurrent and adjuvant TMZ was tolerable in selected patients with a T1-weighted enhancing tumor <6 cm. They defined the high-dose volume to be the surgical cavity and residual tumor with a 5-mm margin. Median survival in this study was 16.2 months. One patient experienced vision loss in the left eye 7 months after IMRT. Four patients underwent repeat surgery for suspected tumor recurrence 6 to 12 months after IMRT, three had radionecrosis. In another study, Floyd et al. (87) treated 20 patients with GBM adjuvantly such that a dose of 50 Gy was delivered in 5-Gy daily fractions within 2 weeks to enhancing primary disease, residual tumor, or surgical cavity. Simultaneously, 30 Gy was prescribed in 3-Gy daily fractions to surrounding edema. The treatment duration was thus reduced from 6 to 2 weeks. Three patients developed radiation necrosis requiring reoperation. The median overall survival was 7 months after treatment completion and all recurrences were found to be within 2 cm of the operative bed.

It is still unclear whether hypofractionated radiation will improve patient outcome in GBM, as the patterns of failure are still predominantly local. This approach, while maintaining tolerability and toxicity, may allow for decreasing treatment time by at least 1 to 2 weeks or more which would be of a significant benefit by itself in this poor survival group. The combination of TMZ and hypofractionation requires further exploration. As GBM patients become increasingly longer term survivors, the potential late effects of hypofractionated radiation, particularly when given with concurrent chemotherapy, have yet to be fully understood.

RADIOIMMUNOTHERAPY (RIT)

RIT is a form of targeted therapy which uses an antibody labeled with a radionuclide to deliver cytotoxic radiation to a target cell (88). It has been widely used in the management of refractory lymphomas and leukemia. An antibody with a high specificity for a tumor-associated antigen is used to deliver a lethal dose of radiation to the tumor cells. The ability for the antibody to specifically bind to a tumor-associated antigen increases the dose delivered to the tumor cells while decreasing the dose to normal tissues. Tumor cell killing can be mediated by a variety of radionuclides, including high-energy beta-emitters such as Y^{90} and I^{131} (89). An alternative choice is to use the low-energy electron emissions of I^{125} (90).

Reardon and colleagues from Duke University (91,92) have reported on the use of mAb 81C6, a murine immunoglobulin glycoprotein-2b that binds an epitope within the fibronectin region of tenascin, which is abundantly expressed in HGG but not in normal brain. They studied this in both the setting of the initial management (91) and with recurrence of malignant gliomas (92). In a phase II study 120 milliCuries (mCi) of I^{131}-labeled 81C6 was injected directly into the surgically created resection cavity of 33 patients (GBM = 27) with previously untreated malignant gliomas (91). The average absorbed dose to a 2 cm interface from I^{131}-labeled 81C6 was 48 Gy (range, 24 to 116 Gy). Patients then received conventional external-beam RT followed by a year of alkylator-based chemotherapy. Median survival for all patients and those with GBM was 21.7 and 19.9 months, respectively. Eleven patients remain alive at a median follow-up of 23.3 months. Toxicity was acceptable with only one patient requiring reoperation for radionecrosis. The average whole-body dose was 0.58 Gy (range, 0.24–1.28 Gy). They concluded that the median survival achieved with I^{131}-labeled 81C6 compared favorably with either I^{125} interstitial brachytherapy or SRS and was associated with a significantly lower rate of reoperation for radionecrosis.

In another phase II study by Reardon et al. (92), 100 mCi of I^{131}-m81C6 was injected directly into the surgically created resection cavity (SCRC) of 43 patients (WHO Gr 4 = 34, Gr 3 = 8) with recurrent malignant gliomas. The average absorbed dose to a 2-cm interface around the surgical cavity was 46 Gy (range, 18–186 Gy). Median overall survival for patients with grade 4 and grade 3 tumors was 16 and 24.8 months, respectively. Toxicity was acceptable with no patient requiring a reoperation for radionecrosis.

Researchers from Drexel University have evaluated the use of I^{125}-labeled IgG2A monoclonal antibody 425 (I^{125}-MAb 425) against epidermal growth factor receptor (EGFR) in the management of HGG. Their research was based on the premise that in cancers, such as brain gliomas, EGFR expression is enhanced on malignant tissues or cell lines compared with the normal counterparts (93,94). In a phase II study, 180 patients diagnosed with malignant gliomas (GBM = 118) were treated as outpatients with an average of three weekly intravenous or intraarterial injections of radiolabeled MAb 425 given 2 to 4 weeks after EBRT to a median dose of 61.2 Gy. The mean total dose after the three infusions was 140 mCi. Overall median survival for patients with GBM and anaplastic astrocytomas was 13.4 and 50.9 months, respectively. Toxicities from administration of I^{125}-MAb 425 were minimal. A phase III randomized trial evaluating the role of I^{131}-labeled antitenascin murine monoclonal antibody (Neuradiab; Bradmer Pharmaceuticals, Inc, Toronto, ON, Canada) in combination with RT and TMZ versus RT and TMZ alone in newly diagnosed patients with GBM is currently ongoing.

BRACHYTHERAPY

Brachytherapy (derived from the Greek word *brachys*, meaning "short distance") is the branch of radiation oncology that utilizes radioisotopes to deliver a high-dose of radiation, locally. It is further classified into temporary and permanent implants. Depending on the technique and isotope it is either intracavitary or interstitial. This modality can be used to deliver boost doses of radiation to primary brain tumors after completion of EBRT or for salvage at recurrence. The rationale for adding brachytherapy as part of the treatment schedule is similar to that of SRS with the goal of dose escalation.

The most commonly used isotopes are permanent or temporary I^{125} or temporary Ir^{192}. Permanent implants are placed at the time of craniotomy and resection while the temporary implants involve the placement of a catheter in the resection cavity, which can then be loaded with the radioisotope. Gliasite RT system (Cytyc Surgical Products) is an intracavitary device which consists of an inflatable balloon at the end of a closed catheter (Figure 2). Iotrex™ (I^{125} solution) is infused into the balloon through an access port. A typical radiation prescription is to deliver 40 to 60 Gy to a depth of 5 to 10 mm from the balloon surface over 4 to 6 days.

Clinical results in high-grade gliomas have been variable with some authors suggesting that any benefit seen is likely due to a selection bias (95) whereas others suggesting that selection bias alone does not account for the improved survival (96). In a comparative study, Wen et al. (97) evaluated 56 patients with GBM treated with stereotactic brachytherapy as part of their initial therapy after surgery and limited field external beam RT. The control group consisted of 40 patients with similar clinical and radiologic features who qualified the criteria for but did not receive brachytherapy. Brachytherapy was delivered with temporarily implanted high-activity I^{125} sources, giving

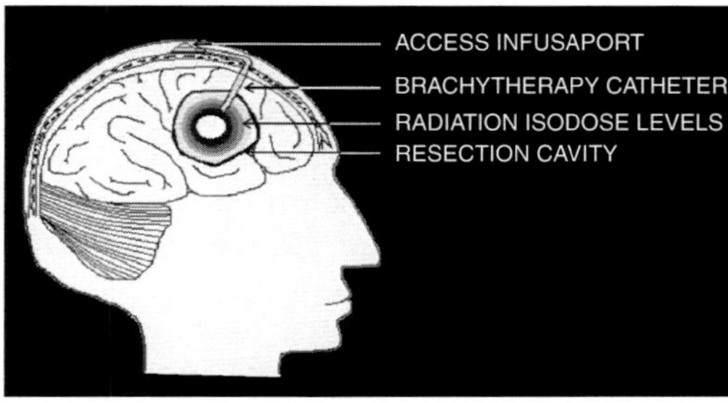

FIGURE 2 Gliasite RT system.

an additional 50 Gy to the tumor bed after which the implant and the catheters were removed. The volume treated was the enhancing region seen on CT plus a 5 mm margin in all three dimensions. Median survival for patients undergoing brachytherapy was 18 months compared with 11 months for the matched brachytherapy control group ($P < .0007$). Survival rates at 1, 2, and 3 years after diagnosis were 83%, 34%, and 27%, respectively, for patients receiving brachytherapy and were significantly increased compared with survival rates of 40%, 12.5%, and 9%, respectively, for the control subjects. Thirty-six patients (64%) underwent reoperation for symptomatic radiation necrosis from 3 to 42 months (median, 11 months) after brachytherapy. The median survival of patients undergoing reoperation was 22 months compared with 13 months for those who did not have further surgery ($P < .02$). The authors concluded that brachytherapy may improve local tumor control and prolong survival when used in the initial treatment of selected patients with GBM.

To clarify these issues and to prospectively evaluate the role of this modality, two randomized clinical trials have been conducted in HGG. The trial from Princess Margaret Hospital (98) randomized 140 patients to EBRT alone or to EBRT followed by brachytherapy implant. Histology was GBM in 89% patients. EBRT consisted of 50 Gy in 25 fractions. In the brachytherapy arm, patients received an additional 60 Gy to the enhancing tumor using high-activity I^{125} sources. The median survival was 13.2 months in the EBRT arm and 13.8 months in the EBRT + brachytherapy arm (P = ns). The second trial was performed by the Brain Tumor Cooperative Group, Study 87–01 (99). Two hundred and seventy patients were randomized after surgery to EBRT + BCNU or to an interstitial I^{125} implant followed by EBRT+BCNU. The brachytherapy implant was designed to deliver a total dose of 60 Gy at 40 cGy/hr to the residual enhancing tumor. Median survival was 68.1 weeks in the brachytherapy arm and 58.9 weeks in the arm without brachytherapy. This difference of approximately 9 weeks showed a trend but did not reach statistical significance ($P = .101$). It is felt that the inhomogeneity associated with the I^{125} implant and the technical challenges might have had a negative effect. The results from the two randomized trials do not support the routine use of this modality in the initial treatment of HGG.

Brachytherapy has also been used in the recurrence setting to deliver a highly conformal dose to the target. This is especially important since most of these patients would have received prior EBRT. A summary of studies using various modalities of brachytherapy both in the initial and recurrent setting are presented in Table 4. Toxicity data has been variably reported depending on the modality used with rates of 10% to 25% and include minor wound infections, neurologic decline requiring steroids to more severe radiation necrosis (98,100,101). Comparative studies evaluating the role of SRS versus brachytherapy in the recurrence setting have found that though the patterns of failure and survival of patients are similar after either modality, the risk of reoperation might be lower with SRS (41).

■ PARTICLE THERAPY

Historical Perspective

In 1946, Robert Wilson (110) first proposed the idea that protons could provide superior dose distributions to photons and thus could be used for medical purposes. The first clinical use of a proton beam occurred at Berkeley, USA, in 1954 (111), then at Uppsala, Sweden, in 1957. At the Harvard cyclotron facility (MGH), Dr. Kjellberg and colleagues used protons to treat pituitary adenomas in early 1960s (112). Fractionated therapy with protons soon followed by Dr. Suit and colleagues in the 1970s (113,114). The world's first hospital-based proton center opened at the Loma Linda University Medical Center in 1990. Protons were not the only particles investigated for therapeutic purposes with interest also seen in pi-mesons, helium ions, and carbon ions. To date there are nine operational proton facilities in the USA and several more planned in the near future.

Advantages of Particle Therapy

The most important advantage of particles compared to photons is the ability to irradiate tumor at any depth in the human body with the least amount of dose to the surrounding normal tissues (integral dose). A finite path length along with the fact that the maximum dose deposition occurs close to the end of its track (Bragg peak) is a clear physical advantage over photons. Preferential sparing of structures just beyond the tumor can be achieved by modulating the position of the Bragg peak and achieving virtually no exit dose. The entrance integral dose is also lower than with photons. Due to these advantages, intracranial lesions have been considered for management by particle therapy. A comparative plan of

TABLE 4 Studies of brachytherapy in the management of malignant gliomas

Author (Year)	Videtic et al. (1999) (102)	Patel et al. (2000) (103)	Videtic et al. (2001) (96)	Chang et al. (2003) (104)	Tatter et al. (2003) (105)	Larson et al. (2003) (106)	Chan et al. (2005) (101)	Welsh et al. (2007) (100)	Chen et al. (2007) (107)	Darakchiev et al. (2008) (108)	Wernicke et al. (2010) (109)
Study type	R (Init.)	R (Rec)	R (Init.)	RMP	P (Rec)	R (Rec)	R (Rec)	R (Init.)	P (Init.)	P (Init.)	P (Init.+Rec)
n	72 analyzed	40	52 implant	28	21	38 (37: analyzed)	24	20	18	34	10
Median age (yrs)	52	50	57.5	51	48.4	47	48.1	59	50	53	56
Histology	AA: 22; GBM: 53	GBM: 40	GBM: 52	GBM: 28	GBM: 15; AA: 5; AO: 1	GBM: 38	GBM: 24	GBM: 20	GBM: 18	GBM: 34	GBM:4; AO/AA: 2, Oth: 4
Surgery	Bx: 15; PR/GTR: 59; U: 1	GTR: 22; STR: 18	Bx: 9; PR/GTR: 44	Bx: 1; GTR: 17; STR: 10	21	Surg (NOS)–all	GTR: 22; STR: 2	Surg (NOS)–all	Bx: 7	GTR: 29; STR: 5	GTR: 6; STR: 4
Median target vol (range) (cc)	–	47.3	15.5 (0.8–78)	17.5 (6.5–41.6)	–	25(3–68)	–	–	18.6 (4.4–41.2)	34 (8–90)	–
Previous EBRT (Gy)	50.4–54	60	50.4–54	60 (50–66)	–	60 (59.4–72)	59.8 (55.8–64.8)	Brachy prior to EBRT: 60	Brachy prior to EBRT: 60	–	PBI: 60; WBRT: 37.5
EBRT to brachy time (wks)	–	–	–	1–4	–	39	–	2	4	–	–
Brachy modality	LDR, I: 125 seeds	I: 125 perm.	LDR, I: 125 seeds	HDR, Ir: 192	LDR, GliaSite	I: 125 perm.	LDR, GliaSite	Gliasite boost (initial Rx)	GTR+ I: 125 brachy+ EBRT	Surg+I: 125 brachy+ BCNU wafers	LDR, GliaSite
Median dose (range) (Gy)	103.68*	120–160	103.68*	30 (18–30)	40–60	300 (100–500)	53.1	50 (84–130)	400 (200–600)	~120	52.0
No. of Fx/ daily freq	–	–	–	10/twice	–	–	–	–	1Gy bid. 5days /wk	–	–
Chemo	–	21 pts	NR	18%	11 pts	24 pts	62%	50%	NR	27 pts	60%
Median follow-up (mos)	All:13.5; AA: 29; GBM: 12.6	14.8	11	28.7	21.8 patient yrs	35	21.8	36	–	14.8	38
Median survival from initial diag (mos)	AA: 38; GBM: 17	NR	NR	19.5	NR	24.5	23.3	–	114	–	–
Median survival from RX (mos)	AA: NR; GBM: NR	47	16	12.5	12.7 (GBM: 8; AA/AO: 17.9)	13	9.1	11.4	–	17.3	14
Overall survival	5 yr (All)–23%; 2 yr AA–58%, GBM–40%; 5 yr AA–40%, GBM–17.5%	6 mos–72%	2 yr: 42%;5 yr: 17.5%	1 yr: 89%; 2 yr: 61%	–	–	–	–	–	1yr: 66%; 2yr: 23%	–

Gy = gray, cc = cubic centimeters, wks = weeks, mos = months, yr = year, OS = overall survival, G = grade of tumor; G1 = grade 1, G2 = grade 2, G3 = grade 3, G4 = grade 4,
*Cumulative dose.

Abbreviations: Bx = biopsy, GTR = gross total resection, STR = subtotal resection, PR = partial resection, U = uncertain, Surg (NOS) = Surgery (not otherwise specified), RCT = randomized control trial, P = prospective, R = retrospective, RMP = retrospective matched pair study, Oth = others, Rec = recurrence.

protons versus IMRT is shown in Figure 3. Note the decrease in the integral dose to the surrounding normal brain parenchyma with comparable coverage of the target. This approach offered the potential for dose escalation to the tumor while differentially sparing the normal tissues as a means of improving the therapeutic ratio. Carbon ions are additionally felt to have a biological advantage over photon therapy with a higher relative biological effectiveness (RBE of 2–5 depending on cell line and end point) (115–117), relatively less dependence on oxygen availability in hypoxic and anoxic tumors and reduced cell cycle phase dependence.

Since its initial use in pituitary adenomas, proton therapy has been applied to various other intracranial lesions like arteriovenous malformations, vestibular schwannomas, and gliomas. Several dosimetric comparison studies have shown the superiority of protons to photons (118–123).

Low-Grade Gliomas (LGGs)

Patients with LGG have a relatively long survival due to the nature of slow disease progression. The role of upfront RT in this disease has been to prolong progression-free survival (EORTC 22845) (124). Studies evaluating the radiation dose–response relationship have concluded that within a dose range of 45 to 65 Gy, the progression-free and overall survival are similar (125,126). An accepted standard dose is 50 to 54 Gy given at 1.8 Gy per fraction. In one trial of 45 versus 59.4 Gy (EORTC 22844) (126), there was deterioration in quality of life with significantly more fatigue/malaise and insomnia immediately after RT and in leisure time and emotional functioning at 7 to 15 months after randomization (127). In another intergroup trial by Shaw et al. (125) of 50.4 versus 64.8 Gy, the 2-year rate of grade 3 to 5 radiation necrosis was 2.5% versus 5%.

The only randomized trial evaluating upfront versus delayed RT, the EORTC 22845 did not assess the quality-of-life parameters and it is not clear if there is associated clinical deterioration with progressive disease or from early RT. A major factor that goes into the decision making of administering RT is the potential for neurocognitive toxicity especially in the long-term survivors (128,129). Patients with 1p/19q codeletion when compared to LGG patients without the codeletion experience a longer median survival (11.9 vs. 8.1 years) and higher 5-year progression-free survival (84% vs. 48%) (130). EORTC has defined a scoring system for high-risk LGG patients who may benefit the most from early RT (131). Age ≥ 40 years, astrocytoma histology subtype, largest diameter of the tumor ≥ 6 cm, tumor crossing the midline, and presence of neurologic deficit before surgery were unfavorable prognostic factors for survival. Presence of up to two of these factors identifies the low-risk group, whereas a higher score identifies high-risk

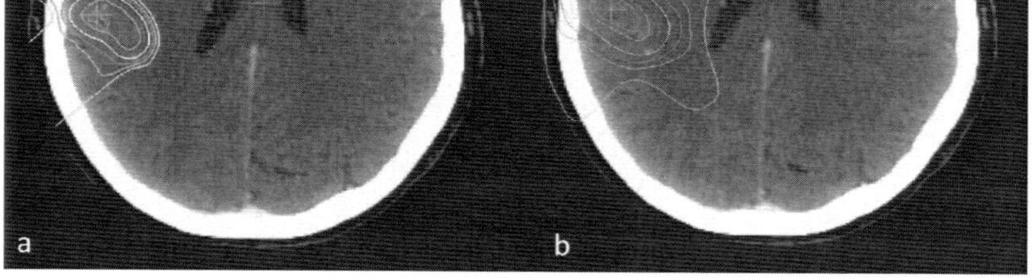

FIGURE 3 Comparative plan of (a) protons versus (b) IMRT. (a) Three-field proton plan with equal weighting and (b) IMRT plan with four equally weighted dynamic conformal arcs using 4 mm MLC leaves (270 arc degrees). Both plans are for a dose of 16 Gy normalized to the 95% isodose line.

patients. It should be noted that more than 90% of failures occur at the original site of disease despite being treated with adjuvant RT (132,133).

Proton therapy is an effective means of targeting tumor while reducing dose to surrounding critical structures and normal brain parenchyma. Whereas upfront RT has been shown to improve progression-free survival in LGG patients (124), concerns of radiation-associated adverse effects drives many patients to avoid RT at the time of diagnosis. Proton therapy poses an opportunity to offer a quality-of-life benefit to patients both as a therapy for their disease and as a treatment modality that minimizes excess radiation dose to the surrounding normal brain tissue. Progression is often associated with new focal neurological deficits or cognitive impairments. Hence it might be more beneficial to evaluate neurological deterioration as the primary end point and not overall survival. This data was not reported in the above trials and remains to be answered. A clinically significant reduction in toxicity may translate to increased use of upfront radiation therapy and a promising new way to manage the LGG patient population. Proton therapy is also felt to have a significantly lower risk of secondary malignancies as compared to photons (134,135).

The role of dose escalation with proton/photon RT in LGGs was assessed in a prospective phase I/II trial conducted at MGH (136). Twenty patients with grade 2/4 (n = 7) and grade 3/4 (n = 13) gliomas, according to the Daumas-Duport classification, were treated to 68.2 Gy (RBE) to gross tumor in grade 2 lesions and 79.7 Gy (RBE) in grade 3 lesions. Fractionation was conventional, with 1.8 to 1.92 Gy (RBE) delivered daily. Three patients with grade 2 lesions died from tumor recurrence, whereas two of the four survivors had evidence of radiation necrosis. Eight of 10 patients with grade 3 lesions died from tumor recurrence. Tumor recurrence was neither prevented nor noticeably delayed relative to published series on photon irradiation. Dose escalation using this fractionation scheme and total dose delivered failed to improve outcome for patients with grade 2 and 3 gliomas.

High-Grade Gliomas

In another phase II study from MGH, Fitzek et al. (12) evaluated 23 patients with GBM to assess whether dose escalation to 90 Gy (RBE) with conformal protons and photons in accelerated fractionation would improve local tumor control and patient survival. Median survival was 20 months. All patients developed new areas of gadolinium enhancement during the follow-up period. Histological examination of tissues obtained at biopsy, resection, or autopsy was conducted in 15 of 23 patients. Radiation necrosis was demonstrated only in seven patients, and their survival was significantly longer than that of patients with recurrent tumor (P = .01). Tumor regrowth occurred most commonly in areas that received doses of 60 to 70 Gy (RBE) or less; recurrent tumor was found in only one case in the 90 Gy (RBE) volume. Although a dose of 90 Gy (RBE) was effective in preventing local tumor recurrences, such high doses were associated with high rates of radiation necrosis and associated neurological symptoms.

In vitro data for the treatment of gliomas cell lines with carbon ions have shown superior killing effect compared to photons (116). A combination of carbon ion RT and TMZ has also been evaluated and has shown an additive effect in GBM cell lines (115).

The first clinical study evaluating a carbon ion boost in patients with GBM was recently published by Mizoe et al. (137) from Chiba, Japan. Forty-eight patients with histologically confirmed malignant gliomas (16 AA and 32 GBM) were enrolled in this phase I/II clinical study. The treatment involved the application of 50 Gy/25 fractions/5 weeks of photon RT with nimustine hydrochloride (ACNU), followed by carbon ion RT at 8 fractions/2 weeks. Carbon ion boost was applied with stepwise increasing total doses up to 24.8 Gy (RBE). Median overall survival in patients with GBM was 17 months with most benefit seen with a higher boost dose.

Ongoing Trials in Particle Therapy

Multiple centers are currently conducting parallel trials to characterize the late radiation effects in LGG (WHO II) patients treated with proton radiation therapy. The hypothesis is that protons can offer the same therapeutic efficacy as conventional photon radiation delivery but at a lower risk of radiation-related adverse effects. If the results are encouraging then a national trial comparing state of the art IMRT versus protons could potentially be considered.

In a randomized phase II study, CLEOPATRA Trial (138) at HIT, Germany, a carbon ion boost will be compared to a proton boost applied to the macroscopic tumor after surgery at primary diagnosis in patients with GBM applied after standard radiochemotherapy with TMZ up to 50 Gy. In the experimental arm, a carbon ion boost will be applied to the macroscopic tumor up to a total dose of 18 Gy (RBE) in 6 fractions at a single dose of 3 Gy (RBE). In the standard arm, a proton boost will be applied up to a total dose 10 Gy (RBE) in 5 single fractions of 2 Gy (RBE). The primary end point will be overall survival and the secondary objectives are progression-free survival, toxicity, and safety. This is the first study to evaluate the effect of carbon ion RT within multimodality treatment of primary GBM in a randomized trial comparing this innovative treatment with the treatment standard of photon RT with TMZ.

The HIT group has also undertaken a randomized phase I/II study to evaluate carbon ion RT versus FSRT in patients with recurrent or progressive gliomas, called the CINDERELLA trial (117). In the phase I part of the trial, the recommended dose (RD) of carbon ion radiotherapy will be determined in a dose escalation scheme. Patients will be treated within seven increasing dose regimens starting at 10 × 3 Gy (RBE) up to 16×3 Gy (RBE). In the subsequent randomized phase II part, the RD will be evaluated in the experimental arm and compared to the standard arm of FSRT 36 Gy in 18 fractions. The Cinderella trial is the first study to evaluate carbon ion RT for recurrent gliomas and to compare this treatment to photon FSRT in a randomized setting.

■ CONCLUSIONS

Malignant gliomas are inherently infiltrating neoplasms as seen on pathological and magnetic resonance spectroscopy studies. Dose escalation has unfortunately not shown to impact the patterns of local failure to date. The use of advanced radiation modalities represents innovation on the part of the radiation oncologist in treating this fatal disease. Though the results reported with advanced techniques by several groups have been encouraging, the overall survival is still dismal. With better understanding of glioma biology, new biological imaging developing, and emergence of several molecular targeted therapies, a reassessment on the role of advanced RT techniques by well-designed clinical trials is warranted. Till then, the search for the magic bullet continues.

■ REFERENCES

1. Chang SD, Main W, Martin DP, Gibbs IC, Heilbrun MP. An analysis of the accuracy of the CyberKnife: a robotic frameless stereotactic radiosurgical system. *Neurosurgery.* 2003;52(1):140–6; discussion 146.
2. Lutz W, Winston KR, Maleki N. A system for stereotactic radiosurgery with a linear accelerator. *Int J Radiat Oncol Biol Phys.* 1988;14(2):373–381.
3. Yeung D, Palta J, Fontanesi J, Kun L. Systematic analysis of errors in target localization and treatment delivery in stereotactic radiosurgery (SRS). *Int J Radiat Oncol Biol Phys.* 1994;28(2):493–498.
4. Yu C, Luxton G, Jozsef G, Apuzzo ML, Petrovich Z. Dosimetric comparison of three photon radiosurgery techniques for an elongated ellipsoid target. *Int J Radiat Oncol Biol Phys.* 1999;45(3):817–826.
5. Yu C, Jozsef G, Apuzzo ML, Petrovich Z. Dosimetric comparison of CyberKnife with other radiosurgical modalities for an ellipsoidal target. *Neurosurgery.* 2003;53(5):1155–62; discussion 1162.
6. Weber DC, Bogner J, Verwey J, et al. Proton beam radiotherapy versus fractionated stereotactic radiotherapy for uveal melanomas: A comparative study. *Int J Radiat Oncol Biol Phys.* 2005;63(2):373–384.
7. Baumert BG, Norton IA, Lomax AJ, Davis JB. Dose conformation of intensity-modulated stereotactic photon beams, proton beams, and intensity-modulated proton beams for intracranial lesions. *Int J Radiat Oncol Biol Phys.* 2004;60(4):1314–1324.
8. Walker MD, Strike TA, Sheline GE. An analysis of dose-effect relationship in the radiotherapy of malignant gliomas. *Int J Radiat Oncol Biol Phys.* 1979;5(10):1725–1731.
9. Bleehen NM, Stenning SP. A Medical Research Council trial of two radiotherapy doses in the treatment of grades 3 and 4 astrocytoma. The Medical Research Council Brain Tumour Working Party. *Br J Cancer.* 1991;64(4):769–774.
10. Hochberg FH, Pruitt A. Assumptions in the radiotherapy of glioblastoma. *Neurology.* 1980;30(9):907–911.
11. Gaspar LE, Fisher BJ, Macdonald DR, et al. Supratentorial malignant glioma: patterns of recurrence and implications for external beam local treatment. *Int J Radiat Oncol Biol Phys.* 1992;24(1):55–57.
12. Fitzek MM, Thornton AF, Rabinov JD, et al. Accelerated fractionated proton/photon irradiation to 90 cobalt gray equivalent for glioblastoma multiforme: results of a phase II prospective trial. *J Neurosurg.* 1999;91(2):251–260.
13. Lee SW, Fraass BA, Marsh LH, et al. Patterns of failure following high-dose 3-D conformal radiotherapy for high-grade astrocytomas: a quantitative dosimetric study. *Int J Radiat Oncol Biol Phys.* 1999;43(1):79–88.
14. Chan JL, Lee SW, Fraass BA, et al. Survival and failure patterns of high-grade gliomas after three-dimensional conformal radiotherapy. *J Clin Oncol.* 2002;20(6):1635–1642.
15. Brown JM, Koong AC. High-dose single-fraction radiotherapy: exploiting a new biology? *Int J Radiat Oncol Biol Phys.* 2008;71(2):324–325.
16. Garcia-Barros M, Paris F, Cordon-Cardo C, et al. Tumor response to radiotherapy regulated by endothelial cell apoptosis. *Science.* 2003;300(5622):1155–1159.

17. Andisheh B, Brahme A, Bitaraf MA, Mavroidis P, Lind BK. Clinical and radiobiological advantages of single-dose stereotactic light-ion radiation therapy for large intracranial arteriovenous malformations. Technical note. *J Neurosurg.* 2009;111(5):919–926.

18. Fuks Z, Kolesnick R. Engaging the vascular component of the tumor response. *Cancer Cell.* 2005;8(2):89–91.

19. Shaw E, Scott C, Souhami L, et al. Single dose radiosurgical treatment of recurrent previously irradiated primary brain tumors and brain metastases: final report of RTOG protocol 90–05. *Int J Radiat Oncol Biol Phys.* 2000;47(2):291–298.

20. Shehata MK, Young B, Reid B, et al. Stereotatic radiosurgery of 468 brain metastases < or =2 cm: implications for SRS dose and whole brain radiation therapy. *Int J Radiat Oncol Biol Phys.* 2004;59(1):87–93.

21. Flickinger JC, Niranjan A, Lunsford DL. Dose selection in stereotactic radiosurgery. In: Szeifert GT, Kondziolka D, Levivier M, Lunsford LD (eds). *Radiosurgery and Pathological Fundamentals,* vol. 20, ch. 3. Prog Neurol Surg. Basel: Karger; 2007:28–42.

22. Loeffler JS, Alexander E 3rd, Shea WM, et al. Radiosurgery as part of the initial management of patients with malignant gliomas. *J Clin Oncol.* 1992;10(9):1379–1385.

23. Sarkaria JN, Mehta MP, Loeffler JS, et al. Radiosurgery in the initial management of malignant gliomas: survival comparison with the RTOG recursive partitioning analysis. Radiation Therapy Oncology Group. *Int J Radiat Oncol Biol Phys.* 1995;32(4):931–941.

24. Curran WJ Jr, Scott CB, Horton J, et al. Recursive partitioning analysis of prognostic factors in three Radiation Therapy Oncology Group malignant glioma trials. *J Natl Cancer Inst.* 1993;85(9):704–710.

25. Irish WD, Macdonald DR, Cairncross JG. Measuring bias in uncontrolled brain tumor trials–to randomize or not to randomize? *Can J Neurol Sci.* 1997;24(4):307–312.

26. Curran WJ Jr, Scott CB, Weinstein AS, et al. Survival comparison of radiosurgery-eligible and -ineligible malignant glioma patients treated with hyperfractionated radiation therapy and carmustine: a report of Radiation Therapy Oncology Group 83–02. *J Clin Oncol.* 1993;11(5):857–862.

27. Souhami L, Seiferheld W, Brachman D, et al. Randomized comparison of stereotactic radiosurgery followed by conventional radiotherapy with carmustine to conventional radiotherapy with carmustine for patients with glioblastoma multiforme: report of Radiation Therapy Oncology Group 93–05 protocol. *Int J Radiat Oncol Biol Phys.* 2004;60(3):853–860.

28. Kondziolka D, Flickinger JC, Bissonette DJ, Bozik M, Lunsford LD. Survival benefit of stereotactic radiosurgery for patients with malignant glial neoplasms. *Neurosurgery.* 1997;41(4):776–83; discussion 783.

29. Mehta MP, Masciopinto J, Rozental J, et al. Stereotactic radiosurgery for glioblastoma multiforme: report of a prospective study evaluating prognostic factors and analyzing long-term survival advantage. *Int J Radiat Oncol Biol Phys.* 1994;30(3):541–549.

30. Gannett D, Stea B, Lulu B, Adair T, Verdi C, Hamilton A. Stereotactic radiosurgery as an adjunct to surgery and external beam radiotherapy in the treatment of patients with malignant gliomas. *Int J Radiat Oncol Biol Phys.* 1995;33(2):461–468.

31. Shrieve DC, Alexander E 3rd, Black PM, et al. Treatment of patients with primary glioblastoma multiforme with standard postoperative radiotherapy and radiosurgical boost: prognostic factors and long-term outcome. *J Neurosurg.* 1999;90(1):72–77.

32. Nwokedi EC, DiBiase SJ, Jabbour S, Herman J, Amin P, Chin LS. Gamma knife stereotactic radiosurgery for patients with glioblastoma multiforme. *Neurosurgery.* 2002;50(1):41–6; discussion 46.

33. Prisco FE, Weltman E, de Hanriot RM, Brandt RA. Radiosurgical boost for primary high-grade gliomas. *J Neurooncol.* 2002;57(2):151–160.

34. Smith KA, Ashby LS, Gonzalez LF, et al. Prospective trial of gross-total resection with Gliadel wafers followed by early postoperative Gamma Knife radiosurgery and conformal fractionated radiotherapy as the initial treatment for patients with radiographically suspected, newly diagnosed glioblastoma multiforme. *J Neurosurg.* 2008;109 Suppl:106–117.

35. Dirks P, Bernstein M, Muller PJ, Tucker WS. The value of reoperation for recurrent glioblastoma. *Can J Surg.* 1993;36(3):271–275.

36. Harsh GRt, Levin VA, Gutin PH, et al. Reoperation for recurrent glioblastoma and anaplastic astrocytoma. *Neurosurgery.* 1987;21:615–621.

37. Brandes AA, Pasetto LM, Monfardini S. New drugs in recurrent high grade gliomas. *Anticancer Res.* 2000;20(3B):1913–1920.

38. Brem H, Piantadosi S, Burger PC, et al. Placebo-controlled trial of safety and efficacy of intraoperative controlled delivery by biodegradable polymers of chemotherapy for recurrent gliomas. The Polymer-brain Tumor Treatment Group. *Lancet.* 1995;345(8956):1008–1012.

39. Chamberlain MC, Tsao-Wei DD. Salvage chemotherapy with cyclophosphamide for recurrent, temozolomide-refractory glioblastoma multiforme. *Cancer.* 2004;100(6):1213–1220.

40. Chua SL, Rosenthal MA, Wong SS, et al. Phase 2 study of temozolomide and Caelyx in patients with recurrent glioblastoma multiforme. *Neuro-oncology.* 2004;6(1):38–43.

41. Shrieve DC, Alexander E 3rd, Wen PY, et al. Comparison of stereotactic radiosurgery and brachytherapy in the treatment of recurrent glioblastoma multiforme. *Neurosurgery.* 1995;36(2):275–82; discussion 282.

42. Chamberlain MC, Barba D, Kormanik P, Shea WM. Stereotactic radiosurgery for recurrent gliomas. *Cancer.* 1994;74(4):1342–1347.

43. Hall WA, Djalilian HR, Sperduto PW, et al. Stereotactic radiosurgery for recurrent malignant gliomas. *J Clin Oncol.* 1995;13(7):1642–1648.

44. Selch MT, DeSalles A, Goetsch SJ, et al. Single-fraction radiosurgery for primary and recurrent malignant gliomas. *J Radiosurgery*. 1998;1:155–168.

45. Sanghavi S, Skrupky R, Badie B, et al. Recurrent malignant gliomas treated with radiosurgery. *J Radiosurgery*. 1999;2:119–125.

46. Larson DA, Prados M, Lamborn KR, et al. Phase II study of high central dose Gamma Knife radiosurgery and marimastat in patients with recurrent malignant glioma. *Int J Radiat Oncol Biol Phys*. 2002;54(5):1397–1404.

47. Sarkar A, Pollock BE, Brown PD, Gorman DA. Evaluation of gamma knife radiosurgery in the treatment of oligodendrogliomas and mixed oligodendroastrocytomas. *J Neurosurg*. 2002;97(5 Suppl):653–656.

48. Combs SE, Widmer V, Thilmann C, Hof H, Debus J, Schulz-Ertner D. Stereotactic radiosurgery (SRS): treatment option for recurrent glioblastoma multiforme (GBM). *Cancer*. 2005;104(10):2168–2173.

49. Mahajan A, McCutcheon IE, Suki D, et al. Case-control study of stereotactic radiosurgery for recurrent glioblastoma multiforme. *J Neurosurg*. 2005;103(2):210–217.

50. Hsieh PC, Chandler JP, Bhangoo S, et al. Adjuvant gamma knife stereotactic radiosurgery at the time of tumor progression potentially improves survival for patients with glioblastoma multiforme. *Neurosurgery*. 2005;57(4):684–92; discussion 684.

51. Patel M, Siddiqui F, Jin JY, et al. Salvage reirradiation for recurrent glioblastoma with radiosurgery: radiographic response and improved survival. *J Neurooncol*. 2009;92(2):185–191.

52. Pouratian N, Crowley RW, Sherman JH, Jagannathan J, Sheehan JP. Gamma Knife radiosurgery after radiation therapy as an adjunctive treatment for glioblastoma. *J Neurooncol*. 2009;94(3):409–418.

53. Hulshof MC, Schimmel EC, Andries Bosch D, González González D. Hypofractionation in glioblastoma multiforme. *Radiother Oncol*. 2000;54(2):143–148.

54. Cardinale R, Won M, Choucair A, et al. A phase II trial of accelerated radiotherapy using weekly stereotactic conformal boost for supratentorial glioblastoma multiforme: RTOG 0023. *Int J Radiat Oncol Biol Phys*. 2006;65(5):1422–1428.

55. Baumert BG, Brada M, Bernier J, et al. EORTC 22972–26991/MRC BR10 trial: fractionated stereotactic boost following conventional radiotherapy of high grade gliomas. Clinical and quality-assurance results of the stereotactic boost arm. *Radiother Oncol*. 2008;88(2):163–172.

56. Baumert BG, Lutterbach J, Bernays R, Davis JB, Heppner FL. Fractionated stereotactic radiotherapy boost after post-operative radiotherapy in patients with high-grade gliomas. *Radiother Oncol*. 2003;67(2):183–190.

57. Grosu AL, Weber WA, Franz M, et al. Reirradiation of recurrent high-grade gliomas using amino acid PET (SPECT)/CT/MRI image fusion to determine gross tumor volume for stereotactic fractionated radiotherapy. *Int J Radiat Oncol Biol Phys*. 2005;63(2):511–519.

58. Jain RK, di Tomaso E, Duda DG, Loeffler JS, Sorensen AG, Batchelor TT. Angiogenesis in brain tumours. *Nat Rev Neurosci*. 2007;8(8):610–622.

59. Lamszus K, Ulbricht U, Matschke J, Brockmann MA, Fillbrandt R, Westphal M. Levels of soluble vascular endothelial growth factor (VEGF) receptor 1 in astrocytic tumors and its relation to malignancy, vascularity, and VEGF-A. *Clin Cancer Res*. 2003;9(4):1399–1405.

60. Sathornsumetee S, Cao Y, Marcello JE, et al. Tumor angiogenic and hypoxic profiles predict radiographic response and survival in malignant astrocytoma patients treated with bevacizumab and irinotecan. *J Clin Oncol*. 2008;26(2):271–278.

61. Plate KH, Breier G, Weich HA, Risau W. Vascular endothelial growth factor is a potential tumour angiogenesis factor in human gliomas in vivo. *Nature*. 1992;359(6398):845–848.

62. Vredenburgh JJ, Desjardins A, Herndon JE 2nd, et al. Phase II trial of bevacizumab and irinotecan in recurrent malignant glioma. *Clin Cancer Res*. 2007;13(4):1253–1259.

63. Beal K, Abrey LE, Gutin PH. Antiangiogenic agents in the treatment of recurrent or newly diagnosed glioblastoma: analysis of single-agent and combined modality approaches. *Radiat Oncol*. 2011;6:2.

64. Gutin PH, Iwamoto FM, Beal K, et al. Safety and efficacy of bevacizumab with hypofractionated stereotactic irradiation for recurrent malignant gliomas. *Int J Radiat Oncol Biol Phys*. 2009;75(1):156–163.

65. Laing RW, Warrington AP, Graham J, Britton J, Hines F, Brada M. Efficacy and toxicity of fractionated stereotactic radiotherapy in the treatment of recurrent gliomas (phase I/II study). *Radiother Oncol*. 1993;27(1):22–29.

66. Cardinale RM, Schmidt-Ullrich RK, Benedict SH, Zwicker RD, Han DC, Broaddus WC. Accelerated radiotherapy regimen for malignant gliomas using stereotactic concomitant boosts for dose escalation. *Radiat Oncol Investig*. 1998;6(4):175–181.

67. Nieder C, Nestle U, Walter K, et al. Hypofractionated stereotactic radiotherapy for malignant glioma: A phase I/II study. *J Radiosurgery*. 1999;2:107–111.

68. Lederman G, Wronski M, Arbit E, et al. Treatment of recurrent glioblastoma multiforme using fractionated stereotactic radiosurgery and concurrent paclitaxel. *Am J Clin Oncol*. 2000;23(2):155–159.

69. Ernst-Stecken A, Ganslandt O, Lambrecht U, Sauer R, Grabenbauer G. Survival and quality of life after hypofractionated stereotactic radiotherapy for recurrent malignant glioma. *J Neurooncol*. 2007;81(3):287–294.

70. Schwer AL, Damek DM, Kavanagh BD, et al. A phase I dose-escalation study of fractionated stereotactic radiosurgery in combination with gefitinib in patients with recurrent malignant gliomas. *Int J Radiat Oncol Biol Phys*. 2008;70(4):993–1001.

71. Fokas E, Wacker U, Gross MW, Henzel M, Encheva E, Engenhart-Cabillic R. Hypofractionated stereotactic reirradiation of recurrent glioblastomas: a beneficial treatment

option after high-dose radiotherapy? *Strahlenther Onkol.* 2009;185(4):235–240.

72. Henke G, Paulsen F, Steinbach JP, et al. Hypofractionated reirradiation for recurrent malignant glioma. *Strahlenther Onkol.* 2009;185(2):113–119.

73. Fogh SE, Andrews DW, Glass J, et al. Hypofractionated stereotactic radiation therapy: an effective therapy for recurrent high-grade gliomas. *J Clin Oncol.* 2010;28(18):3048–3053.

74. Hermanto U, Frija EK, Lii MJ, Chang EL, Mahajan A, Woo SY. Intensity-modulated radiotherapy (IMRT) and conventional three-dimensional conformal radiotherapy for high-grade gliomas: does IMRT increase the integral dose to normal brain? *Int J Radiat Oncol Biol Phys.* 2007;67(4):1135–1144.

75. Murshed H, Liu HH, Liao Z, et al. Dose and volume reduction for normal lung using intensity-modulated radiotherapy for advanced-stage non-small-cell lung cancer. *Int J Radiat Oncol Biol Phys.* 2004;58(4):1258–1267.

76. Nutting CM, Bedford JL, Cosgrove VP, Tait DM, Dearnaley DP, Webb S. A comparison of conformal and intensity-modulated techniques for oesophageal radiotherapy. *Radiother Oncol.* 2001;61(2):157–163.

77. Pirzkall A, Carol M, Lohr F, Höss A, Wannenmacher M, Debus J. Comparison of intensity-modulated radiotherapy with conventional conformal radiotherapy for complex-shaped tumors. *Int J Radiat Oncol Biol Phys.* 2000;48(5):1371–1380.

78. Cheng JC, Wu JK, Huang CM, et al. Dosimetric analysis and comparison of three-dimensional conformal radiotherapy and intensity-modulated radiation therapy for patients with hepatocellular carcinoma and radiation-induced liver disease. *Int J Radiat Oncol Biol Phys.* 2003;56(1):229–234.

79. Cozzi L, Fogliata A, Bolsi A, Nicolini G, Bernier J. Three-dimensional conformal vs. intensity-modulated radiotherapy in head-and-neck cancer patients: comparative analysis of dosimetric and technical parameters. *Int J Radiat Oncol Biol Phys.* 2004;58(2):617–624.

80. Huang E, Teh BS, Strother DR, et al. Intensity-modulated radiation therapy for pediatric medulloblastoma: early report on the reduction of ototoxicity. *Int J Radiat Oncol Biol Phys.* 2002;52(3):599–605.

81. Narayana A, Yamada J, Berry S, et al. Intensity-modulated radiotherapy in high-grade gliomas: clinical and dosimetric results. *Int J Radiat Oncol Biol Phys.* 2006;64(3):892–897.

82. Thilmann C, Zabel A, Grosser KH, Hoess A, Wannenmacher M, Debus J. Intensity-modulated radiotherapy with an integrated boost to the macroscopic tumor volume in the treatment of high-grade gliomas. *Int J Cancer.* 2001;96(6):341–349.

83. Panet-Raymond V, Souhami L, Roberge D, et al. Accelerated hypofractionated intensity-modulated radiotherapy with concurrent and adjuvant temozolomide for patients with glioblastoma multiforme: a safety and efficacy analysis. *Int J Radiat Oncol Biol Phys.* 2009;73(2):473–478.

84. Sultanem K, Patrocinio H, Lambert C, et al. The use of hypofractionated intensity-modulated irradiation in the treatment of glioblastoma multiforme: preliminary results of a prospective trial. *Int J Radiat Oncol Biol Phys.* 2004;58(1):247–252.

85. Morganti AG, Balducci M, Salvati M, et al. A phase I dose-escalation study (ISIDE-BT-1) of accelerated IMRT with temozolomide in patients with glioblastoma. *Int J Radiat Oncol Biol Phys.* 2010;77(1):92–97.

86. Chen C, Damek D, Gaspar LE, et al. Phase I trial of hypofractionated intensity-modulated radiotherapy with temozolomide chemotherapy for patients with newly diagnosed glioblastoma multiforme. *Int J Radiat Oncol Biol Phys.* 2011;81(4):1066–1074.

87. Floyd NS, Woo SY, Teh BS, et al. Hypofractionated intensity-modulated radiotherapy for primary glioblastoma multiforme. *Int J Radiat Oncol Biol Phys.* 2004;58(3):721–726.

88. Milenic DE, Brady ED, Brechbiel MW. Antibody-targeted radiation cancer therapy. *Nat Rev Drug Discov.* 2004;3(6):488–499.

89. Hofer KG, Hughes WL. Radiotoxicity of intranuclear tritium, 125 iodine and 131 iodine. *Radiat Res.* 1971;47(1):94–101.

90. Martin RF, Haseltine WA. Range of radiochemical damage to DNA with decay of iodine-125. *Science.* 1981;213(4510):896–898.

91. Reardon DA, Akabani G, Coleman RE, et al. Phase II trial of murine (131)I-labeled antitenascin monoclonal antibody 81C6 administered into surgically created resection cavities of patients with newly diagnosed malignant gliomas. *J Clin Oncol.* 2002;20(5):1389–1397.

92. Reardon DA, Akabani G, Coleman RE, et al. Salvage radioimmunotherapy with murine iodine-131-labeled antitenascin monoclonal antibody 81C6 for patients with recurrent primary and metastatic malignant brain tumors: phase II study results. *J Clin Oncol.* 2006;24(1):115–122.

93. Libermann TA, Nusbaum HR, Razon N, et al. Amplification, enhanced expression and possible rearrangement of EGF receptor gene in primary human brain tumours of glial origin. *Nature.* 1985;313(5998):144–147.

94. von Deimling A, Louis DN, von Ammon K, et al. Association of epidermal growth factor receptor gene amplification with loss of chromosome 10 in human glioblastoma multiforme. *J Neurosurg.* 1992;77(2):295–301.

95. Florell RC, Macdonald DR, Irish WD, et al. Selection bias, survival, and brachytherapy for glioma. *J Neurosurg.* 1992;76(2):179–183.

96. Videtic GM, Gaspar LE, Zamorano L, Stitt LW, Fontanesi J, Levin KJ. Implant volume as a prognostic variable in brachytherapy decision-making for malignant gliomas stratified by the RTOG recursive partitioning analysis. *Int J Radiat Oncol Biol Phys.* 2001;51(4):963–968.

97. Wen PY, Alexander E 3rd, Black PM, et al. Long term results of stereotactic brachytherapy used in the

initial treatment of patients with glioblastomas. *Cancer.* 1994;73(12):3029–3036.

98. Laperriere NJ, Leung PM, McKenzie S, et al. Randomized study of brachytherapy in the initial management of patients with malignant astrocytoma. *Int J Radiat Oncol Biol Phys.* 1998;41(5):1005–1011.

99. Selker RG, Shapiro WR, Burger P, et al.; Brain Tumor Cooperative Group. The Brain Tumor Cooperative Group NIH Trial 87–01: a randomized comparison of surgery, external radiotherapy, and carmustine versus surgery, interstitial radiotherapy boost, external radiation therapy, and carmustine. *Neurosurgery.* 2002;51(2):343–55; discussion 355.

100. Welsh J, Sanan A, Gabayan AJ, et al. GliaSite brachytherapy boost as part of initial treatment of glioblastoma multiforme: a retrospective multi-institutional pilot study. *Int J Radiat Oncol Biol Phys.* 2007;68(1):159–165.

101. Chan TA, Weingart JD, Parisi M, et al. Treatment of recurrent glioblastoma multiforme with GliaSite brachytherapy. *Int J Radiat Oncol Biol Phys.* 2005;62(4):1133–1139.

102. Videtic GM, Gaspar LE, Zamorano L, et al. Use of the RTOG recursive partitioning analysis to validate the benefit of iodine-125 implants in the primary treatment of malignant gliomas. *Int J Radiat Oncol Biol Phys.* 1999;45(3):687–692.

103. Patel S, Breneman JC, Warnick RE, et al. Permanent iodine-125 interstitial implants for the treatment of recurrent glioblastoma multiforme. *Neurosurgery.* 2000;46(5):1123–8; discussion 1128.

104. Chang CN, Chen WC, Wei KC, et al. High-dose-rate stereotactic brachytherapy for patients with newly diagnosed glioblastoma multiformes. *J Neurooncol.* 2003;61(1):45–55.

105. Tatter SB, Shaw EG, Rosenblum ML, et al.; New Approaches to Brain Tumor Therapy Central Nervous System Consortium. An inflatable balloon catheter and liquid 125I radiation source (GliaSite Radiation Therapy System) for treatment of recurrent malignant glioma: multicenter safety and feasibility trial. *J Neurosurg.* 2003;99(2):297–303.

106. Larson DA, Suplica JM, Chang SM, et al. Permanent iodine 125 brachytherapy in patients with progressive or recurrent glioblastoma multiforme. *Neuro-oncology.* 2004;6(2):119–126.

107. Chen AM, Chang S, Pouliot J, et al. Phase I trial of gross total resection, permanent iodine-125 brachytherapy, and hyperfractionated radiotherapy for newly diagnosed glioblastoma multiforme. *Int J Radiat Oncol Biol Phys.* 2007;69(3):825–830.

108. Darakchiev BJ, Albright RE, Breneman JC, Warnick RE. Safety and efficacy of permanent iodine-125 seed implants and carmustine wafers in patients with recurrent glioblastoma multiforme. *J Neurosurg.* 2008;108(2):236–242.

109. Wernicke AG, Sherr DL, Schwartz TH, et al. The role of dose escalation with intracavitary brachytherapy in the treatment of localized CNS malignancies: outcomes and toxicities of a prospective study. *Brachytherapy.* 2010;9(1):91–99.

110. WILSON RR. Radiological use of fast protons. *Radiology.* 1946;47(5):487–491.

111. Boone ML, Lawrence JH, Connor WG, Morgado R, Hicks JA, Brown RC. Introduction to the use of protons and heavy ions in radiation therapy: historical perspective. *Int J Radiat Oncol Biol Phys.* 1977;3:65–69.

112. Kjellberg RN, Shintani A, Frantz AG, Kliman B. Proton-beam therapy in acromegaly. *N Engl J Med.* 1968;278(13):689–695.

113. Suit H, Goitein M, Munzenrider J, et al. Evaluation of the clinical applicability of proton beams in definitive fractionated radiation therapy. *Int J Radiat Oncol Biol Phys.* 1982;8(12):2199–2205.

114. Munzenrider JE, Austin-Seymour M, Blitzer PJ, et al. Proton therapy at Harvard. *Strahlentherapie.* 1985;161(12):756–763.

115. Combs SE, Bohl J, Elsasser T, et al. Radiobiological evaluation and correlation with the local effect model (LEM) of carbon ion radiation therapy and temozolomide in glioblastoma cell lines. *Int J Radiat Biol.* 2009;85(2):126–137.

116. Iwadate Y, Mizoe J, Osaka Y, Yamaura A, Tsujii H. High linear energy transfer carbon radiation effectively kills cultured glioma cells with either mutant or wild-type p53. *Int J Radiat Oncol Biol Phys.* 2001;50(3):803–808.

117. Combs SE, Burkholder I, Edler L, et al. Randomised phase I/II study to evaluate carbon ion radiotherapy versus fractionated stereotactic radiotherapy in patients with recurrent or progressive gliomas: the CINDERELLA trial. *BMC Cancer.* 2010;10:533.

118. Bolsi A, Fogliata A, Cozzi L. Radiotherapy of small intracranial tumours with different advanced techniques using photon and proton beams: a treatment planning study. *Radiother Oncol.* 2003;68(1):1–14.

119. Baumert BG, Lomax AJ, Miltchev V, Davis JB. A comparison of dose distributions of proton and photon beams in stereotactic conformal radiotherapy of brain lesions. *Int J Radiat Oncol Biol Phys.* 2001;49(5):1439–1449.

120. Lin R, Hug EB, Schaefer RA, Miller DW, Slater JM, Slater JD. Conformal proton radiation therapy of the posterior fossa: a study comparing protons with three-dimensional planned photons in limiting dose to auditory structures. *Int J Radiat Oncol Biol Phys.* 2000;48(4):1219–1226.

121. Fuss M, Poljanc K, Miller DW, et al. Normal tissue complication probability (NTCP) calculations as a means to compare proton and photon plans and evaluation of clinical appropriateness of calculated values. *Int J Cancer.* 2000;90(6):351–358.

122. Miralbell R, Lomax A, Russo M. Potential role of proton therapy in the treatment of pediatric medulloblastoma/primitive neuro-ectodermal tumors: spinal theca irradiation. *Int J Radiat Oncol Biol Phys.* 1997;38(4):805–811.

123. Mock U, Georg D, Bogner J, Auberger T, Pötter R. Treatment planning comparison of conventional, 3D conformal, and intensity-modulated photon (IMRT) and proton therapy for paranasal sinus carcinoma. *Int J Radiat Oncol Biol Phys.* 2004;58(1):147–154.

124. van den Bent MJ, Afra D, de Witte O, et al.; EORTC Radiotherapy and Brain Tumor Groups and the UK Medical Research Council. Long-term efficacy of early versus delayed radiotherapy for low-grade astrocytoma and oligodendroglioma in adults: the EORTC 22845 randomised trial. *Lancet.* 2005;366(9490):985–990.

125. Shaw E, Arusell R, Scheithauer B, et al. Prospective randomized trial of low- versus high-dose radiation therapy in adults with supratentorial low-grade glioma: initial report of a North Central Cancer Treatment Group/Radiation Therapy Oncology Group/Eastern Cooperative Oncology Group study. *J Clin Oncol.* 2002;20(9):2267–2276.

126. Karim AB, Maat B, Hatlevoll R, et al. A randomized trial on dose-response in radiation therapy of low-grade cerebral glioma: European Organization for Research and Treatment of Cancer (EORTC) Study 22844. *Int J Radiat Oncol Biol Phys.* 1996;36(3):549–556.

127. Kiebert GM, Curran D, Aaronson NK, et al. Quality of life after radiation therapy of cerebral low-grade gliomas of the adult: results of a randomised phase III trial on dose response (EORTC trial 22844). EORTC Radiotherapy Co-operative Group. *Eur J Cancer.* 1998;34(12):1902–1909.

128. Douw L, Klein M, Fagel SS, et al. Cognitive and radiological effects of radiotherapy in patients with low-grade glioma: long-term follow-up. *Lancet Neurol.* 2009;8(9):810–818.

129. Olson JD, Riedel E, DeAngelis LM. Long-term outcome of low-grade oligodendroglioma and mixed glioma. *Neurology.* 2000;54(7):1442–1448.

130. Jenkins RB, Blair H, Ballman KV, et al. A t(1;19)(q10;p10) mediates the combined deletions of 1p and 19q and predicts a better prognosis of patients with oligodendroglioma. *Cancer Res.* 2006;66(20):9852–9861.

131. Pignatti F, van den Bent M, Curran D, et al.; European Organization for Research and Treatment of Cancer Brain Tumor Cooperative Group; European Organization for Research and Treatment of Cancer Radiotherapy Cooperative Group. Prognostic factors for survival in adult patients with cerebral low-grade glioma. *J Clin Oncol.* 2002;20(8):2076–2084.

132. Pu AT, Sandler HM, Radany EH, et al. Low grade gliomas: preliminary analysis of failure patterns among patients treated using 3D conformal external beam irradiation. *Int J Radiat Oncol Biol Phys.* 1995;31(3):461–466.

133. Rudoler S, Corn BW, Werner-Wasik M, et al. Patterns of tumor progression after radiotherapy for low-grade gliomas: analysis from the computed tomography/magnetic resonance imaging era. *Am J Clin Oncol.* 1998;21(1):23–27.

134. Miralbell R, Lomax A, Cella L, Schneider U. Potential reduction of the incidence of radiation-induced second cancers by using proton beams in the treatment of pediatric tumors. *Int J Radiat Oncol Biol Phys.* 2002;54(3):824–829.

135. Newhauser WD, Fontenot JD, Mahajan A, et al. The risk of developing a second cancer after receiving craniospinal proton irradiation. *Phys Med Biol.* 2009;54(8):2277–2291.

136. Fitzek MM, Thornton AF, Harsh G 4th, et al. Dose-escalation with proton/photon irradiation for Daumas-Duport lower-grade glioma: results of an institutional phase I/II trial. *Int J Radiat Oncol Biol Phys.* 2001;51(1):131–137.

137. Mizoe JE, Tsujii H, Hasegawa A, et al.; Organizing Committee of the Central Nervous System Tumor Working Group. Phase I/II clinical trial of carbon ion radiotherapy for malignant gliomas: combined X-ray radiotherapy, chemotherapy, and carbon ion radiotherapy. *Int J Radiat Oncol Biol Phys.* 2007;69(2):390–396.

138. Combs SE, Kieser M, Rieken S, et al. Randomized phase II study evaluating a carbon ion boost applied after combined radiochemotherapy with temozolomide versus a proton boost after radiochemotherapy with temozolomide in patients with primary glioblastoma: the CLEOPATRA trial. *BMC Cancer.* 2010;10:478.

Biomarkers for Malignant Gliomas

Erica Hlavin Bell and Deliang Guo*

Department of Radiation Oncology, Comprehensive Cancer Center, The Ohio State University Medical Center, Columbus, OH

ABSTRACT

High-grade gliomas frequently exhibit elevated levels of heterogeneity and resistance to both radiation and chemotherapy. In order to enhance clinical outcomes in this often fatal disease, an increased understanding of the molecular profile of glioma subpopulations, mechanisms of resistance, and biomarkers is absolutely essential. This chapter will review currently known genetic, epigenetic, and metabolic biomarkers of malignant gliomas. Specifically, common tumor suppressor and oncogene alterations, such as IDH, 1p/19q, Rb, PTEN, p53, PDGF, EGFR, and PI3K/Akt, will be discussed in detail with regard to their presence in gliomas, evidence of biomarker status, and their possible roles in a clinical setting. Furthermore, metabolic reprogramming has been found to promote GBM malignant growth. Recent studies have demonstrated that PI3K/Akt/SREBP-1 plays a key role in integrating oncogenic signaling and metabolic networks. Here, we will additionally summarize recent advances in the understanding of metabolism in GBM, including glycolysis, glutaminolysis, lipogenesis, and cholesterol metabolism.

Keywords: glioma, prognostic biomarkers, predictive biomarkers, cancer metabolism

INTRODUCTION

Gliomas represent about half of all diagnosed adult brain tumors (1). Malignant gliomas include all high-grade gliomas, such as anaplastic astrocytoma (WHO grade III) and glioblastoma multiforme (GBM) (WHO grade IV). Although significant advancements have been made within brain tumor research in the last decade, the prognosis for GBM patients remains dismal (~12–15 months). High-grade gliomas display high levels of heterogeneity and are often resistant to both radiation and chemotherapy. In order to significantly improve the outcome in patients, many investigators, including The Cancer Genome Atlas (TCGA), have made discovering novel molecular biomarkers of malignant gliomas, a top priority. Ideally, these biomarkers will aid clinicians in diagnosis of glioma patients, and also help facilitate decisions of personalized therapy modalities for patients harboring malignant gliomas based on molecular criteria in association with histopathological characteristics. Furthermore, identifying novel biomarkers will help elucidate key proteins involved in gliomagenesis and treatment resistance. This chapter will review currently known genetic, epigenetic, and metabolic biomarkers of malignant gliomas (see Figure 1). For a more clinically focused review of biomarkers and gliomas, refer to our previously published chapter (2).

*Corresponding author, Assistant Professor, Department of Radiation Oncology, Comprehensive Cancer Center, The Ohio State University Medical Center, Tzagournis Medical Research Facility 514B, 410 W 12th Ave, Columbus, OH 43210

E-mail address: deliang.guo@osumc.edu

Radiation Medicine Rounds 3:2 (2012) 339–358.

DOI: 10.5003/2151–4208.3.2.339

Molecular Biomarker	Putative Biomarker Status
1p/19q co-deletion	diagnostic, prognostic, predictive
IDH1/2 mutation	diagnostic, prognostic
p53	diagnostic
Rb/p16/CDK4	p16-prognostic?
PDGFR	prognostic
EGFR/NFKBIA	diagnostic (EGFR), prognostic (NFKBIA), predictive (EGFR)
VEGF	prognostic?
PTEN	prognostic, predictive
PI3K/AKT	prognostic
MAPK	prognostic, predictive
Wnt/Hedgehog pathways	prognostic
MGMT methylation	prognostic, predictive
miRNAs	prognostic, predictive
SREBP-1/ACC/FASN	prognostic?, predictive?

FIGURE 1 Current putative molecular biomarkers in malignant gliomas. The most common molecular alterations in malignant gliomas and their corresponding proposed biomarker statuses are listed.

■ GENETIC BIOMARKERS

IDH1/2 Mutations

NADP-dependent isocitrate dehydrogenase (IDH) is an essential enzyme within the citric acid cycle as it catalyzes the conversion of isocitrate into α-ketoglutarate. Its isozymes IDH1 and IDH2 are additionally implicated in a variety of metabolic processes such as signal transduction, lipid synthesis, and oxidative stress (3). Gliomas with IDH mutations were first described in 2008 when a genome-wide analysis was conducted on GBM tissue (3–5). IDH1 and IDH2 mutations represent one of the first somatic genetic alterations in metabolic enzymes identified in gliomas, thus suggesting the importance of metabolic reprogramming in tumorigenesis (4). In low-grade brain tumors, IDH mutations are common genetic alterations arising from the astrocytic and oligodendroglial lineage, which is surprising given their large genetic differences. These mutations are also commonly identified in secondary GBMs (6,7). Presently, IDH1 and IDH2 mutations are used as diagnostic markers for diffuse WHO grade II and III gliomas and secondary GBMs (3,6).

Interestingly, there is evidence to suggest that genetic mutations within the IDH gene, specifically the $IDH1^{R132H/S}$ mutations, are among the earliest formed mutations and occur in ~40% of gliomas (5,8). IDH mutations are seen in more than 70% and 50% of WHO grade II and III, respectively (5,9,10). Additional studies identified IDH1 gene mutations in approximately 80% of diffuse astrocytomas and 85% of secondary GBMs. In contrast, only 5% of primary GBMs carry an IDH mutation (7,9). Histopathologically, tumors harboring an IDH mutation appear to have less necrosis than oligodendroglial features. IDH1/2 mutations are often identified concomitantly with 1p19q codeletions or p53 mutations (3,6). These tumors also tend to highly correlate with O_6-methyl guanine DNA methyltransferase (MGMT) promoter methylation (8,11) and CpG island methylator phenotype (G-CIMP) (12). Recently, a study showed that the IDH1 mutation is sufficient for establishment of the glioma hypermethylator phenotype (13). Furthermore, the majority of the tumors with IDH mutations mutually expressed the proneural signature, which is associated with improved survival (11). IDH mutations also appear to be mutually exclusive of epidermal growth factor receptor (EGFR) amplification (8).

The molecular mechanism involved with IDH mutations and tumorigenesis remains elusive. IDH1 mutations have been revealed to lead to increased formation of 2-hydroxyglutarate (2HG), which can directly inhibit adenosine 5′ triphosphate synthase, thereby altering essential mitochondrial processes (3,4,6). Consequently, this can cause selective pressure in the cell and promote metabolic adaptation and a shift toward aerobic glycolysis. This metabolic shift may provide a growth advantage in an increased proliferative state (4). Recently, 2HG produced by mutant IDH has been demonstrated to inhibit histone demethylation in immortalized astrocytes and resulted in hyperhistone methylation (14). Further hypotheses on the role of IDH mutations in gliomagenesis that are being investigated are its involvement in angiogenesis, glucose transport, glycolysis, and inhibition of apoptosis (3,4). Therefore, 2HG is believed to be a potential therapeutic target, a putative serum biomarker for cancers harboring IDH1 and IDH2 mutations, and a potential response biomarker. Intriguingly, there is supportive proof that D-2HG may be visualized via magnetic resonance spectroscopy, which could significantly aid in diagnosis and therapy delivery (4).

It is evident that glioma patients containing IDH mutations display a prognostic advantage (3,6). For example, somatic mutations at codon 132 were present in 18 of 149 (12%) GBMs and positively correlated with survival as the overall survival was 31 months compared to 15 months in patients without IDH mutations (6). IDH mutations can be used as a diagnostic tool because they can help differentiate between lower grade gliomas, and secondary GBM from primary GBM. Even though IDH is a useful diagnostic and prognostic tool, it currently does not appear to be able to predict responsiveness to a particular type of therapy (3). Therefore, future clinical trials examining IDH mutations need to be implemented to determine its role as a predictive molecular biomarker.

LOH of 1p/19q

The loss of heterozygosity (LOH) of 1p and 19q is the most common genetic alteration in oligodendrogliomas, occurring in ~40% to 90% of cases (3,6,15,16). Codeletion of 1p/19q is the result of an unbalanced whole-arm translocation between chromosomes 19 and 1 and occurs as an early event in the majority of oligodendrogliomas and anaplastic oligodendrogliomas (8). LOH of 1p/19q is also found in 20% to 30% of mixed glial tumors (17) and <10% of diffuse astrocytic gliomas (3). LOH of 1p/19q also occurs in oligoastrocytomas and anaplastic oligoastrocytomas (8). Deletions involving 1p and 19q are uncommon in GBM, but have been identified in a small percentage of cases (18). Intriguingly, 1p/19q loss confers a favorable response to chemotherapy, radiation, and survival (15,19). Although the regions of chromosomes and 1p and 19q have been mapped, the tumor-suppressor genes as well as genes that confer prolonged survival at this position are yet to be elucidated.

The first observation of a favorable prognosis of patients harboring 1p/19q LOH was within a large percentage of patients with recurrent anaplastic oligodendrogliomas (grade III) that responded to chemotherapy. In 1998, Cairncross et al. first identified that the loss of 1p significantly increased sensitivity to procarbazine, lomustine, and vincristine (PCV) treatment (20). This study showed evidence that patients with codeletions had increased survival times. Moreover, loss of 1p/19q has been shown to increase sensitivity to temozolomide (21) and loss of 1p has been shown to increase radiation sensitivity (8,22). The genes on chromosomes 1p and 19q that contribute to a more favorable therapeutic response remain to be determined, and identifying which genes that normally increase resistance to common therapies is essential in order to fully understand resistance mechanisms within gliomas. Due to the overall increased survival of patients with codeletions, it is thought that 1p/19q loss may be a prognostic marker of increased survival rather than a predictive marker of specific therapies. However, a recent study conducted by the Radiation Therapy Oncology Group (RTOG) showed that codeletion of 1p and 19q has both definitive prognostic and predictive values for treatment of adult patients with pure and mixed anaplastic oligodendrogliomas. Specifically, the absence of 1p/19q was associated with a significantly better prognosis and doubling of median survival time when treatment with combined chemotherapy (PCV) and radiation therapy was compared to treatment with radiation therapy alone (23). Furthermore, when treated with PCV plus RT 1p/19q codeletion patients had significantly longer overall survival (14.7 years) compared to 1p/19q codeletion patients treated with radiation alone (7.3 years) suggesting that LOH of 1p/19q also has predictive significance (24).

Of importance is the differentiation between complete and partial loss of chromosome 1p because partial losses occur in astrocytic tumors and are associated with poor outcome in contrast to LOH of 1p/19q. Consequently, some techniques, such as FISH, are not always successful in distinguishing between partial and whole loss of 1p (8). Furthermore, there are common alterations that occur concomitantly with 1p/19q codeletions, such as IDH1 and IDH2 mutations (9). 1p/19q loss has also been shown to be mutually exclusive of p53 mutations, 10q deletions, and amplification of EGFR (19). 1p/19q codeletions are additionally frequently associated with MGMT promoter methylation and the proneural gene-expression profile, which are both associated with a positive prognosis and may help explain why patients respond favorably to chemotherapy (8).

Currently, determining 1p/19q status is part of the standard of care for oligodendroglial tumors. Status of 1p/19q is informative based on the knowledge that patients with oligodendrogliomas containing LOH of 1p/19q will, likely, survive longer and be more responsive to a broad range of therapies.

Other Genetic Variants

Large genome-wide profiling of tumors is currently being conducted at many cancer institutions and within large phase III clinical trials. One recent large study showed that SNPs within telomerase reverse transcriptase (TERT), regulator of telomere elongation helicase 1 (RTEL1), and cyclin-dependent kinase 4 inhibitor B (CDKN2B) were strongly associated with GBM (25,26). Importantly, SNPs that are associated with tumor formation may be able to be identified in patients before tumors can be detected and will likely in the near future be an invaluable diagnostic tool.

■ TUMOR SUPPRESSOR BIOMARKERS

Rb/p16INK4a/CDK4

The retinoblastoma protein, Rb, is a tumor suppressor that is one of the most fundamental proteins responsible for antiproliferative signaling (7). Rb prevents proliferation by inhibiting the G1 to S phase transition and DNA replication (7,27). Under normal conditions, Rb is inactivated by cyclin D1 and CDK4 and CDK6 complexes so that DNA synthesis may proceed. p16INK4a is an additional protein, encoded from the CDKN2A gene, that is a regulator of the Rb pathway and a tumor-suppressor gene as it negatively regulates CDK4 and CDK6, thereby preventing cell cycle progression and DNA synthesis (7,27).

Alterations of the Rb pathway are common in high-grade gliomas (7). Tumor progression from low-grade gliomas to anaplastic astrocytomas (grade III) is typically characterized by common mutations, such as p16 or Rb mutations and amplification or overexpression of CDK4 (7,28). Deletion or mutation of the Rb gene occurs in approximately 30% and 13% to 25% of grade II and III astrocytomas, respectively (15). Alterations of the Rb gene occur in ~40% of secondary GBM cases as well (15). The frequency of Rb mutations in all high-grade gliomas is numerous and is estimated to occur in ~25% of all cases (7). Deletion or mutation of p16INK4A as a consequence of loss of chromosome 9p or hypermethylation occurs in approximately 12% to 60% of grade III AA tumors (15). In primary GBM, loss of p16 has been reported in ~20% to 50% of cases (29,30). Although the Rb pathway alterations are very common in gliomas, how these putative biomarkers will translate into the clinic remains elusive. However, a recent study showed that p16 mutations were strong prognostic indicators of overall survival in grade IV patients treated with TMZ (31).

NFκB Inhibitor α

NFκB inhibitor α (NFκBIA) represses NFκB, thereby inhibiting signaling in the NFκB and EGFR pathways. Recently, Bredel et al. examined 790 human GBM cases for deletions, mutations, or expression of NFκBIA and EGFR and correlated the molecular findings to outcome data in 570 patients (32). This study demonstrated that NFκBIA is often deleted (~25%), but not mutated in GBMs. Additionally, it was also found that deletion of NFκBIA and amplification of EGFR appeared to be mutually exclusive (32). Most deletions occurred in non-classical subtypes of GBM and were inversely correlated with EGFR alterations. The conclusion from this study was that low-expression levels of NFκBIA were associated with decreased survival and had similar clinical outcomes to patients with EGFR amplifications (32). Interestingly, when patients were stratified for both NFκBIA and MGMT expression there was a very strong correlation with survival suggesting that a two-gene stratification scheme may be better than using either NFκBIA or MGMT expression alone (32).

Phosphatase and Tensin Homolog

Phosphatase and tensin homolog (PTEN) is a tumor suppressor and negative regulator of the PI3K/Akt pathway. PTEN dephosphorylates PIP3 and once PTEN is lost, PIP3 levels accumulate and lead to constitutive PI3K/Akt signaling and activation (33). As a result, alterations of PTEN are associated with increased cell growth and poor prognosis (15,31,34). PTEN mutations are found in ~8% of oligodendrogliomas and there is evidence that the presence of this mutation in patients is associated with poor prognosis in oligodendrogliomas as well (35). PTEN downregulation occurs in approximately 50% of grade II and grade III oligodendrogliomas, which appears to be primarily a consequence of promoter methylation (36,37). In grade II and III astrocytomas, PTEN promoter hypermethylation occurs in ~43% to 67% of cases (36,37). In GBM, PTEN is deleted due to LOH of chromosome 10q in ~50% to 70% of primary cases (38,39). Methylation of the PTEN promoter in GBM has also been observed (36). In many cases, loss of PTEN (~50% of high-grade gliomas) results in unregulated PI3K/Akt signaling and upregulation of mammalian target of rapamycin (mTOR) signaling, which increases protein translation

(7,40). PTEN alterations also commonly occur in the classical glioma expression subtype (11). Presently, PTEN is thought to be a negative prognostic molecular biomarker as patients with loss of PTEN have decreased survival. However, in recent years PTEN has been shown to be a predictive biomarker of certain targeted therapies, such as PARP inhibitors (41,42).

TP53

p53 is a tumor-suppressor protein that is encoded by the gene *TP53,* which was identified in 1989. The *TP53* tumor-suppressor gene was later identified to be responsible for chromosome 17 alterations in GBM (27). p53 is essential in a large number of critical processes that regulate normal cell function, such as cell cycle control, DNA damage response, cell death, differentiation, and inhibition of angiogenesis. Thus, p53 is commonly referred to as the "guardian of the genome (7)". p53 is important in the G1/S checkpoint whereby activated p53 can increase expression of p21, a CDK2 inhibitor, resulting in cell cycle arrest (27). Alterations of p53 can lead to an unregulated cell cycle and uncontrolled proliferation resulting in tumorigenesis.

Since low-grade astrocytomas often possess inactivating mutations of p53, it is thought that these mutations are characteristic mutations of low-grade gliomas. Alterations of p53 also occur in secondary GBM that arise from lower grade gliomas (28). p53 mutations occur in grade II astrocytomas (35%–60%), grade III astrocytomas (~50%), primary GBM (~30%), and secondary GBM (~60%–65%) (15,30,37). Additionally, in a specific study p53 mutations were found in ~44% and ~13% of grade II oligoastrocytoma and oligodendroglioma cases, respectively (37). Overexpression of p53 has also been observed in ~50% of GBM cases (29). Surprisingly, tumors that have 1p/19q codeletions do not contain p53 mutations (7,28). A negative regulator of p53, MDM2, has also been reported to be amplified or mutated in anaplastic astrocytoma (13%–43%) and in GBM (~10%–27%) (15,29). p53 mutations are also commonly associated with the mesenchymal glioma subtype, which displays the worst prognosis (11). Currently, p53 has not been determined to be predictive or prognostic (43). However, it does have a role in the diagnostic setting as it can help distinguish low-grade gliomas from high-grade gliomas.

■ ONCOGENE BIOMARKERS

Platelet-Derived Growth Factor

Platelet-derived growth factor (PDGF) plays an important role in cell migration, cell proliferation, and angiogenesis. Both the levels of PDGF and PDGFRs are important in angiogenesis and gliomagenesis (15,28). Amplification of PDGFRα occurs in ~7% of oligodendroglial tumors and up to 30% of astrocytic tumors have been shown to have amplified PDGFRα and/or PDGFRβ (15). PDGFRα and PDGFRβ amplification also occurs in ~25% of primary GBM and ~60% of secondary GBM. Due to its frequency, amplification of PDGF appears to be a key regulator of gliomagenesis, and overexpression or amplification of PDGFR has been identified to be a potential prognostic biomarker as it has been shown to associate with survival data (44). Imatinib, a tyrosine kinase inhibitor (TKI) of PDGFR, c-abl, and c-kit, is being investigated in clinical trials to assess its efficacy in malignant gliomas.

Epidermal Growth Factor Receptor

EGFR along with other receptor tyrosine kinases (RTKs) play a significant role in gliomagenesis (see Figure 2). The EGFR pathway normally activates the transcription factor of k-light polypeptide gene enhancer in B-cells (NFκB) to promote transcription

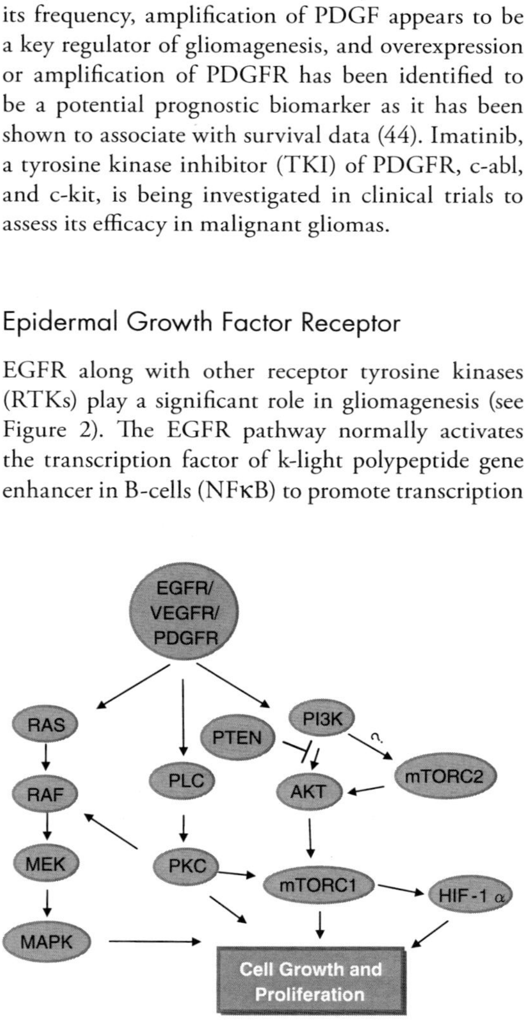

FIGURE 2 Growth factor signaling pathways in malignant gliomas. Multiple growth factors bind and activate receptor tyrosine kinases and their respective signaling cascades leading to increased cell growth and proliferation.

of DNA. Recently, three EGFR polymorphisms have been described as having a transcriptional regulatory function. This study further implicated EGFR 191C/A and $CA_{(n)}$ repeat polymorphisms as risk factors for gliomas. Furthermore, their work suggests EGFR polymorphism 191C/A is a prognostic marker in GBM (45).These polymorphisms may help to determine glioma susceptibility as well as possibly be used to stratify patients based on molecular characteristics for individualized treatment strategies.

EGFR additionally promotes gliomagenesis and is another common molecular alteration of GBM (7). In the mid-1980s it was shown that extra copies of chromosome 7 led to EGFR amplification/overexpression in some glioma tissue (27). EGFR promotes proliferation, invasion and angiogenesis, induces resistance to apoptosis, and may mediate radiation resistance (15,30). In primary GBM, EGFR amplification at 7p12 is the most common amplified and overexpressed gene occurring in ~30%–70% of cases (3,7,15,29). In addition, EGFRvIII is the most important mutated RTK receptor in GBM (3,28). The EGFRvIII mutation arises from loss of exons 2 and 7 and occurs in ~50% of GBM cases that overexpress EGFR (3). EGFRvIII leads to loss of the ligand-binding domain, which induces constitutive activation of EGFR and the PI3K/Akt pathway (6,28). Intriguingly, EGFRvIII receptors display a more invasive phenotype than those with wild-type EGFR (7). One of the main molecular distinctions between primary and secondary GBMs is that primary GBMs tend to have more EGFR amplifications than secondary GBMs, where it occurs in only 5% to 8% of cases (7,28–30). EGFR amplifications also occur in ~15% of anaplastic astrocytomas (15,30).

Several studies using EGFR TKIs, such as gefitinib and erlotinib, have shown some antitumor activity in patients with GBM. However, EGFR inhibitor monotherapy has shown only minor results for patients with recurrent GBM (46–48). The efficacy of EGFR TKIs remains controversial for newly diagnosed GBM, although few patients have been reported to respond dramatically to EGFR inhibitors. Due to the discrepancy of overexpression of EGFR in GBMs (up to 50%) and the low-response rate (~10%–20%) using EGFR TKIs, it is hypothesized that other molecular alterations may predict patient sensitivity such as EGFR downstream effectors (49). Consequently, the predictive and prognostic use of EGFR remains to be fully elucidated as there are many studies that are contradicting in the literature. For example, total levels of EGFR were shown to have no prognostic value in newly diagnosed GBM in a large patient set from multiple RTOG trials (50). On the other hand, there are multiple studies that have showed EGFR overexpression is associated with adverse outcome (see [50] for complete review). A recent report from RTOG 0211 showed that activation of Akt signaling, a downstream effector of EGFR, correlated with adverse outcome when GBM patients were treated with Gefitinib and radiation, whereas EGFR expression did not correlate with survival (51). Due to the high percentage of GBM cases with EGFR/PI3K/Akt dysregulation, targeted therapy of EGFR may be a helpful treatment for a subpopulation of glioma patients (43).

Vascular Endothelial Growth Factor and Its Receptors

Vascular endothelial growth factor (VEGF) and its receptors (VEGFR) are critical in angiogenesis and therefore, are essential components in the development and progression of GBM. In a recent study, 17 SNPs in VEGF and 27 in VEGFR were found in the blood of 154 patients with GBM (52). However, only two SNPs found in VEGFR2 were significantly associated with survival and could not be confirmed in an additional dataset. With the addition of bevacizumab, a monoclonal antibody toward VEGF, to the approved drug list for recurrent GBM, identifying the underlying mechanisms of VEGF in GBM is essential as is determining if any genetic alterations of VEGF can serve as molecular biomarkers.

VEGF is considered to be the driving factor of angiogenesis in astrocytic gliomas and VEGF expression appears to increase with grade and progression. For example, VEGF has been identified in 40% of grade II astrocytomas and approximately 65% of high-grade astrocytomas (53). It is not surprising that GBM has high levels of VEGF because it is recognized as a highly angiogenic tumor (54). Moreover, VEGF expression appears to significantly correlate with survival, thus VEGF is thought to be a possible prognostic factor in patients with gliomas (53). A new class of targeted therapy includes antiangiogenic agents that target VEGF. Bevacizumab, a humanized monoclonal antibody that recognizes and blocks VEGF, was approved by the FDA as a second-line or salvage treatment of GBM. Recent recurrent GBM studies have shown that bevacizumab improved progression-free survival, but several severe side effects have also been reported, such as intracranial hemorrhage, gastrointestinal perforation, and thromboembolic complications (55–57). At this time, RTOG is conducting a phase III trial (RTOG 0825) of conventional concurrent chemoradiation and adjuvant TMZ plus bevacizumab versus conventional concurrent chemoradiation and adjuvant TMZ in patients with newly diagnosed GBM. The results from this study are eagerly awaited as this trial will determine the efficacy of adding bevacizumab to the current standard of care for GBM. Furthermore, multiple molecular analyses of RTOG 0825 tissue are planned, including genome-wide profiling to identify and validate novel molecular biomarkers for GBM patients.

PI3K/Akt/mTOR

PI3K/Akt signaling is an important mediator of cell growth and proliferation. Its hyperactivation is frequent in a broad range of cancer types, including gliomas, and is associated with poor prognosis in glioma patients (7). Multiple growth factor receptors, such as EGFR, exert their proliferation effects through activation of the PI3K/Akt pathway, which is constitutively activated in ~70%–88% of GBM patients and is associated with mutations or deletions in the tumor-suppressor gene PTEN (58,59). mTOR is downstream of Akt, which regulates protein biosynthesis, ribosome biogenesis, and the transcription of essential genes involved in cell proliferation (7,60). mTOR inhibitors have been shown to significantly decrease PI3K/Akt/mTOR downstream signaling and combined mTOR and EGFR inhibition has demonstrated synergistic effects in GBM xenografts, as well as shown a partial response in a small patient cohort (58,61). Activation of the PI3K/mTOR pathway also occurs in most adult low-grade gliomas (60). Activation of PI3K was first shown to be associated with decreased survival in gliomas in 2004 (62). This particular study demonstrated that expression of PI3K, p70S6K, and p-Akt negatively correlated with survival in gliomas of all grades (62). Therefore, the use of selective PI3K, Akt, or mTOR inhibitors in the treatment of gliomas may become a valuable therapy choice in multimodality treatment regimens.

MAPK/BRAF

The mitogen-activated protein kinase (MAPK) pathway is one of the most important signal transduction pathways involved in gliomagenesis. It is stimulated by mitogens and pro-inflammatory cytokines, such as TGF-β, and stimulates the downstream activation of RAS and phosphorylation of MAPK by mitogen-activated protein kinase kinase (MEK). Phosphorylated MAPK then activates nuclear transcription factors, such as genes involved in cell cycle progression, apoptosis, cell differentiation, and cell migration (7,30). The MAPK pathway is often activated in gliomas; however, the activation is thought to be due to unregulated RTK or integrin activation rather than mutations (7). Additionally, activation of the proto-oncogene BRAF has been shown to cause upregulation of the MAPK pathway. Increased activation of BRAF, most commonly by gene duplication and fusion, has recently been identified as a primary genetic alteration in pilocytic astrocytomas. It occurs in ~60%–80% of pilocytic astrocytoma cases (3). The rate-limiting step of RAS activation is farnesylation, which explains the use of farnesyltransferase inhibitors in gliomas. Two separate farnesyltransferase inhibitors, tipifarnib and lonafarnib, have led to mixed results in clinical trials (63,64).

In another recent article, it was identified that ERK, also known as MAPK, is also activated in astrocytomas. In GBM, nuclear staining of pERK/pMAPK was identified to be a favorable prognostic marker in the presence of an IDH1-R132H mutation (65). This is one of only a very few studies that have differentiated between nuclear and cytoplasmic concentrations as proteins can be spatially regulated. MAPK proteins appear to be both potential predictive and prognostic molecular biomarkers. For example, another study showed phosphorylated MAPK was found to be inversely correlated with survival and associated with increased radiation resistance in GBM (66). Therefore, the exact significance of MAPK as a biomarker remains to be determined, specifically in relation to different histopathological grades and other mutations in gliomas.

β-Catenin /Gli1

Recently, β-catenin and Gli1 have been identified as prognostic markers in glioblastoma (67). This study showed that β-catenin and Gli1 are better prognostic markers of shorter survival than Ki67, p53, and EGFR (67). β-catenin and Gli1 are critical components of the Wnt signaling pathway and the hedgehog signaling pathway, respectively. β-catenin is an integral component of the Wnt signaling pathway, which is critical for the formation of cadherin-based cell-cell adhesions, contact inhibition, and cell proliferation

(68). Gli proteins are critical downstream transcription factors in the sonic hedgehog signaling pathway and have been shown to be involved in embryonic development, cell proliferation, and glioma stem cell renewal. The hedgehog signaling pathway is also activated in multiple types of cancer contributing to tumorigenesis. In addition, sonic hedgehog signaling is also connected with other signaling pathways that contribute to cancer progression (69). Given that β-catenin and Gli1 are strong indicators of shortened survival, β-catenin and Gli1 are likely involved in GBM malignancy. Therefore, inhibiting members of the Wnt and hedgehog pathways may potentially be a successful therapeutic strategy for GBM patients.

Notch1

Notch1 has also recently been shown to be upregulated in glioma and associated with tumorigenesis (70). Signaling of Notch1 is important for angiogenesis, cell proliferation, differentiation, and apoptosis. In this recent study, Notch1 mRNA and protein were increased in glioma tissue compared to normal adjacent tissue and normal brain tissue. It was also identified that Notch1 expression increases with grade, therefore it is likely important in progression of gliomas and may potentially serve as a diagnostic and therapeutic target (70,71). Notch1 is also known to interact with other glioma-signaling pathways, such as PI3K, NFκB, EGFR, and Wnt. Another recent study has showed that Notch1 is a prognostic factor for patients with gliomas. Specifically, in this study increased Notch1 protein expression correlated with lower overall survival in a multivariate analysis suggesting Notch1 as an independent prognostic factor in gliomas (71).

Other Oncogene Markers

Another possible prognostic biomarker of glioma that has been identified is replication protein A (RPA) (72). RPA is an important protein during replication as it binds and stabilizes single-stranded DNA. Expression of RPA2 in this study was identified to be an independent prognostic factor in grade IV gliomas as well as other astrocytomas. Additionally, this study showed that expression of RPA1, RPA2, and cyclins D2 and D3 increases with tumor grade and therefore, these proteins are all important in the progression of malignant gliomas (72).

NDGR2 is an additional possible prognostic biomarker of astrocytomas (73). NDGR2 is a protein involved in the N-myc downstream-regulated gene family and is involved in cell proliferation and differentiation. Protein and mRNA levels of NDGR2 have recently been shown to be downregulated in astrocytomas and lower expression levels tend to correlate with a higher grade. Furthermore, NDGR2 levels negatively correlate with survival data, which is to be expected since expression levels seem to decrease with malignant progression (73). Therefore, NDGR2 could potentially be used as a diagnostic and/or prognostic biomarker of gliomas.

Genome-Wide Expression Profile of Glioma Subtypes

In 2006, Aldape and colleagues defined three subtypes of high-grade gliomas: proneural, mesenchymal, and proliferative (74). Within these subtypes, the proneural subtype showed longer survival than mesenchymal and proliferative subtypes (74). Recently large-scale profiling has been conducted on gliomas within TCGA, which included a priority for glioblastoma. These large-scale gene-expression profile studies have identified transcriptional profiles that reveal the underlying tumor biology for particular subtypes of gliomas. Furthermore, these profiles can be used for tumor classification and to predict patient outcome and treatment sensitivity. Verhaak et al., in 2010, further classified GBM into four subtypes using the TCGA database based on gene-expression patterns: classical, proneural, mesenchymal, and neural (75). This expanded on the study by Aldape and colleagues as Verhaak and colleagues confirmed two of the subtypes previously found, but then two new subtypes were identified in their recent study.

The classical gene-expression profile is distinguished by abnormally high levels of EGFR, lack of TP53 classical mutations, PTEN loss or mutation, CDKN2A loss, and activation of notch, and sonic hedgehog pathways. The classical phenotype also displayed the longest survival with aggressive treatment; therefore, this GBM subtype is predictive of aggressive therapy (75). In contrast, proneural tumors have high levels of TP53 mutations. Also, the proneural subtype has the highest levels of mutations in the IDH1 gene as well as increased levels of PDGFRA. Interestingly, the average age of patients with the proneural profile was significantly younger than the other three subtypes and the genes commonly mutated in the proneural subtype have been previously associated with secondary GBM. Additionally, these patients often had longer survival suggesting that patients harboring this tumor subtype have a prognostic advantage and in this study most known secondary GBM patients did display the proneural phenotype. Furthermore, proneural tumors did not show an increased survival benefit from receiving aggressive treatment (75). The mesenchymal profile is unique in that it contains the highest frequency of NF1 mutations of all of the subtypes as well as frequent mutations in PTEN and TP53. There was also an additional survival benefit in patients with the mesenchymal group with aggressive treatment, thus suggesting this profile can be used as a predictive biomarker. The neural subgroup has many of the same gene alterations of the other subtypes, but is differentiated by expressing many genes that are important for normal brain cells (75). Intriguingly, patients harboring neural tumors tend to be older than the other subtypes of GBM. Tumors with neural phenotype responded to aggressive therapy, but not to the extent of the classical and mesenchymal subtypes (75). These large-scale studies show that comprehensive molecular classifiers can be used as predictive and prognostic biomarkers to predict survival and treatment response. In addition, Gravendeel et al. using a large series of 276 gliomas (grade I–IV) showed that gene-expression profile stratification was a better predictor of survival than histology (76). However, these molecular classifications have yet to be fully analyzed in low-grade gliomas.

■ EPIGENETIC BIOMARKERS

O_6-Methyl Guanine DNA Methyltransferase Gene

MGMT encodes a direct reversal DNA repair protein that removes the alkyl groups from the O_6 position of guanine that are commonly produced by chemotherapeutic alkylating agents. MGMT is one of the principal enzymes involved in DNA repair and is a suicide enzyme, which requires de novo synthesis of MGMT to replenish the enzyme. Therefore, the MGMT promoter needs to be functional if DNA repair is to take place as the MGMT protein needs to be constantly replenished in the presence of DNA damage. Downregulation of the MGMT promoter by hypermethylation of a CpG island in a 5′ region of the gene and subsequent decrease of MGMT protein commonly occurs in gliomas (77). Importantly, the level of MGMT promoter methylation has been shown to correlate with the sensitivity of malignant gliomas to alkylating agents (3). Hypermethylation of the promoter of MGMT has been identified in ~10% of grade II astrocytomas, ~30% of oligoastrocytomas, and ~60% of oligodendroglioma cases (37). In GBM, MGMT methylation was identified in ~35% of primary GBM and ~75% of secondary GBM cases (15). However, the MGMT promoter methylation frequencies vary widely. Another report identified the presence of MGMT promoter methylation in ~70% of cases, which includes ~80% in grade II gliomas, ~70% in grade III gliomas, and ~60% in GBM. Intriguingly, the methylation status of MGMT promoter was not significantly associated with 1p/19q loss, nor was there any significant association of promoter methylation with EGFR amplification or *TP53* mutation.

The critical trial published in 2005 by Stupp et al. showed with a median follow-up of 28 months, that the median survival was 14.6 months with RT plus TMZ versus 12.1 months with RT alone. The 2-year overall survival was 26.5% with RT plus TMZ and 10.4% with RT alone (78), whereas the 5-year overall analysis showed 9.8% with RT and TMZ, versus 1.9% with RT alone (79). Additionally, patients whose tumor had a methylated MGMT gene promoter had improved survival with an overall survival of 21.7 months compared to 12.7 months for patients with unmethylated MGMT (80). Although initially it was thought that the benefit of MGMT promoter hypermethylation only applied to alkylating agents, a recent study suggested that decreased MGMT confers sensitivity to radiation alone as well (81). Therefore, the status of MGMT as a prognostic and/or predictive biomarker remains to be completely elucidated (3).

Glioma-CpG Island Methylator Phenotype

Not only has gene expression and genomic data been evaluated on a genome-wide scale, in 2010 Noushmehr et al. studied genome-wide methylation alterations in 272 TCGA glioblastoma tumors (82). This study identified a subtype of GBM that displayed hypermethylation of a large number of genes. Thus, they further described this phenotype as glioma-CpG island methylator phenotype (G-CIMP). Additionally, it was demonstrated that the G-CIMP tumors displayed the proneural expression subtype and therefore, the G-CIMP subtype is also more common among lower grade gliomas. Additionally, the G-CIMP profile is tightly associated with IDH1 mutations, specific copy-number alterations, and has higher levels of survival than tumors with a non G-CIMP profile (82). It will be important in the future to uncouple G-CIMP and IDH1 for clinical purposes,; however, it is apparent that the G-CIMP subtype is a likely prognostic biomarker.

Other Methylation/Acetylation Markers

Other whole genome integrative analyses of methylation and overall survival have been done on patients treated with surgery, radiotherapy, and TMZ (STUPP protocol) (12). This study with 50 patients identified six CpG sites that associate with overall survival, including Sox10 which is a protein involved in embryonic development and cell fate. Although this study needs to be validated, it shows that genome-wide profiling is currently underway in multiple studies and will eventually identify the role the methylome has in gliomagenesis, survival, and treatment response. Another study identified that a known cancer gene, POTE ankyrin domain family, member H (POTEH), is commonly hypomethylated in gliomas and increased POTEH expression was shown to negatively correlate with survival (83). An additional study showed that hypermethylation of two HOX genes (HOXA9 and 10) can be used as a prognostic factor in GBM patients. HOX genes are transcription factors that are key regulators of embryonic development, cell–cell interactions, and cell growth and differentiation (84). Histone modifications have also begun to receive attention as biomarkers in gliomas. In 2010, Liu et al. reported a recursive partitioning analysis that classified patients based on four histone modifications: H3K9Ac, H3K4diMe, H3K18Ac, and H4K20triMe (85). This study showed that all of the classified groups had significantly different progression-free and overall survival values suggesting that histone modifications may play a prognostic role in gliomas (85). Thus, epigenetic alterations, such as changes in methylation and acetylation, appear to play an important role in malignant glioma diagnosis and prognosis.

miRNAs

MicroRNAs (miRNAs) are short (~22 nt) RNA molecules that target mRNAs whose 3′ untranslated regions have one or more regions of partial complementarity and usually results in degradation or repression of the mRNA transcript. During the initiation and progression of cancer, miRNAs have been found to modulate cell proliferation, survival, tumor angiogenesis, invasion, and metastasis. In recent years, miRNAs have been at the forefront of biomarker studies, especially in gliomas.

MiR-21 was the first oncomir to be discovered in GBM and was shown to target important gliomagenesis genes, such as PTEN. Additionally, it was shown that miR-221 and 222 are overexpresssed in cancers that included GBM (86). Other miRNAs, such as miR-26a, let7, miR-124, and miR-137 are thought to play a role in gliomagenesis as well (87). In a recent study, seven miRNAs were found to have significantly different expression profiles in astrocytomas when compared to the normal adjacent brain tissue (88). Three of the miRNAs in this study correlated with survival analysis. Specifically, low expression of miR-181b or 106a or high expression of miR-21 was significantly associated with poor patient survival. This study demonstrated that miRNA profiling may play a dominant role in glioma biomarker studies in the future (88). Another study showed that miR-182 can be used as a prognostic marker in gliomas. In particular, 5-year survival was ~52% in patients with low miR-182 expression compared to ~7% in patients with high expression (89). MiRNA-196 was also shown to be upregulated in GBM compared to anaplastic astrocytomas and also showed prognostic significance (90). Additional studies have shown that miRNAs can also play a predictive role in brain tumors. One such study showed that miR-181 can help predict response to concomitant chemotherapy (RT + TMZ) in GBM patients (91). MiR-34a also has been shown to confer chemosensitivity to cisplatin and mitomycin C through modulation of MAGE-A and p53 in medulloblastoma (92).

Importantly, changes in miRNAs can also be detected in fluids, such as blood and cerebrospinal fluid. Two recent studies have looked at these fluids for miRNA signatures in glioblastoma patients (93,94). Although the initial results are promising, further investigations are essential before translation into the clinic could occur. Therefore, because there is no current peripheral fluid biomarker for GBM many investigators are currently looking for molecular characteristics that can be identified in blood that can aid in early detection, prognosis, and prediction of response to different therapy modalities.

■ METABOLIC BIOMARKERS

Metabolic reprogramming is a hallmark of cancer (95). Genetic mutation or amplification activates oncogenic growth signaling to cooperatively regulate glucose, glutamine, and lipid metabolism to orchestrate the bioenergetics and biosynthesis process and facilitate cancer cell malignant growth (96–99). Addictive glycolysis is a main feature of cancer cells in an aerobic condition (Warburg effect) (100). Recently, exacerbated lipogenesis has been revealed as a common characteristic in multiple cancers (101). Glucose and glutamine metabolism intermediates are the main resources for de novo biosynthesis of lipids, which processes are revealed to be tightly mediated by sterol regulatory element-binding protein-1 (SREBP-1), a master transcription factor that controls lipid metabolism (Figure 3) (102–104). Intriguingly, cancer cells have been revealed to import a large amount of cholesterol through upregulating low-density lipoprotein (LDL) receptor (LDLR) to support its rapid growth, which is also mediated by SREBP-1 (105). Here, we summarize recent insights in cancer metabolism in glioma, and introduce several new metabolic markers, and discuss their potential for molecular targeted therapy in glioma.

Glycolytic Markers

HK2

Hexokinase-2 (HK2) is an important mediator of aerobic glycolysis, which phosphorylates glucose as the first step of the glycolytic pathway (106). HK2 has been revealed to be highly expressed in GBM and is crucial for the Warburg effect. In contrast, hexokinase-1 (HK1) is predominantly expressed in normal brain and low-grade gliomas to regulate oxidative glucose metabolism (107). Overexpressing HK2 in GBM cells led to increased proliferation and intracranial growth. Conversely, genetic knockdown of HK2 in GBM cells was shown to restore oxidative glucose metabolism, decrease tumor growth, and enhance mice survival in an intracranial model (107,108). These data suggest that targeting of HK2 to modulate the Warburg effect is a novel therapeutic strategy to treat GBM.

Lipogenesis Markers

SREBP-1

SREBPs are key transcription factors that regulate lipogenesis and lipid uptake (109). In mammals, there are two SREBP genes, SREBP-1 and -2 (110,111). The SREBP-1 gene produces two isoforms 1a and 1c encoded from different promoters, which mainly regulate fatty acid synthesis pathway (109–112). SREBP-2 is shown to mainly regulate cholesterol synthesis (110,112,113). However, there is significant overlap in regulation of lipid metabolism by SREBP-1 and -2 (112–114). SREBPs activities are tightly controlled by endogenous sterol levels (109). They associate with insulin-induced gene (Insig) and are retained in the endoplasmic reticulum membrane when cellular sterol levels are sufficient. Once sterols level drop, SREBPs will dissociate from Insig and be escorted to Golgi by SREBP cleavage activating protein, then to be cleaved by site-1 and site-2 proteases (S1P and S2P) sequentially and release their N-terminus in order to act as transcription factors, which then enter into the nucleus to promote lipogenesis genes and LDLR expression (109,110).

Recently, SREBP-1 activity and its N-terminus levels were shown to be upregulated by PI3K/Akt signaling (115,116). In GBM, SREBP-1 was revealed to be highly expressed in tumor tissues, and its N-terminus is abundant in the nucleus. Consistent with SREBP-1 levels, SREBP-1 downstream target genes acetyl-CoA carboxylase (ACC) and fatty acid synthase (FASN) levels are also high in GBM tumor tissues (102). Furthermore, the levels of SREBP-1/ACC/FAS are tightly correlated with p-EGFR and p-Akt levels in GBM patients. By using isogenic cell lines, upregulation of SREBP-1 by EGFR was revealed to be mediated by PI3K/Akt signaling (Figure 3) (102,115). However, the molecular mechanism of how PI3K/Akt signaling regulates SREBP-1 is still not clear. There are two possible mechanisms for the regulation of SREBP-1. One is that SREBP-1 activity is maintained by Akt through inhibiting GSK3β activated ubiquitin ligase Fbw7 (F-box and WD repeat domain-containing 7)-mediated degradation of its nuclear form (117–119); another explanation is mTORC1 could phosphorylate lipin 1, a phosphatidic acid phosphatase, to control SREBP-1 nucleus localization and its stability (Figure 3) (120,121). These two distinct observations for the regulation of SREBP-1 probably originate from using different tissue-derived mammalian cell lines. In studies using normal tissue cell lines like retinal pigment epithelial cells, NIH3T3, hepatocytes, and mouse embryonic fibroblasts, SREBP-1 mRNA, and protein levels are sensitive to mTORC1 inhibition (116,120–122). However, in cancer cells, it is much more complicated. A recent study shows that inhibiting mTORC1 using rapamycin has little effect on SREBP-1 nucleus localization and its abundance in GBM patient tissues, but inhibiting its

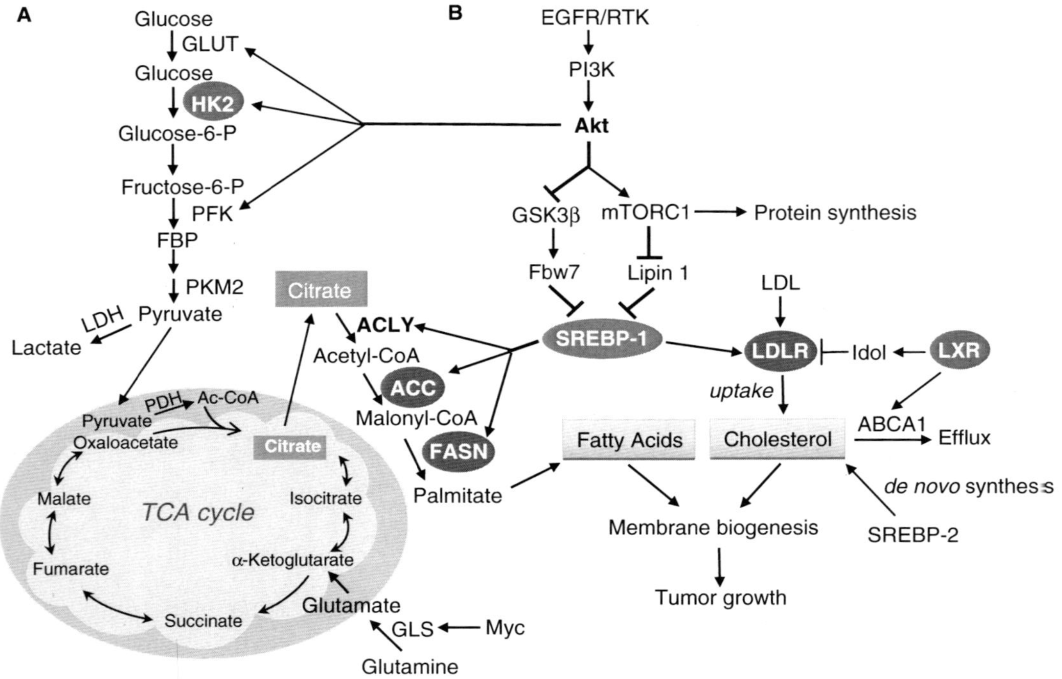

FIGURE 3 The regulation of metabolism in cancer. (A) The scheme at left side shows glycolysis is stimulated by PI3K/Akt signaling via promoting GLUT translocation and activating HK2 and PKM2 to produce pyruvate. Thus, further converting pyruvate into lactate by LDH or promoting the entrance of pyruvate into the mitochondria, which is regulated by PDH in order to integrate pyruvate into the TCA cycle and produce citrate as a precursor for lipid synthesis. Glutamine is then incorporated into the TCA cycle through glutaminolysis regulated by the Myc oncogene, to provide an additional energy source for cell growth, and also to produce citrate as a precursor for lipid synthesis through reductive carboxylation. (B) The scheme at right side shows that SREBP-1 plays an integral role in mediating oncogenic signaling RTK/PI3K/Akt to fatty acid synthesis and cholesterol uptake. SREBP-1 directly regulates ACLY, ACC, and FASN to promote fatty acid synthesis, and upregulates LDLR to enhance cholesterol uptake. Activation of LXR stimulates ABCA1 expression and promotes cholesterol efflux, also reduces LDLR levels via upregulating Idol, a ubiquitin ligase E3. ABCA1 = ATP-binding cassette transporter member 1; ACC = acetyl-CoA carboxylase; ACLY = ATP citrate lyase; EGFR = epidermal growth factor receptor; FASN = fatty acid synthase; FBP = fructose-1,6-bisphosphate; Fbw 7 = F-box and WD repeat domain-containing 7; GLS = glutaminase; GLUT = glucose transporter; HK2 = hexokinase-2; Idol = inducible degrader of LDLR; LDH = lactate dehydrogenase; LDL = low-density lipoprotein; LDLR = low-density lipoprotein receptor; LXR = liver X receptor; PDH = pyruvate dehydrogenase; PFK = phosphofructokinase; PKM2 = pyruvate kinase M2; RTK = receptor tyrosine kinase; SREBP-1 = sterol regulatory element-binding protein-1; SREBP-2 = sterol regulatory element-binding protein-2; TCA cycle = tricarboxylic acid cycle.

upstream regulators like EGFR, PI3K, and Akt significantly decreases SREBP-1 N-terminal fragment as well as diminishes its abundance in the nucleus (102). These data suggest that different molecules beyond mTORC1, but under PI3K/Akt signaling are involved in SREBP-1 regulation (Figure 1).

Recently, targeting metabolic alteration has emerged as a new strategy to treat cancer (108,123,124). SREBP-1, a central regulator to integrate PI3K/Akt signaling regulated glucose metabolism and c-Myc regulated glutamine metabolism to fatty acid synthesis (Figure 1) (96,102,125,126), has been shown to be a promising druggable target in cancer treatment. Pharmacological and genetic inhibition of SREBP-1 significantly suppressed tumor cell growth and resulted in cell death (102). These data demonstrate that SREBP-1 is a key molecular target in cancers. Therefore, developing specific inhibitors to target SREBP-1 could become a new therapeutic strategy to treat GBM.

ACC and FASN

Cancer cells are addictive to de novo fatty acid synthesis to form new membranes, particularly for lipid raft formation (101,127,128). Its upstream source is originated from glucose and glutamine (95,101). Through entering mitochondria, glycolytic intermediate pyruvate and glutamine intermediate glutamate via reductive carboxylation both convert to citrate, which is then released into cytoplasm and lysed to acetyl-CoA by ATP citrate lyase (ACLY) as a precursor for lipid synthesis (129,130). Then, ACC catalyzes the irreversible carboxylation of acetyl-CoA to produce malonyl-CoA (131,132), which is then incorporated with acetyl-CoA to form long-chain saturated fatty acid, palmitate, by FASN (Figure 1) (101,133). Palmitate can be elongated or desaturated to produce diverse fatty acids, which could incorporate into phospholipid for cell membrane formation, form triglycerides for energy storage, enter into mitochondria for energy production, acyl-modify proteins for posttranslational modification or be used as intermediates for the synthesis of hormones (101,133,134).

In SREBP-1 regulated fatty acid synthesis pathway, ACLY, ACC, and FASN have been revealed to be highly expressed in multiple cancer subtypes (101,102,130,135). Inhibition of these molecules has shown a significant reduction of cancer cell growth in vitro and in vivo (130,136–138). Pharmacological and genetic inhibition of ACLY, the enzyme that regulates the first step to synthesize fatty acid, has been shown to significantly inhibit cancer cell growth in vitro and in vivo (130,136). ACC, the enzyme to control the rate-limiting step of fatty acid synthesis, is highly expressed in GBM patient tissues (102). Inhibition of ACC was shown to significantly suppress GBM cell growth (139). FASN at the terminal step in the de novo synthesis of fatty acids plays a key role in tumor malignant growth. It has been shown to be elevated in the majority of cancers including prostate, breast, GBM, and ovarian (101,102,135). Inhibition of FASN significantly suppressed GBM cell growth in vitro and in vivo (102). Taken together, these data strongly indicate that targeting SREBP-1 regulated fatty acid synthesis pathway is a promising strategy in cancer treatment.

Cholesterol Metabolism Markers

LDLR

Cholesterol is a critical component of cellular membrane. It maintains membrane integrity and fluidity (140). Cholesterol homeostasis is critical to sustain cellular physiology function. It is tightly regulated by uptake, de novo synthesis, and efflux (110,141,142). SREBPs and nuclear receptor liver X receptor (LXR) are major players to control cellular cholesterol balance (142,143). A recent study uncovered that activated EGFR/PI3K signaling promotes cholesterol uptake through upregulating LDLR, which was revealed to be mediated by SREBP-1 (see Figure 3) (105). This study demonstrated that depriving cells of cholesterol results in cell death and could be a novel therapeutic strategy to treat cancer.

LDL is a major cholesterol carrier, which transports cholesterol from liver to the rest of the body (144). When cellular cholesterol levels decrease, LDLR expression will be enhanced and inserted in the cellular membrane with coated clathrin pitch, and its extracellular domain can bind LDL. Subsequently, the cell will endocytose LDL and deliver it to the lysosome, in which LDL will be hydrolyzed by lipases and release free cholesterol for cell utilization (145,146). Given that LDLR is highly upregulated in GBM, and its critical role for cholesterol uptake (102,147), it is likely that LDLR could be a promising molecular target. Further genetic and pharmacological inhibition of LDLR should be tested in GBM cells and tumor xenograft models to determine its function in tumorigenesis, and to provide the rationale for developing a specific inhibitor or antibody to block LDLR-mediated cholesterol uptake and test its anticancer effect.

LXR

LXR is a nuclear receptor, and plays an important role to control cellular cholesterol levels. When endogenous cholesterol levels increase, oxysterol levels will elevate, which then enter into the nucleus and bind LXR to promote its target gene transcription, such as ATP-binding cassette, subfamily A (ABCA1), or subfamily G (ABCG1). These genes are cholesterol transporters, which will remove cholesterol to the outside of cells in order to maintain cellular cholesterol homeostasis (142,148). Many studies have shown that activating LXR by its synthetic agonists GW3965 and T9091317 significantly reduces atherosclerosis lesions in mice models through increasing cholesterol efflux (149). Recently, activating LXR by its agonist GW3965 has been shown to significantly inhibit GBM cell growth and lead to cell death in vitro and in vivo through elevating ABCA1-mediated cholesterol efflux (see Figure 3) (105,150,151)

LXR has emerged as a promising druggable target in cancer therapy through reducing cellular cholesterol levels (105). However, activation of LXR by its agonists unfortunately stimulates SREBP-1 gene expression and enhances fatty acid synthesis, which could compromise the efficacy of LXR agonist in cancer treatment (152). To enhance the efficacy of LXR agonist in cancer treatment, combining it with inhibitors of enzymes in the fatty acid synthesis pathway would be a powerful strategy in suppressing tumor growth and overcome this resistance mechanism. However, considering the potential toxicity due to the combination of multiple drugs, it could be a better strategy to develop a novel LXR agonist with a low effect on SREBP-1 expression to treat cancer.

Notably, Tontonoz's group recently observed that activation of LXR significantly reduces LDLR levels via an inducible degrader of LDLR (Idol), a ubiquitin ligase E3 (153). In GBM cells, activation of LXR also significantly increases Idol expression and reduces LDLR levels, and overexpressing Idol in GBM cells dramatically reduces LDLR and induces cell death in combination with GW3965 treatment (102). Overall, these studies indicate that reducing cellular cholesterol levels via activation of LXR is mediated by two mechanisms, which are through ABCA1-mediated cholesterol efflux and through reducing LDL uptake via degradation of LDLR (see Figure 3). These data strongly indicate that LXR is a promising molecular target in GBM treatment. Taken together, targeting lipid metabolism may open a new window to treat GBM and may overcome the resistance of cancer cells to many common chemotherapy drugs.

■ CONCLUSIONS

As our understanding of the molecular pathways of malignant gliomas increases with the identification and validation of novel glioma biomarkers, multiple new targets and stratification criteria will be developed. Thus, the uniform approach to treatment of malignant gliomas will likely make a critical shift in the near future. Therefore, identifying the mechanisms of therapy resistance will also allow the use of targeted therapies that are individualized for each patient's unique resistance mechanisms. Following treatment efficacy throughout the standard course of therapy with novel fluid biomarkers will additionally allow therapy to be adjusted for resistance mechanisms in "real time" within the clinic.

In summary, elucidating our understanding of malignant glioma subpopulations that benefit from each targeted therapy will lead to individualized therapy modalities with significantly increased efficacy. Therefore, we expect that using a more targeted therapeutic approach will aid in circumventing the current limitations in the treatment of malignant gliomas and result in increased clinical outcomes for these patients.

■ REFERENCES

1. Siker ML, Chakravarti A, Mehta MP. Should concomitant and adjuvant treatment with temozolomide be used as standard therapy in patients with anaplastic glioma? *Crit Rev Oncol Hematol.* 2006;60(2):99–111.
2. Hlavin Bell E, Hadziahmetovic M, Chakravarti A. Evolvement of molecular biomarkers in targeted therapy of malignant gliomas. In: Abujamra AL, ed. *Brain Tumors—Current and Emerging Therapeutic Strategies.* 2011. Croatia: InTech.
3. Riemenschneider MJ, Jeuken JW, Wesseling P, Reifenberger G. Molecular diagnostics of gliomas: state of the art. *Acta Neuropathol.* 2010;120(5):567–584.
4. Yen KE, Bittinger MA, Su SM, Fantin VR. Cancer-associated IDH mutations: biomarker and therapeutic opportunities. *Oncogene.* 2010;29(49):6409–6417.
5. Parsons DW, Jones S, Zhang X, et al. An integrated genomic analysis of human glioblastoma multiforme. *Science.* 2008;321(5897):1807–1812.
6. Jansen M, Yip S, Louis DN. Molecular pathology in adult gliomas: diagnostic, prognostic, and predictive markers. *Lancet Neurol.* 2010;9(7):717–726.
7. Fischer I, Aldape K. Molecular tools: biology, prognosis, and therapeutic triage. *Neuroimaging Clin N Am.* 2010;20(3):273–282.
8. Ducray F, Idbaih A, Wang XW, Cheneau C, Labussiere M, Sanson M. Predictive and prognostic factors for gliomas. *Expert Rev Anticancer Ther.* 2011;11(5):781–789.
9. Yan H, Parsons DW, Jin G, et al. IDH1 and IDH2 mutations in gliomas. *N Engl J Med.* 2009;360(8):765–773.
10. Sanson M, Marie Y, Paris S, et al. Isocitrate dehydrogenase 1 codon 132 mutation is an important prognostic biomarker in gliomas. *J Clin Oncol.* 2009;27(25):4150–4154.
11. DeAngelis LM, Mellinghoff IK. Virchow 2011 or how to ID(H) human glioblastoma. *J Clin Oncol.* 2011;29(34):4473–4474.
12. Etcheverry A, Aubry M, de Tayrac M, et al. DNA methylation in glioblastoma: impact on gene expression and clinical outcome. *BMC Genomics.* 2010;11:701.
13. Turcan S, Rohle D, Goenka A, et al. IDH1 mutation is sufficient to establish the glioma hypermethylator phenotype. *Nature.* 2012;483(7390):479–483.
14. Lu C, Ward PS, Kapoor GS, et al. IDH mutation impairs histone demethylation and results in a block to cell differentiation. *Nature.* 2012;483(7390):474–478.

15. Gladson CL, Prayson RA, Liu WM. The pathobiology of glioma tumors. *Annu Rev Pathol.* 2010;5:33–50.

16. Cairncross G, Jenkins R. Gliomas with 1p/19q codeletion: a.k.a. oligodendroglioma. *Cancer J.* 2008;14(6):352–357.

17. Aldape K, Burger PC, Perry A. Clinicopathologic aspects of 1p/19q loss and the diagnosis of oligodendroglioma. *Arch Pathol Lab Med.* 2007;131(2):242–251.

18. Smith JS, Perry A, Borell TJ, et al. Alterations of chromosome arms 1p and 19q as predictors of survival in oligodendrogliomas, astrocytomas, and mixed oligoastrocytomas. *J Clin Oncol.* 2000;18(3):636–645.

19. Nutt CL. Molecular genetics of oligodendrogliomas: a model for improved clinical management in the field of neurooncology. *Neurosurg Focus.* 2005;19(5):E2.

20. Cairncross JG, Ueki K, Zlatescu MC, et al. Specific genetic predictors of chemotherapeutic response and survival in patients with anaplastic oligodendrogliomas. *J Natl Cancer Inst.* 1998;90(19):1473–1479.

21. Kouwenhoven MC, Kros JM, French PJ, et al. 1p/19q loss within oligodendroglioma is predictive for response to first line temozolomide but not to salvage treatment. *Eur J Cancer.* 2006;42(15):2499–2503.

22. Bauman GS, Ino Y, Ueki K, et al. Allelic loss of chromosome 1p and radiotherapy plus chemotherapy in patients with oligodendrogliomas. *Int J Radiat Oncol Biol Phys.* 2000;48(3):825–830.

23. Cairncross G, Berkey B, Shaw E, et al.; Intergroup Radiation Therapy Oncology Group Trial 9402. Phase III trial of chemotherapy plus radiotherapy compared with radiotherapy alone for pure and mixed anaplastic oligodendroglioma: Intergroup Radiation Therapy Oncology Group Trial 9402. *J Clin Oncol.* 2006;24(18):2707–2714.

24. Cairncross JGW, Shaw E, Jenkins RB, et al. Chemotherapy plus radiotherapy (CT-RT) versus RT alone for patients with anaplastic oligodendroglioma: long-term results of the RTOG 9402 phase III study. *J Clin Oncol.* 2012;30(suppl):abstr 2008b.

25. Wrensch M, Jenkins RB, Chang JS, et al. Variants in the CDKN2B and RTEL1 regions are associated with high-grade glioma susceptibility. *Nat Genet.* 2009;41(8):905–908.

26. Keller A, Harz C, Matzas M, et al. Identification of novel SNPs in glioblastoma using targeted resequencing. *PLoS ONE.* 2011;6(6):e18158.

27. Van Meir EG, Hadjipanayis CG, Norden AD, Shu HK, Wen PY, Olson JJ. Exciting new advances in neuro-oncology: the avenue to a cure for malignant glioma. *CA Cancer J Clin.* 2010;60(3):166–193.

28. Noda SE, El-Jawahri A, Patel D, Lautenschlaeger T, Siedow M, Chakravarti A. Molecular advances of brain tumors in radiation oncology. *Semin Radiat Oncol.* 2009;19(3):171–178.

29. Kim B, Myung JK, Seo JH, et al. The clinicopathologic values of the molecules associated with the main pathogenesis of the glioblastoma. *J Neurol Sci.* 2010;294(1–2):112–118.

30. Sulman EP, Guerrero M, Aldape K. Beyond grade: molecular pathology of malignant gliomas. *Semin Radiat Oncol.* 2009;19(3):142–149.

31. Ang C, Guiot MC, Ramanakumar AV, Roberge D, Kavan P. Clinical significance of molecular biomarkers in glioblastoma. *Can J Neurol Sci.* 2010;37(5):625–630.

32. Bredel M, Scholtens DM, Yadav AK, et al. NFKBIA deletion in glioblastomas. *N Engl J Med.* 2011;364(7):627–637.

33. Maehama T, Dixon JE. The tumor suppressor, PTEN/MMAC1, dephosphorylates the lipid second messenger, phosphatidylinositol 3,4,5-trisphosphate. *J Biol Chem.* 1998;273(22):13375–13378.

34. Ermoian RP, Furniss CS, Lamborn KR, et al. Dysregulation of PTEN and protein kinase B is associated with glioma histology and patient survival. *Clin Cancer Res.* 2002;8(5):1100–1106.

35. Sasaki H, Zlatescu MC, Betensky RA, Ino Y, Cairncross JG, Louis DN. PTEN is a target of chromosome 10q loss in anaplastic oligodendrogliomas and PTEN alterations are associated with poor prognosis. *Am J Pathol.* 2001;159(1):359–367.

36. Wiencke JK, Zheng S, Jelluma N, et al. Methylation of the PTEN promoter defines low-grade gliomas and secondary glioblastoma. *Neuro-oncology.* 2007;9(3):271–279.

37. Bourne TD, Schiff D. Update on molecular findings, management and outcome in low-grade gliomas. *Nat Rev Neurol.* 2010;6(12):695–701.

38. Fujisawa H, Reis RM, Nakamura M, et al. Loss of heterozygosity on chromosome 10 is more extensive in primary (de novo) than in secondary glioblastomas. *Lab Invest.* 2000;80(1):65–72.

39. Ohgaki H, Dessen P, Jourde B, et al. Genetic pathways to glioblastoma: a population-based study. *Cancer Res.* 2004;64(19):6892–6899.

40. Zoncu R, Efeyan A, Sabatini DM. mTOR: from growth signal integration to cancer, diabetes and ageing. *Nat Rev Mol Cell Biol.* 2011;12(1):21–35.

41. McEllin B, Camacho CV, Mukherjee B, et al. PTEN loss compromises homologous recombination repair in astrocytes: implications for glioblastoma therapy with temozolomide or poly(ADP-ribose) polymerase inhibitors. *Cancer Res.* 2010;70(13):5457–5464.

42. Dedes KJ, Wetterskog D, Mendes-Pereira AM, et al. PTEN deficiency in endometrioid endometrial adenocarcinomas predicts sensitivity to PARP inhibitors. *Sci Transl Med.* 2010;2(53):53ra75.

43. Tabatabai G, Stupp R, van den Bent MJ, et al. Molecular diagnostics of gliomas: the clinical perspective. *Acta Neuropathol.* 2010;120(5):585–592.

44. Toedt G, Barbus S, Wolter M, et al. Molecular signatures classify astrocytic gliomas by IDH1 mutation status. *Int J Cancer.* 2011;128(5):1095–1103.

45. Costa BM, Viana-Pereira M, Fernandes R, et al. Impact of EGFR genetic variants on glioma risk and patient outcome. *Cancer Epidemiol Biomarkers Prev.* 2011;20(12):2610–2617.

46. Rich JN, Reardon DA, Peery T, et al. Phase II trial of gefitinib in recurrent glioblastoma. *J Clin Oncol.* 2004;22(1):133–142.

47. Prados MD, Chang SM, Butowski N, et al. Phase II study of erlotinib plus temozolomide during and after radiation therapy in patients with newly diagnosed glioblastoma multiforme or gliosarcoma. *J Clin Oncol.* 2009;27(4):579–584.

48. van den Bent MJ, Brandes AA, Rampling R, et al. Randomized phase II trial of erlotinib versus temozolomide or carmustine in recurrent glioblastoma: EORTC brain tumor group study 26034. *J Clin Oncol.* 2009;27(8):1268–1274.

49. Mellinghoff IK, Wang MY, Vivanco I, et al. Molecular determinants of the response of glioblastomas to EGFR kinase inhibitors. *N Engl J Med.* 2005;353(19):2012–2024.

50. Chakravarti A, Seiferheld W, Tu X, et al. Immunohistochemically determined total epidermal growth factor receptor levels not of prognostic value in newly diagnosed glioblastoma multiforme: report from the Radiation Therapy Oncology Group. *Int J Radiat Oncol Biol Phys.* 2005;62(2):318–327.

51. Chakravarti A, Wang M, Mischel P, et al. An update on correlative molecular endpoints from RTOG 0211: phase I/II study of gefitinib + radiation for newly diagnosed glioblastoma patients. *Int J Radiat Oncol Biol Phys.* 2008;72(1):S9–S10.

52. Sjöström S, Wibom C, Andersson U, et al. Genetic variations in VEGF and VEGFR2 and glioblastoma outcome. *J Neurooncol.* 2011;104(2):523–527.

53. Oehring RD, Miletic M, Valter MM, et al. Vascular endothelial growth factor (VEGF) in astrocytic gliomas–a prognostic factor? *J Neurooncol.* 1999;45(2):117–125.

54. Ahluwalia MS, Gladson CL. Progress on antiangiogenic therapy for patients with malignant glioma. *J Oncol.* 2010;2010:689018.

55. Friedman HS, Vredenburgh JJ, Desjardins A, et al. A phase I study of sunitinib plus irinotecan in the treatment of patients with recurrent malignant glioma. *ASCO Annual Meeting,* May 2009. Orlando, FL: *J Clin Oncol* 2009;27(suppl; abstr e13024).

56. Vredenburgh JJ, Desjardins A, Reardon DA, et al. Bevacizumab (BEV) in combination with temozolomide (TMZ) and radiation therapy (XRT) followed by BEV, TMZ, and irinotecan for newly diagnosed glioblastoma multiforme (GBM). *ASCO Annual Meeting,* 2010. San Diego, CA: *J Clin Oncol* 2010;28:15s(suppl; abstr 2023).

57. Lai A, Tran A, Nghiemphu PL, et al. Phase II study of bevacizumab plus temozolomide during and after radiation therapy for patients with newly diagnosed glioblastoma multiforme. *J Clin Oncol.* 2011;29(2):142–148.

58. Kreisl TN, Lassman AB, Mischel PS, et al. A pilot study of everolimus and gefitinib in the treatment of recurrent glioblastoma (GBM). *J Neurooncol.* 2009;92(1):99–105.

59. Cancer Genome Atlas Research Network. Comprehensive genomic characterization defines human glioblastoma genes and core pathways. *Nature.* 2008;455(7216):1061–1068.

60. McBride SM, Perez DA, Polley MY, et al. Activation of PI3K/mTOR pathway occurs in most adult low-grade gliomas and predicts patient survival. *J Neurooncol.* 2010;97(1):33–40.

61. Goudar RK, Shi Q, Hjelmeland MD, et al. Combination therapy of inhibitors of epidermal growth factor receptor/vascular endothelial growth factor receptor 2 (AEE788) and the mammalian target of rapamycin (RAD001) offers improved glioblastoma tumor growth inhibition. *Mol Cancer Ther.* 2005;4(1):101–112.

62. Chakravarti A, Zhai G, Suzuki Y, et al. The prognostic significance of phosphatidylinositol 3-kinase pathway activation in human gliomas. *J Clin Oncol.* 2004;22(10):1926–1933.

63. Lustig R, Mikkelsen T, Lesser G, et al.; New Approaches to Brain Tumor Therapy CNS Consortium. Phase II preradiation R115777 (tipifarnib) in newly diagnosed GBM with residual enhancing disease. *Neuro-oncology.* 2008;10(6):1004–1009.

64. Cloughesy TF, Wen PY, Robins HI, et al. Phase II trial of tipifarnib in patients with recurrent malignant glioma either receiving or not receiving enzyme-inducing antiepileptic drugs: a North American Brain Tumor Consortium Study. *J Clin Oncol.* 2006;24(22):3651–3656.

65. Saetta AA, Levidou G, El-Habr EA, et al. Expression of pERK and pAKT in human astrocytomas: correlation with IDH1-R132H presence, vascular endothelial growth factor, microvascular characteristics and clinical outcome. *Virchows Arch.* 2011;458(6):749–759.

66. Pelloski CE, Lin E, Zhang L, et al. Prognostic associations of activated mitogen-activated protein kinase and Akt pathways in glioblastoma. *Clin Cancer Res.* 2006;12(13):3935–3941.

67. Rossi M, Magnoni L, Miracco C, et al. ß-catenin and Gli1 are prognostic markers in glioblastoma. *Cancer Biol Ther.* 2011;11(8):753–761.

68. Fu Y, Zheng S, An N, et al. ß-catenin as a potential key target for tumor suppression. *Int J Cancer.* 2011;129(7):1541–1551.

69. Onishi H, Katano M. Hedgehog signaling pathway as a therapeutic target in various types of cancer. *Cancer Sci.* 2011;102(10):1756–1760.

70. Jiang L, Wu J, Chen Q, Hu X, Li W, Hu G. Notch1 expression is upregulated in glioma and is associated with tumor progression. *J Clin Neurosci.* 2011;18(3):387–390.

71. Li J, Cui Y, Gao G, Zhao Z, Zhang H, Wang X. Notch1 is an independent prognostic factor for patients with glioma. *J Surg Oncol.* 2011;103(8):813–817.

72. Kanakis D, Levidou G, Gakiopoulou H, et al. Replication protein A: a reliable biologic marker of prognostic and therapeutic value in human astrocytic tumors. *Hum Pathol.* 2011;42(10):1545–1553.

73. Li L, Wang J, Shen X, et al. Expression and prognostic value of NDRG2 in human astrocytomas. *J Neurol Sci.* 2011;308(1–2):77–82.

74. Phillips HS, Kharbanda S, Chen R, et al. Molecular subclasses of high-grade glioma predict prognosis, delineate a pattern of disease progression, and resemble stages in neurogenesis. *Cancer Cell.* 2006;9(3):157–173.

75. Verhaak RG, Hoadley KA, Purdom E, et al.; Cancer Genome Atlas Research Network. Integrated genomic analysis identifies clinically relevant subtypes of glioblastoma characterized by abnormalities in PDGFRA, IDH1, EGFR, and NF1. *Cancer Cell.* 2010;17(1):98–110.

76. Gravendeel LA, Kouwenhoven MC, Gevaert O, et al. Intrinsic gene expression profiles of gliomas are a better predictor of survival than histology. *Cancer Res.* 2009;69(23):9065–9072.

77. Gerson SL. MGMT: its role in cancer aetiology and cancer therapeutics. *Nat Rev Cancer.* 2004;4(4):296–307.

78. Stupp R, Mason WP, van den Bent MJ, et al.; European Organisation for Research and Treatment of Cancer Brain Tumor and Radiotherapy Groups; National Cancer Institute of Canada Clinical Trials Group. Radiotherapy plus concomitant and adjuvant temozolomide for glioblastoma. *N Engl J Med.* 2005;352(10):987–996.

79. Stupp R, Hegi ME, Mason WP, et al.; European Organisation for Research and Treatment of Cancer Brain Tumour and Radiation Oncology Groups; National Cancer Institute of Canada Clinical Trials Group. Effects of radiotherapy with concomitant and adjuvant temozolomide versus radiotherapy alone on survival in glioblastoma in a randomised phase III study: 5-year analysis of the EORTC-NCIC trial. *Lancet Oncol.* 2009;10(5):459–466.

80. Hegi ME, Diserens AC, Gorlia T, et al. MGMT gene silencing and benefit from temozolomide in glioblastoma. *N Engl J Med.* 2005;352(10):997–1003.

81. Rivera AL, Pelloski CE, Gilbert MR, et al. MGMT promoter methylation is predictive of response to radiotherapy and prognostic in the absence of adjuvant alkylating chemotherapy for glioblastoma. *Neuro-oncology.* 2010;12(2):116–121.

82. Noushmehr H, Weisenberger DJ, Diefes K, et al.; Cancer Genome Atlas Research Network. Identification of a CpG island methylator phenotype that defines a distinct subgroup of glioma. *Cancer Cell.* 2010;17(5):510–522.

83. Liu X, Tang H, Zhang Z, et al. POTEH hypomethylation, a new epigenetic biomarker for glioma prognosis. *Brain Res.* 2011;1391:125–131.

84. Di Vinci A, Casciano I, Marasco E, et al. Quantitative methylation analysis of HOXA3, 7, 9, and 10 genes in glioma: association with tumor WHO grade and clinical outcome. *J Cancer Res Clin Oncol.* 2012;138(1):35–47.

85. Liu BL, Cheng JX, Zhang X, et al. Global histone modification patterns as prognostic markers to classify glioma patients. *Cancer Epidemiol Biomarkers Prev.* 2010;19(11):2888–2896.

86. Ciafrè SA, Galardi S, Mangiola A, et al. Extensive modulation of a set of microRNAs in primary glioblastoma. *Biochem Biophys Res Commun.* 2005;334(4):1351–1358.

87. Purow B. The elephant in the room: do microRNA-based therapies have a realistic chance of succeeding for brain tumors such as glioblastoma? *J Neurooncol.* 2011;103(3):429–436.

88. Zhi F, Chen X, Wang S, et al. The use of hsa-miR-21, hsa-miR-181b and hsa-miR-106a as prognostic indicators of astrocytoma. *Eur J Cancer.* 2010;46(9):1640–1649.

89. Jiang L, Mao P, Song L, et al. miR-182 as a prognostic marker for glioma progression and patient survival. *Am J Pathol.* 2010;177(1):29–38.

90. Guan Y, Mizoguchi M, Yoshimoto K, et al. MiRNA-196 is upregulated in glioblastoma but not in anaplastic astrocytoma and has prognostic significance. *Clin Cancer Res.* 2010;16(16):4289–4297.

91. Slaby O, Lakomy R, Fadrus P, et al. MicroRNA-181 family predicts response to concomitant chemoradiotherapy with temozolomide in glioblastoma patients. *Neoplasma.* 2010;57(3):264–269.

92. Weeraratne SD, Amani V, Neiss A, et al. miR-34a confers chemosensitivity through modulation of MAGE-A and p53 in medulloblastoma. *Neuro-oncology.* 2011;13(2):165–175.

93. Baraniskin A, Kuhnhenn J, Schlegel U, et al. Identification of microRNAs in the cerebrospinal fluid as biomarker for the diagnosis of glioma. *Neuro-oncology.* 2012;14(1):29–33.

94. Roth P, Wischhusen J, Happold C, et al. A specific miRNA signature in the peripheral blood of glioblastoma patients. *J Neurochem.* 2011;118(3):449–457.

95. Vander Heiden MG, Cantley LC, Thompson CB. Understanding the Warburg effect: the metabolic requirements of cell proliferation. *Science.* 2009;324(5930):1029–1033.

96. DeBerardinis RJ, Lum JJ, Hatzivassiliou G, Thompson CB. The biology of cancer: metabolic reprogramming fuels cell growth and proliferation. *Cell Metab.* 2008;7(1):11–20.

97. Cairns RA, Harris I, McCracken S, Mak TW. Cancer cell metabolism. *Cold Spring Harb Symp Quant Biol.* 2011;76:299–311.

98. Metallo CM, Gameiro PA, Bell EL, et al. Reductive glutamine metabolism by IDH1 mediates lipogenesis under hypoxia. *Nature.* 2012;481(7381):380–384.

99. Mullen AR, Wheaton WW, Jin ES, et al. Reductive carboxylation supports growth in tumour cells with defective mitochondria. *Nature.* 2012;481(7381):385–388.

100. Koppenol WH, Bounds PL, Dang CV. Otto Warburg's contributions to current concepts of cancer metabolism. *Nat Rev Cancer.* 2011;11(5):325–337.

101. Menendez JA, Lupu R. Fatty acid synthase and the lipogenic phenotype in cancer pathogenesis. *Nat Rev Cancer.* 2007;7(10):763–777.

102. Guo D, Prins RM, Dang J, et al. EGFR signaling through an Akt-SREBP-1-dependent, rapamycin-resistant pathway sensitizes glioblastomas to antilipogenic therapy. *Sci Signal.* 2009;2(101):ra82.

103. Wang X, Sato R, Brown MS, Hua X, Goldstein JL. SREBP-1, a membrane-bound transcription factor released by sterol-regulated proteolysis. *Cell.* 1994;77(1):53–62.

104. Yokoyama C, Wang X, Briggs MR, et al. SREBP-1, a basic-helix-loop-helix-leucine zipper protein that controls

transcription of the low density lipoprotein receptor gene. *Cell.* 1993;75(1):187–197.

105. Guo D, Reinitz F, Youssef M, et al. An LXR agonist promotes glioblastoma cell death through inhibition of an EGFR/AKT/SREBP-1/LDLR-dependent pathway. *Cancer Discov.* 2011;1(5):442–456.

106. Pedersen PL. Warburg, me and Hexokinase 2: Multiple discoveries of key molecular events underlying one of cancers' most common phenotypes, the "Warburg Effect," i.e., elevated glycolysis in the presence of oxygen. *J Bioenerg Biomembr.* 2007;39(3):211–222.

107. Wolf A, Agnihotri S, Munoz D, Guha A. Developmental profile and regulation of the glycolytic enzyme hexokinase 2 in normal brain and glioblastoma multiforme. *Neurobiol Dis.* 2011;44(1):84–91.

108. Wolf A, Agnihotri S, Micallef J, et al. Hexokinase 2 is a key mediator of aerobic glycolysis and promotes tumor growth in human glioblastoma multiforme. *J Exp Med.* 2011;208(2):313–326.

109. Horton JD, Goldstein JL, Brown MS. SREBPs: activators of the complete program of cholesterol and fatty acid synthesis in the liver. *J Clin Invest.* 2002;109(9):1125–1131.

110. Brown MS, Goldstein JL. The SREBP pathway: regulation of cholesterol metabolism by proteolysis of a membrane-bound transcription factor. *Cell.* 1997;89(3):331–340.

111. Osborne TF, Espenshade PJ. Evolutionary conservation and adaptation in the mechanism that regulates SREBP action: what a long, strange tRIP it's been. *Genes Dev.* 2009;23(22):2578–2591.

112. Horton JD, Shimomura I, Ikemoto S, Bashmakov Y, Hammer RE. Overexpression of sterol regulatory element-binding protein-1a in mouse adipose tissue produces adipocyte hypertrophy, increased fatty acid secretion, and fatty liver. *J Biol Chem.* 2003;278(38):36652–36660.

113. Horton JD, Shah NA, Warrington JA, et al. Combined analysis of oligonucleotide microarray data from transgenic and knockout mice identifies direct SREBP target genes. *Proc Natl Acad Sci USA.* 2003;100(21):12027–12032.

114. Jeon TI, Osborne TF. SREBPs: metabolic integrators in physiology and metabolism. *Trends Endocrinol Metab.* 2012;23(2):65–72.

115. Porstmann T, Griffiths B, Chung YL, et al. PKB/Akt induces transcription of enzymes involved in cholesterol and fatty acid biosynthesis via activation of SREBP. *Oncogene.* 2005;24(43):6465–6481.

116. Li S, Brown MS, Goldstein JL. Bifurcation of insulin signaling pathway in rat liver: mTORC1 required for stimulation of lipogenesis, but not inhibition of gluconeogenesis. *Proc Natl Acad Sci USA.* 2010;107(8):3441–3446.

117. Sundqvist A, Ericsson J. Transcription-dependent degradation controls the stability of the SREBP family of transcription factors. *Proc Natl Acad Sci USA.* 2003;100(24):13833–13838.

118. Bengoechea-Alonso MT, Ericsson J. SREBP in signal transduction: cholesterol metabolism and beyond. *Curr Opin Cell Biol.* 2007;19(2):215–222.

119. Sundqvist A, Bengoechea-Alonso MT, Ye X, et al. Control of lipid metabolism by phosphorylation-dependent degradation of the SREBP family of transcription factors by SCF(Fbw7). *Cell Metab.* 2005;1(6):379–391.

120. Porstmann T, Santos CR, Griffiths B, et al. SREBP activity is regulated by mTORC1 and contributes to Akt-dependent cell growth. *Cell Metab.* 2008;8(3):224–236.

121. Peterson TR, Sengupta SS, Harris TE, et al. mTOR complex 1 regulates lipin 1 localization to control the SREBP pathway. *Cell.* 2011;146(3):408–420.

122. Düvel K, Yecies JL, Menon S, et al. Activation of a metabolic gene regulatory network downstream of mTOR complex 1. *Mol Cell.* 2010;39(2):171–183.

123. Maschek G, Savaraj N, Priebe W, et al. 2-deoxy-D-glucose increases the efficacy of adriamycin and paclitaxel in human osteosarcoma and non-small cell lung cancers in vivo. *Cancer Res.* 2004;64(1):31–34.

124. Dang CV, Hamaker M, Sun P, Le A, Gao P. Therapeutic targeting of cancer cell metabolism. *J Mol Med.* 2011;89(3):205–212.

125. DeBerardinis RJ, Mancuso A, Daikhin E, et al. Beyond aerobic glycolysis: transformed cells can engage in glutamine metabolism that exceeds the requirement for protein and nucleotide synthesis. *Proc Natl Acad Sci USA.* 2007;104(49):19345–19350.

126. Deberardinis RJ, Sayed N, Ditsworth D, Thompson CB. Brick by brick: metabolism and tumor cell growth. *Curr Opin Genet Dev.* 2008;18(1):54–61.

127. Menendez JA, Vellon L, Lupu R. Targeting fatty acid synthase-driven lipid rafts: a novel strategy to overcome trastuzumab resistance in breast cancer cells. *Med Hypotheses.* 2005;64(5):997–1001.

128. Menendez JA, Colomer R, Lupu R. Why does tumor-associated fatty acid synthase (oncogenic antigen-519) ignore dietary fatty acids? *Med Hypotheses.* 2005;64(2):342–349.

129. Hardwick DC. The fate of acetyl groups derived from glucose in the isolated perfused goat udder. *Biochem J.* 1966;99(1):228–231.

130. Bauer DE, Hatzivassiliou G, Zhao F, Andreadis C, Thompson CB. ATP citrate lyase is an important component of cell growth and transformation. *Oncogene.* 2005;24(41):6314–6322.

131. GANGULY J. Studies on the mechanism of fatty acid synthesis. VII. Biosynthesis of fatty acids from malonyl CoA. *Biochim Biophys Acta.* 1960;40:110–118.

132. Gregolin C, Ryder E, Kleinschmidt AK, Warner RC, Lane MD. Molecular characteristics of liver acetyl CoA carboxylase. *Proc Natl Acad Sci USA.* 1966;56(1):148–155.

133. Menendez JA, Lupu R, Colomer R. Obesity, fatty acid synthase, and cancer: serendipity or forgotten causal linkage? *Mol Genet Metab.* 2005;84(3):293–295.

134. Wellen KE, Hatzivassiliou G, Sachdeva UM, Bui TV, Cross JR, Thompson CB. ATP-citrate lyase links cellular metabolism to histone acetylation. *Science.* 2009;324(5930):1076–1080.

135. Yoon S, Lee MY, Park SW, et al. Up-regulation of acetyl-CoA carboxylase alpha and fatty acid synthase by human epidermal growth factor receptor 2 at the translational level in breast cancer cells. *J Biol Chem.* 2007;282(36):26122–26131.

136. Hatzivassiliou G, Zhao F, Bauer DE, et al. ATP citrate lyase inhibition can suppress tumor cell growth. *Cancer Cell.* 2005;8(4):311–321.

137. Vazquez-Martin A, Colomer R, Brunet J, Menendez JA. Pharmacological blockade of fatty acid synthase (FASN) reverses acquired autoresistance to trastuzumab (Herceptin by transcriptionally inhibiting 'HER2 super-expression' occurring in high-dose trastuzumab-conditioned SKBR3/Tzb100 breast cancer cells. *Int J Oncol.* 2007;31(4):769–776.

138. Chuang HY, Chang YF, Hwang JJ. Antitumor effect of orlistat, a fatty acid synthase inhibitor, is via activation of caspase-3 on human colorectal carcinoma-bearing animal. *Biomed Pharmacother.* 2011;65(4):286–292.

139. Beckers A, Organe S, Timmermans L, et al. Chemical inhibition of acetyl-CoA carboxylase induces growth arrest and cytotoxicity selectively in cancer cells. *Cancer Res.* 2007;67(17):8180–8187.

140. Maxfield FR, van Meer G. Cholesterol, the central lipid of mammalian cells. *Curr Opin Cell Biol.* 2010;22(4):422–429.

141. Brown MS, Goldstein JL. A receptor-mediated pathway for cholesterol homeostasis. *Science.* 1986;232(4746):34–47.

142. Zelcer N, Tontonoz P. Liver X receptors as integrators of metabolic and inflammatory signaling. *J Clin Invest.* 2006;116(3):607–614.

143. Raghow R, Yellaturu C, Deng X, Park EA, Elam MB. SREBPs: the crossroads of physiological and pathological lipid homeostasis. *Trends Endocrinol Metab.* 2008;19(2):65–73.

144. Segrest JP, Jones MK, De Loof H, Dashti N. Structure of apolipoprotein B-100 in low density lipoproteins. *J Lipid Res.* 2001;42(9):1346–1367.

145. Goldstein JL, Brown MS. The LDL receptor. *Arterioscler Thromb Vasc Biol.* 2009;29(4):431–438.

146. Brown MS, Ho YK, Goldstein JL. The low-density lipoprotein pathway in human fibroblasts: relation between cell surface receptor binding and endocytosis of low-density lipoprotein. *Ann N Y Acad Sci.* 1976;275:244–257.

147. Rudling MJ, Angelin B, Peterson CO, Collins VP. Low density lipoprotein receptor activity in human intracranial tumors and its relation to the cholesterol requirement. *Cancer Res.* 1990;50(3):483–487.

148. Calkin AC, Tontonoz P. Liver x receptor signaling pathways and atherosclerosis. *Arterioscler Thromb Vasc Biol.* 2010;30(8):1513–1518.

149. Joseph SB, McKilligin E, Pei L, et al. Synthetic LXR ligand inhibits the development of atherosclerosis in mice. *Proc Natl Acad Sci USA.* 2002;99(11):7604–7609.

150. Chuu CP, Lin HP. Antiproliferative effect of LXR agonists T0901317 and 22*-hydroxycholesterol on multiple human cancer cell lines. *Anticancer Res.* 2010;30(9):3643–3648.

151. Mehrotra A, Kaul D, Joshi K. LXR-a selectively reprogrammes cancer cells to enter into apoptosis. *Mol Cell Biochem.* 2011;349(1–2):41–55.

152. Schultz JR, Tu H, Luk A, et al. Role of LXRs in control of lipogenesis. *Genes Dev.* 2000;14(22):2831–2838.

153. Zelcer N, Hong C, Boyadjian R, Tontonoz P. LXR regulates cholesterol uptake through Idol-dependent ubiquitination of the LDL receptor. *Science.* 2009;325(5936):100–104.

Index

Page numbers with "*f*" and "*t*" denote figures and tables, respectively.